Nursing and Clinical Informatics:
Socio-Technical Approaches

Bettina Staudinger
University for Health Sciences, Medical Informatics and Technology, Austria

Victoria Höß
University for Health Sciences, Medical Informatics and Technology, Austria

Herwig Ostermann
University for Health Sciences, Medical Informatics and Technology, Austria

Medical Information Science REFERENCE

MEDICAL INFORMATION SCIENCE REFERENCE

Hershey · New York

Director of Editorial Content: Kristin Klinger
Director of Production: Jennifer Neidig
Managing Editor: Jamie Snavely
Assistant Managing Editor: Carole Coulson
Typesetter: Chris Hrobak
Cover Design: Lisa Tosheff
Printed at: Yurchak Printing Inc.

Published in the United States of America by
Information Science Reference (an imprint of IGI Global)
701 E. Chocolate Avenue, Suite 200
Hershey PA 17033
Tel: 717-533-8845
Fax: 717-533-8661
E-mail: cust@igi-global.com
Web site: http://www.igi-global.com

and in the United Kingdom by
Information Science Reference (an imprint of IGI Global)
3 Henrietta Street
Covent Garden
London WC2E 8LU
Tel: 44 20 7240 0856
Fax: 44 20 7379 0609
Web site: http://www.eurospanbookstore.com

Library of Congress Cataloging-in-Publication Data

Nursing and clinical informatics : socio-technical approaches / Bettina Staudinger, Victoria Hoess, and Herwig Ostermann, editors.
p. ; cm.
Includes bibliographical references and index.
Summary: "This book gives a general overview of the current state of nursing informatics giving particular attention to social, socio-technical, and political basic conditions"--Provided by publisher.
ISBN 978-1-60566-234-3 (h/c)
1. Nursing informatics. 2. Information storage and retrieval systems--Nursing. I. Staudinger, Bettina, 1967- II. Hoess, Victoria. III. Ostermann, Herwig.
[DNLM: 1. Nursing Informatics. 2. Nursing Process. 3. Social Conditions. WY 26.5 N9736 2009]
RT50.5.N858 2009
651.5'04261--dc22

2008033942

British Cataloguing in Publication Data
A Cataloguing in Publication record for this book is available from the British Library.

EDITORIAL ADVISORY BOARD

LIST OF REVIEWERS

Herwig Ostermann, *UMIT, Austria*
Rüdiger Ostermann, *FH Münster, Germany*
Pammla Petrucka, *University of Saskatchewan, Canada*
Stefan Piehler, *UMIT, Austria*
Elizabeth Rogerson, *University of Dundee, UK*
Monika Roth, *UMIT, Austria*
Jerono Rotich, *North Carolina Agricultural & Technical State University, USA*
Martina Schaffenrath-Resi, *UMIT, Austria*
Bettina Staudinger, *UMIT, Austria*
Oskar Staudinger, *S2-Engineering, Austria*
Christa Them, *UMIT, Austria*
Lawrence Tomei, *RMU, USA*
Harald Stummer, *UMIT, Austria*
Werner Auer-Rizzi, *Johannes Kepler Universität, Austria*
Fritz Hoppichler, *A.ö. Krankenhaus der Barmherzigen Brüder, Austria*

Table of Contents

Detailed Table of Contents

The objective of this chapter is to promote public health nursing and community health nursing's role in the new care delivery patterns, with predictive and preventative care models for populations. This entry will broaden the range of information available for informaticists, as their role expands in the new healthcare arena. Articulation with nursing informatics and the 'quality chasm' crossings in US healthcare will assist the informaticists with search and retrieval activities. All players in the healthcare arena will continue to be involved, but probably with a more rational policy-making role.

Experience in nursing practice shows that there are still problems with assessment in computer-based nursing documentation. In addition to nursing documentation an assessment instrument, which captures the needs for care, must also be integrated. The chapter describes different Nursing Assessment Instruments and the advantages of Computer-Based Nursing Process Documentation by using quality criteria for assessment instruments such as validity, sensitivity, specificity, reliability, practicability and the appropriateness of the instrument. Quality criteria for computer-based systems are basically software ergonomic aspects and therefore not part of this study. Each country should choose for itself those specific assessment instruments that capture the needs for care of their clients. The data presented make it possible that facilities are compared (also in regard of reliable cost estimates).

Increasingly, new and extended roles and responsibilities for nurses are being supported through the introduction of clinical decision support systems (CDSS). This chapter provides an overview of research on nurses' use of CDSS, considers the impact of CDSS on nurse decision making and patient outcomes, and explores the socio-technical factors that impact the use of CDSS. The chapter presents the results of a multi-site case study that explored how CDSS are used by nurses in practice in a range of contexts. The study reveals that how a system is used may vary considerably from the original intentions of the system designer.

This chapter will give an overview of the health care related challenges that most newcomer immigrants and refugees encounter as they acculturate into their new environments in Western countries. It will highlight practical tips that can: enhance the caregiver and patient relationships across cultures and across continents; enhance culturally sensitive health care services; and help to create culturally inviting health care environments. It is also evident that, although these newcomers enrich their new nations with their diverse backgrounds, language and cultural differences continues to pose formidable obstacles to their health, health care providers and health system in general. While the patients and providers realize the effects of immigration on the quality and access to health care, they seem to be overwhelmed by the barriers.

This chapter presents the imperatives of mobile technologies in the health care. It presents the contextual overview in development of the diffusion, penetration, and uptake of health related mobile technologies. A consideration of the roles and responsibilities of the diaspora in the embracing of information and communication technologies is emphasized. Key examples of mobile technologies in development to increase understanding and demonstrate promising practices in this emergent field are given.

Computerized patient care documentation (CPD) is a vital part of a Patient Care Information System (PCIS). Studying CPD in a well-established PCIS is useful because problems of system adoption and startup do not interfere with observations. Factors interfering with optimal nursing use of CPD are particularly challenging and of great concern, given today's shortage of nursing manpower. The chapter describes problems and advantages of CPD usage identified by nurses in a series of research interviews. It is shown that explicit consideration of nursing workflow constraints and communication processes is necessary for development of effective nursing documentation systems. Some findings point to a PCIS reconfiguration strategy that is feasible in the short term. Other findings suggest the value of considering mobile and team-oriented technologies in future versions of the PCIS.

Home telehealth, the use of information and communication technologies to deliver and support health care directly to the home, is emerging as an important application for nurses. This chapter provides an overview of home telehealth and how it may be applied to the practical challenges nurses face everyday. We provide a summary of the evidence available to support its use in specific areas and a guide for those thinking of implementing telehealth in their own practice. The future of home telehealth lies in carefully considered and designed research, ongoing education and training and a multidisciplinary approach.

This chapter presents a theoretical framework and research base for the successful transition of an established Master of Science in Nursing program from that of traditional classroom delivery to one that is web-based with no geographic limitations to students. The application of socio-technical systems theory to facilitate creation of a positive learning environment for future nurse leaders is described. Use of social processes and application of technology to optimize learning is explained and the latest research on content presentation and student engagement in an e-learning environment are presented. The chapter gives an understanding of the competencies necessary for students and faculty to be successful in online education.

Concerning nursing resource allocation health service executives have different views about whether systems based on ratios or those based on patient dependency are more accurate. This chapter reports on a statistical analysis of almost 2 million hours of nursing data provided by 22 acute care public and private hospitals in Australia, New Zealand and Thailand. To evaluate both ways an informatics system was used which has the capacity to simultaneously measure nurse patient ratios and nursing workloads by a dependency method of nursing hours per patient day. The results showed that it predicts actual direct nursing care requirements with greater accuracy than ratios for all hospital and patient types, facilitating better allocation of nursing resources and demonstrating that the cost of nursing care would be less for hospitals using that system than for ratios.

A range of new technologies/information systems are being implemented in clinical settings in order to reduce errors associated with the medication administration process. Simulation methods can be used to assess the impact of integrating new technology/information systems into the nurses' work environment prior to full scale implementation of a health technology/information system. Simulations as an evaluative tool emerged from a direct need to assess unintended and intended consequences of health information systems upon nurses' work before systems are fully implemented. Nurse informatician use of simulations to assess and test health technologies/information systems will allow nurses to determine the impact of a new software and/or hardware upon aspects of nurses' work before its implementation to allow for appropriate system modifications.

This chapter explores the potential of a conceptual framework – Hodges' model – both as a socio-technical structure and means to explore such structures of relevance to nursing informatics theory and practice. The model can be applied universally by virtue of its structure and the content which it can encompass. In apprehending this chapter readers will be able to draw, describe and explain the scope of Hodges' model within contemporary health care contexts and the wider global issues presented by the 21st century that influence and shape nursing informatics. Critically, the reader will also gain insight into how socio-technical structures can facilitate cross fertilization of clinical and informatics theory and practice; drawing attention to information as a concept that provides a bridge between socio-technical,

Foreword

While computer systems to document nursing care have been in existence since at least the early 1960's, it was only in the early 1980's that we began to formally define and describe the emerging discipline of nursing informatics. Since those early days, nurses in many parts of the world have taken leading roles in exploring, implementing, researching and promoting the use of a range of increasingly computerised, and increasingly networked, technologies to support the delivery of nursing and all other aspects of healthcare. Nurses and nurse informaticians have long recognised that simple technical and technological solutions will not address the problems of the world's health services, and that socio-technical approaches, that take account of the inter-relationship between the social and the technical factors, are vital for successful system implementation and organisational change.

Even today, though, as we move towards the second decade of the twenty first century, and with the ready availability of countless examples, case studies, and a wealth of supporting theory, governments and organisations, sadly, still try, with predictably disastrous results, to implement purely technical and technological solutions to health and healthcare problems. Which makes the need for a book such as this, that foregrounds the importance of socio-technical approaches, all the more important, and its appearance very timely.

In many countries of the world, similar challenges are being faced, and increasingly, the role of nurses and nurse informaticians in helping to inform the decision-making processes is being recognised. Those nurses themselves need to have a good understanding of the complexity of the socio-technical interactions that affect the design, implementation and evaluation of health information systems. They also need to recognise that, just as nursing itself draws on, and interacts with, a wide range of disciplines for its theory and practice base, so socio-technical approaches similarly require awareness and understanding drawn from many disciplines. The wide range of disciplines addressed in this book can help them in that understanding.

As a nurse with a background in critical care, with its high dependence of technology, I became aware early in my career that simple reliance on technology could never fully address the needs of the patients and their families; nor could technologies introduced without the involvement of the nurses and other health professionals expected to use them ever result in real improvements to care. However, we need to recognise the reality that many technologies exist and are continually being developed that offer potential for improving care in whatever setting the nurse or other health professional may interact with the patient or their family, or may contribute to the promotion of health and prevention of disease at the population level. The application of socio-technical approaches, and consideration of the lessons illustrated in many of the chapters of this book, can help us to come to the right decisions on whether the technologies can provide real benefit.

The various chapters, whose authors come from many different parts of the worlds, recognise the increasingly diverse and often, non-traditional, care settings in which nursing informatics has a role and cover a range of methodological approaches. The increasing importance of interaction at a geographic distance, mediated by technology, to provide care is addressed in the chapters that deal with aspects of telehealth and that explore the delivery of telehealth applications in home and other settings, through a range of technologies, and the impact this might have on nursing roles in different contexts.

Mobile technologies, in particularly phones, handheld digital assistants, and the newer 'smartphones' that combine many technologies and applications in one device, offer significant potential to support improvements in healthcare delivery, especially in low-income and developing countries. The chapter addressing these issues will be of particular interest to anyone interested in exploring leading edge developments.

Education is one area where nursing and technology have long had strong interaction, whether in terms of using technologies to deliver and support education, or in exploration of the technologies as the educational content. It is appropriate, therefore, that several chapters explore a range of perspectives including pedagogical strategies, virtual learning communities and use of technologies such as handheld devices.

The definition of nursing informatics adopted in 1998 by the International Medical Informatics Association's Special Interest Group in Nursing Informatics, states that **nursing informatics is "the integration of nursing, its information, and information management with information processing and communication technology, to support the health of people world wide."** In late 2007, the Yahoo! Education website identified nursing informatics as number one in its "10 hottest emerging careers that you might not know about, but probably should". This book is a valuable resource for both the established nurse informatician and the new recruit that we need to attract to the discipline, with lessons for both in the need for appropriate application of socio-technical approaches to using technology to support the health of people world wide. Hopefully, as a result, we can avoid further repetition of the mistakes of the past, and of the present era.

Peter J. Murray PhD, MSc, CertEd, RN, FBCS CITP
Director and Founding Fellow, Centre for Health Informatics Research and Development (CHIRAD)
Vice President Strategic Planning (Implementation and Communication), International Medical Informatics Association

Lincolnshire, UK

Peter J. Murray *is a founding fellow and director of CHIRAD (Centre for Health Informatics Research and Development), a virtual centre based in the UK, through which he teaches and is research module leader on the MSc in health informatics at University of Winchester, UK and at Walter Sisulu University, South Africa. He has over 25 years healthcare experience, originally as a coronary care nurse before moving into education and health informatics. He has an MSc in nursing, and a PhD in nursing infomatics and educational technology from The Open University, in the UK. His current interests include free/libre and open source software, online education and the use of Web 2.0 technologies, and he has numerous publications and conference presentations on these and other topics. He co-founded the IMIA, EFMI and AMIA Open Source Working Groups, has been UK representative to IMIA (International Medical Informatics Association) and the IMIA Nursing Informatics SIG, and is a member of the IMIA Board, as vice president for Strategic Planning. An online CV can be found at http://www.peter-murray.net*

Preface

The field of Nursing Informatics belongs to one of the fastest growing areas of medical informatics and there are several reasons for this:

1. Through increasing life expectancy and the stronger development of the social system, the area of nursing has been able to gain an overall higher status and therefore a higher degree of professionalism. This has the consequence that fast growing markets can be observed in this area.
2. A professionalization offensive in applied nursing runs parallel with this development, the offensive ultimately being thematically controlled by the nursing sciences. The described Theory-Practice-Gap is currently being attempted to be bridged, on the one hand using knowledge transfer, and standardization on the other.
3. From this there is an increased necessity for the application of Nursing Informatics whereby the operative noosing process has to be supported. On the other, both planning data and data that secure quality can be attained, which can be used for the further organizing of the nursing system in a political and structural respect.

The objective of this publication *Nursing and Clinical Informatics: Socio-Technical Approaches* consists of giving a general overview of the current state of Nursing Informatics, giving particular attention to social, socio-technical, and political basic conditions and additionally to sketch out the main focus of further research and development projects.

Here, it is especially important that the interdisciplinarity of the field of research can be clearly worked out. This means that the core areas of Nursing Informatics, technical feasibility, functionality, and recoverability, form a focal point of the work which will combine the technical components with nursing-relevant areas. On the one hand this affects the political and regulatory influences on the nursing system itself (i.e. the organization of the system and the given scope for structure), and on the other it affects the impact of nursing science, particularly there where nursing is carried out in standardised form.

An essential part of the objective is the internationality. This is because the nursing sciences do portray an internationally active scientific community through the political and legal organisation and social impacts, but the individual nursing systems feature severe deviations. This ultimately presents a particular challenge for Nursing Informatics, especially in the area of function and standardisation demands.

This book is aimed at the scientific community in the area of nursing sciences, system research, and nursing informatics as well as the practitioners and operating authorities of nursing infrastructures. It should reflect the current scientific stand in Nursing Informatics in a general context and therefore serve the scientific community with a basis for further research projects. In addition, this handbook should serve as a concrete foundation of how knowledge transfer can take place, particularly in knowledge transfer from science in practice.

The particular value of this book lies in the fact that it will be a unique international comparative work in the area of Nursing Informatics which covers not only the core areas of Nursing Informatics in a technical and functional respect, but also includes the adjacent governing scientific areas and portrays them in their proper context.

As reference will not only be made to the actual situation, or rather the current state of Nursing Informatics, but also to further research prospects and future trends, this handbook shall also concisely feature the fields of responsibility for future research and research needs in this area.

Accordingly, the represented goals the chapters of this book will be presented shortly.

The first chapter deals with how the range of information furthering the search and retrieval activities of informaticists may be broadened in a context where public health nursing and community health nursing's role underlie a new care delivery pattern.

The second chapter gives an overview of the various Nursing Assessment Instruments and describes the advantages of computer-based nursing process documentation. The evaluation of the documentation is based on quality criteria such as for example validity, practicability, and appropriateness.

Due to the new and extended roles of nurses clinical decision support systems (CDSS) gain importance. Therefore, it seems appropriate to give an overview of current research on nurses' use of CDSS and amongst others, its impact on nurse decision-making.

The book's international orientation also makes it possible (in Chapter IV) to look at the obstacles immigrants face when making use of the immigration country's healthcare as this influences the nursing information systems as well.

The fifth chapter gives a contextual overview of the diffusion, penetration, and uptake of health-related mobile technologies and how these may develop in the future.

As computerized patient care documentation is an integrative part of patient care information systems the sixth chapter describes in a case study problems and advantages associated with this kind of documentation.

Given the increasing importance of home telehealth, the seventh chapter explores the possibilities of use of home telehealth for nurses to face practical challenges.

Nursing informatics also encompasses the way nurses are taught. In this regard, the eighth chapter represents a way of how traditional classroom delivery can be transferred into Web-based instruction, using the example of a master's of science in nursing program.

Nursing resource allocation may be made by applying ratios or based on patient dependency. The ninth chapter explores which one is more accurate and facilitates the allocation of nursing resources.

To determine the impact of a new software and/or hardware upon aspects of nurses' work before its implementation may be tested with simulation methods. The tenth chapter promotes the use of simulation methods as an evaluative tool prior to full-scale implementation of health technology and information systems.

Hodge's model as a conceptual framework is applied to explore structures of relevance to nursing informatics theory and practice. The eleventh chapter reviews the socio-technical literature and venture definitions. It offers ways to reflect upon and construct socio-technical structures.

The second chapter (Chapter XII) that deals with teaching nurses, answers one main question, "how can educators effectively teach the very social discipline of nursing in virtual classrooms" and presents research questions that arise from this exploration.

The thirteenth chapter presents a case study where the implementation of an information system on organizational communication processes in a residence of elderly is researched.

As telemedical consultations via telemedicine or distant medical consultations are increasing, as has already been mentioned, possible roles of nurses in different types of telemedical consultations are discussed in the fourteenth chapter.

The purpose of Chapter XV is to discuss in the context of rural Australia the need for enhanced evidence-based medicine (EBM) by nurses, and how nursing informatics could help.

When instructing nurses, handheld computers are most frequently used, as these devices provide students with information for point of care clinical references. Therefore, the sixteenth chapter gives an overview of the use of handheld computers in nursing and medical education and provides advantages and disadvantages then discusses future directions in this field.

The final chapter also deals with Information Technology in nursing education and discusses the development of use of IT in nursing education including mainstream and emerging technologies.

The diverse and comprehensive coverage of multiple disciplines in the field of nursing informatics in this authoritative handbook will contribute to a better understanding of the complexity of nursing informatics. Furthermore, the contributions included in this handbook will be instrumental in the expansion of the body of knowledge in this vast field.

It is our sincere hope that this publication and its great amount of information and research will assist our research colleagues, all faculty, their students, and our organizational decision makers in enhancing their understanding of this discipline. Perhaps this publication will even inspire its readers to contribute to the current discoveries in this immense field, tapping possibilities to assist humankind in making the world a better place to live for all inhabitants of this universe.

Bettina Staudinger, Victoria Höß, Herwig Ostermann
Editors

Acknowledgment

The editors would not have been able to complete this publication without the contribution of nursing and clinical informatics professionals and academics all over the world. In this context, we would also like to acknowledge particularly the efforts of IMIA nursing informatics group, which encouraged authors to contribute to this book as well as participate in the academic debate triggered by the contributions itself. Moreover, the editors would like to thank all persons – academics as well as professionals – for willingly reviewing chapters in time.

The authors would like to express their gratitude to all persons, whose enthusiasm and academic passion in the field of nursing informatics made this publication possible. First and foremost, we notably want to acknowledge Prof. Roland Staudinger, PhD, head of the Institute for Human and Economic Sciences at University of Health Sciences, Medical Informatics and Technology, Hall/Tyrol, Austria, for providing the editors with the opportunity to benefit from an academically challenging and inspiring environment at the institute. Thanks also to Julia Mosemann, development editor at IGI Global, for her editorial assistance and support with the preparation of the manuscript.

Chapter I
A Treatise on Rural Public Health Nursing

Wanda Sneed
Tarleton State University, USA

ABSTRACT

Nursing informaticists can be leaders in promoting prevention of illness and diseases in the 21st century. Developing an infrastructure for application of preventive and predicative models in healthcare delivery is paramount. This chapter stresses the need for rural regions to develop paradigmatic models for incorporating all aspect of the human ecology domain. While movement in public health nursing is contingent on improvement in public health interconnectivity, nurse informaticists need to develop a classification system for public health nursing, develop databases for evidence–based practice, and incorporate the rural culture in their work. Incorporation of genomics in daily nursing practice will soon be a reality. As consumer-driven healthcare becomes the reality, the platform for healthcare delivery will change. A change to care delivery in a variety of community sites with electronic information exchanges and personal health records will require robust work by informaticists. Remote monitoring devices in clients' homes are another arena which will require a new set of skills for nursing interventionists.

A TREATISE ON RURAL PUBLIC HEALTH NURSING INFORMATICS

Rural public health nursing needs a classification system, an evidence-based practice database, and development of a model for nursing care delivery in rural environments. Nursing informatics is the tool to accomplish these needs. Nursing informatics is the retrieval of data and information to support nursing clinical practice and research and for the equipping of information management systems. In the discipline of nursing, cognitive systems have grown more rapidly than practice. Hence nursing informatics has grown in depth rather than breadth. A number of reasons support this phenomenon. The history of the nursing profession clearly shows an almost continuous evaluation and re-evaluation of the discipline. Socio-cultural factors have been the most recent mover of nursing science (Institute of Medicine [Committee on Quality of Health Care], 2001; Kimball & O'Neil, 2003). Health information technology has transformed the healthcare arena. As a result of information available to the public, a demand for greater accuracy and transparency in health care has thrust nursing to the forefront of evidence-based care and a focused research orientation. In addition, a desire within the discipline for scientific support for practice has evolved into a primary focus on evidence-based practice. Nurse informaticists are needed to integrate scientific research into public health, public health nursing and population care. Nursing informaticists are needed to develop a classification system for public health nursing, community care and rural healthcare.

The objective of this chapter is to promote public health nursing and community health nursing's role in the new care delivery patterns, with predictive and preventative care models for populations. This entry will broaden the range of information available for informaticists, as their role expands in the new healthcare arena. Articulation with nursing informatics and the 'quality chasm' crossings in US healthcare will assist the informaticists with search and retrieval activities.

Nursing has a short history of evidence-based practice, unlike medicine which has garnered support from many sources to make evidence-based practice information readily available. Efforts are occurring to utilize research evidence as well as practice acumen to support evidence-based care in nursing (Berg, Fleischer & Behrens, 2005). Research support for public health/community health nursing comes from multiple sources, including biomedical, pharmacological, toxicological, human genomic, and public health sources.

Human Ecology Domain

Public health sources cover the 'gray literature' of human ecology, i.e., environmental practices, economics, agriculture, nutrition, extreme use of antibiotics, veterinary medicine, and infectious disease profiles. Likewise public health nursing examines the 'gray literature' for evidence-based data. Examples of sources include: The Journal of Urban Health; Smithsonian; Scientific American; Journal of Nutraceuticals; Social Justice; National Center for Complimentary & Alternative Medicine; Human Ecology: An Interdisciplinary Journal. These sources provide evidence from experts in their field, historical data, and research data. The skill of informaticists in searching and retrieving evidence from such diverse sources is needed to formalize a database and web-site dedicated to public health nursing and community health nursing.

The disciplines of nursing and public health have a shared history of health care and illness prevention in the community. Public health nursing needs an information infrastructure, delineation of a language and classification in the Unified Medical Language System (UMLS). This is a momentous task, given the sparsely developed public health informatics sector. Prime concerns in the discipline of public health are the socio-cultural and socio-economic constraints related to the application of primary care and primary prevention activities. The economic concerns have been placed on the national agenda by the American Medical Informatics Association (AMIA), 2007 task force, Healthcare terminologies and classifications: An action agenda for the United States. (2006). A previous publication by the Institute of Medicine (IOM), *The Future of the Public's Health in the Twenty-first Century (2003)* portrayed the problem as a societal responsibility, not just a governmental concern. Public health nurses play a major role in providing care to the populations and aggregates defined as the 'public' and consequently share in the need for building of a core infrastructure in public health.

Public Health

In 2001 the American Medical Informatics Spring Congress on "Developing a National Agenda for Public Health Informatics" discussed the idea of 'delivery of just in time information' (Cimino, 2001) in public health. Current technology barriers and solutions were examined by the presenters and participants. Most agreed on the absence or inadequacy of an electronic infrastructure to provide the needed surveillance. Isolated pockets of technology were identified, but the economic constraints on small, regional public health departments were viewed as paramount. Collaboration to extend nursing and medical care into the community was seen as the focus of current public health efforts. Modest efforts to promote connectivity, introduce primary information web sites and increase interdisciplinary activities have appeared on the horizon (Public Health Informatics Institute, 2006b; Institute of Medicine [Committee on the Future of Rural Health Care], 2005; Tilson & Berkowitz, 2006

In 2006 the Public Health Informatics Institute was designated by the Robert Woods Johnson Foundation as the National Clearing House for grant funding in public health. Two significant and innovative fundings were developed and distributed for public health endeavors in the 21st century. They are titled "Common Ground: Transforming Public Health Information Systems" and a report on collaboration, "Taking Care of Business" (Public Health Informatics Institute, 2006a; Public Health Informatics Institute, 2006b) The grant and conference report are major steps forward in developing and implementing a core for public health informatics. Another major event occurred in late 2007, when the American Medical Informatics Association (AMIA) partnered with the Center for Disease Control (CDC) to launch a 5-year cooperative agreement to advance the public health workforce. AMIA is a world leader in biomedical and health informatics. This organization will be presenting one of the first summits on translational bioinformatics in early 2008 (AMIA, 2007). AMIA will also host the 11th International Congress on Nursing Informatics [N12012] in Canada on June 23-27, 2012 (American Medical Informatics Association, 2007

The development of evidenced-based nursing practice databases and web sites is crucial in the migration to client-centered care. Predictive and preventative healthcare models will become a nurse informaticists issue. In addition, development of paradigmatic models for incorporating all aspects of the human ecology domain area needed. Toxic environmental exposures, unsafe water, infectious disease and nutritional problems are in need of planning for prevention and treatment. The political forces and financial interests shaping healthcare delivery should become primary knowledge, thereby promoting these issues.

RURAL PUBLIC HEALTH NURSING

Public health nursing, nursing informatics and public health are exquisitely interconnected. However, the role of nurses in public health is not always accorded due consideration. Public health nurses have a greater independent role in population health, than just clinical outreach or epidemiological surveillance. Public health nurses provide assurance care, education of populations at-risk for disease, health promotion and lifestyle change information, and case-management of aggregates with chronic disease needs. They also actively participate in control of infectious disease and conduct research. Public health nurses advocate privately and in the political arena for the rights of underprivileged disenfranchised groups.

The community-focused care by nurses includes public health functions, plus the managing and delivery of home care to individuals, families and aggregates. Community health nurses perform community assessments, develop policies for care delivery, and function as school health nurses.

Nurse informaticists have a role to play in rural public health nursing, plus a compelling array of topics to research, develop and implement. These efforts must occur simultaneously, in order to meet the challenges of the future. Public health nurses' need to articulate the changing healthcare delivery patterns, as a joint endeavor with public health, government and private institutes. The new delivery patterns focus on predictive and preventative measures, and tools for population health. Also considered in these delivery patterns are urgent reforms needed in preparedness for terrorism attacks. Population health ultimately translates into individual care delivery. Personal health information with construction of personal health records (PHR's) is a major focus for electronic data retrieval. This is a radical change from the previous climate of physician protected disease information. The previous, and largely current, medical monopoly of episodic, acute, disease oriented care delivery will give-way to greater accuracy and transparency in healthcare, with a client-oriented care atmosphere. Public health nurses currently assess populations at greatest risk and target them for health promotion activities, i.e., healthy diets, exercise, saying 'No' to tobacco use. They function as environmental and occupational spokespersons, protecting the health and minimizing risks. Examples in rural areas include monitoring of field spraying with herbicides and organophosphates and monitoring the pollutions effects of dairy and hog farm runoff. The groundwater in rural areas is frequently contaminated by farm pollution, generally in the form of nitrates (Electronic Research Service/United States Department of Agriculture [ERS/USDA]. 2007). Prevention of illness, such as immunizations for infectious diseases is another primary example of services provided by public health nurses.

Models

The preventative model for care delivery has wide-origins. The World Health Organization (WHO)'s report of 1981 comes from years of data collection and information related to health issues in all countries. In 1988 the Institute of Medicine's report, *The Future of Public Health*, set in motion the ideas for reforming the U.S. healthcare system. Nurse informaticists can be leaders in promoting prevention of illness and diseases in the 21st century. They are well prepared in communications skills and interdisciplinary activities.

The principle preventative model in the U.S. is the public health practice model of primary, secondary and tertiary prevention. This model is comprehensive, basic and based on assessment of known risks and existing hazards. The focus is firstly on education for health promotion, then screening and treatment and follow-thru with management to prevent relapse and complications. Adjunctive to this preventative model are various models and systems of care delivery developed by private centers, academic centers and recently the third-party payers group. These models tend to address managing disease processes to prevent complications. Examples include the chronic care model and the disease management model. The chronic disease model integrates community resources, health system organizations and patient self-management supported by information technology (Bu, Pan, Johnston, Walker, Adler-Milstein, Kendrick, et.al, 2007). The disease management model uses a multidisciplinary team approach to management of a chronic disease, with emphasis on patient self-management. A prime component of this model is information technology support. Disease management is an enhanced version of the medical model, with more evidence-based guidelines and patient involvement.

Some variants of population or group care delivery are not classifiable as models, but involve significant changes in the delivery focus. In the United States several recent innovations demonstrate the changing face of care delivery. The skills of advanced nurse practitioners are used in a reformed environment. One example is a process called *Care in the Express Lane* (Waton, 2007, April) which describes the needs of individuals and how they utilize walk-in client services at mini clinics. This system radically reduces the costs, improves the benefits for common complaints and demonstrates the changing face of care delivery. 'On-site health centers' are another system which provides corporate wellness strategies and illness prevention strategies for large employers and their employees. Examples include the 10,000 employees at Credit Suisse and the 17,000 client visits in 2006 at the Sprint Nextel health center (Basler, 2007). Other walk-in systems include health service centers in grocery stores, pharmacies, and other high traffic areas of a community. These examples address the need for primary care and secondary care (screening) delivered specifically with clients as the focus. The processes of providing preventative care are the rational solution to comprehensive quality care, the reduction of suffering and disability and the choice of newly empowered, electronic-savvy generations.

The design, implementation and evaluation of another new care delivery pattern, e.g., predictive care provision based on genomic profiles will be revolutionary. The Human Genome Project, completed in 2001 formed the basis for identification and control of chronic diseases, gene transmitted diseases, child and adolescent defects and disabilities, infectious diseases and more. Progresses in endeavors for human genome predictions have not been rapidly advanced. Several reasons exist for slow progress. One reason is the lack of trained bioinformatists to analyze and interpret the data which is continuously made available. Another reason pertains to a lack of enthusiasm among care-providers and third-party payers to change an embedded system of acute care. Thirdly, the bioethics of identifying a condition for which no cure or treatment exists remains resolved. Fourthly, the economics of individual genome analysis has hampered advancement. The medical-insurance complex has apparently been waiting for the $1000.00 gene test.

However, a body of information for predictive modeling has emerged. This information is readily available on the Internet. The Center for Disease Control and Prevention provides multiple education programs, seminars, Web Sites, and databases on the subject of genomic data, public health, population health and predictions for the future of healthcare (National Office of Public Health Genomics [CDC], 2007). A focus on population needs, based on consideration of the basic facets of human exposure, can reveal possible patterns of disease (Khoury & Mensah, 2005) and suggest early intervention.

Predictive modeling is not a new concept. Predictive modeling as a group of analytical methods has been used by healthcare plans for decades. In the past, the primary use of predictive modeling has been to (1) reduce financial risk for payors and (2) to identify high risk patients with high cost diseases. The latest vendor push is integrated systems which look at healthcare claims data but also look at data gathered for proactive intervenability. This data collection may begin with an enrollees' self-perception of their health, then, a delineation of behavior and lifestyle and a record of compliance via a personal health record. This is followed with assignment of a healthcare proctor who functions on a one-to-one basis with the enrollee to advise and educate. These models are helpful but not enough, and do not address the science and technology available for patient-centered, patient-directed care based on individual genetic profiles.

Care management with predictive models needs to utilize intelligent communications with enrollees/consumers to positively impact their behavior. Effective data gathering yields information which 'puts a face on the consumer'. More than logistics and a few medical facts are needed. It will be important to know if screening tests were initiated by providers or individuals, what are the age-gender-responsibilities of workers, are there financial difficulties and where is the information about community resources that can assist with payments for healthcare. Consumer/client driven healthcare comes with empowerment and self-management and predictive modeling. Ethically we must provide the consumer with sufficient information to manage their care, as well as decide as a society how to provide for those who make imprudent decisions (Robbins & Brill, 2005). However the out-reach for evidence-based, predictive genomic information will be the revolutionary step to healthcare transformation in the 21st century.

HEALTHCARE DELIVERY PATTERNS

Healthcare savvy, computer oriented consumers are seeking support and guidance for planning their health and future life. They already have access to large amounts of data from the Internet regarding the 'quality chasm' issues identified by the Institute of Medicine (IOM) (Corrigan, J, Kohn, L, & Donaldson, M., 2000; IOM, 2001). These 'quality chasm' issues or gaps in healthcare delivery are caused by a fragmented and poorly organized system that does not utilize its resources efficiently. The needed correction is possible with a new health care system that has the following six attributes: (1) safe care, (2) effective care, (3) patient-centered care, (4) timely care, (5) efficient care and (6) equitable care (IOM, 2001). Appropriate use of technology can improve the safety aspect; evidence-based knowledge and practice will provide effectiveness, and an actual focus on patient-centered care will provide timely proactive interventions. A reduction in redundancy, collaborative care and the use of informatics at the point of care will provide the basis for efficient and equitable care.

Patient-centered, consumer/client driven care requires greater transparency and accountability. No longer is it possible for unquestioning compliance to orders to continue as the norm in healthcare. Quality assurance evaluations of care, healthcare providers, systems and institutions are available on the Internet. Rating systems regarding hospital performance rates, statistics on mortality rates and quality profiles of individual practitioners are readily available. Ratings of insurance plan coverage and responsiveness are posted by governments and private institutions. Healthcare providers, especially those involved in population health have a responsibility to educate individuals, aggregates and countries in quality measures.

A scenario for predictive modeling uses genomic medicine, patient health perception and new care delivery formats. Scenario: The case involves a 25 year old white Anglo woman who is knowledgeable regarding her positive family history of breast cancer. She seeks a physicians' help for predictive testing. Genetic tests exclude BRCA1 and BRCA2 genetic mutations. Further testing demonstrates a spike in metabolic residue from excess hydrogen radical formation, which indicates a beginning pathway to malignancy. Other conventional assessments exclude any breast mass, cysts or abnormalities. She is referred to the advanced nurse practitioner (ANP) for counseling and education. The ANP obtains a detailed history of lifetime environmental exposures, dietary habits, work environments, types of recreational activities, i.e., exposure types in hobbies, and medication usage. The ANP discusses the known exposures to risk factors, specifically xenoestrogens. These include childhood and adolescent exposure to organophosphate chemicals on her parents' farm, swimming in lakes with runoff from the now-defunct chemical-fertilizer plant near her home. The patient is advised to continue yearly physical examinations and genomic assessments. She is provided information on including antioxidants in her diet, e.g., cruciferous vegetables, plus use of alternative biological antioxidants. These antioxidants can be obtained in nutraceutical dosage forms and/or functional foods containing nordihydroguaiaretic acid. The ANP enrolls the client in the healthcare payor's information registry and forwards all existing records to the account. This includes genetic testing results, counseling information and family history genetic algorithm. With client agreement, she also establishes a timeline for notices and reminders of appoints needed. In this scenario the ANP functions as a case manager and clinical specialist with extensive knowledge of genomic testing and interventions for lifestyle behaviors.

The role of nurse informaticists in the new care delivery models needs to be developed beyond the standard data and information storage and management techniques. The 'delivery of just in time information' (Cimino, 2001) should be the goal and the standard. Public health nurses with advanced degrees have the attributes and knowledge to use predictive modeling of genomic data to provide care for populations. The informaticists' has to analyze, model and present the necessary knowledge to enable behavioral interventions for groups of individuals and professionals. The individual may be self-managing their health and desire some assistance. Nursing professionals' need assurance an adequate fund of scientific, evidence-based information exists. This information must be readily available and deliverable to both urban and rural areas. An example of the kinds of genomic information needed by nursing professionals is the text '*Nutrigenomics and Beyond: Informing the Future*' by Institute of Medicine (2007). This text provides further evidence of nutrient-gene and gene-environment interactions. The impact of human nutritional needs, healthy and unhealthy dietary habits, maintenance of a safe food supply and the economics of food production invades most sectors of life. The data and information being developed in this sphere of health and illness may be the most important event of the 21st century.

EVIDENCE-BASED PRACTICE

Evidence-based practice resources are available from a number of entities. These include governmental agencies, universities, academic centers, libraries, veterans system and private vendor organizations. Most of the documents are available via the World Wide Web and in print. The Agency for Healthcare Research and Quality (AHRQ) is one of the oldest and most widely known. AHRQ produces evidence reports and clinical practice guidelines. AHRQ has funded thirteen evidenced-based practice centers, based in technology centers, universities and academic center (AHRQ, 2007). Other governmental sites include the Center for Disease Control and Prevention (CDC) site for public health professionals(CDC, 2007), the Veterans Evidence-Based Research Dissemination Implementation Center (VERDICT, 2007). Private entities have learning resources and websites on the topic of evidence-based practice (Netting the Evidence, 2007). The four databases on evidence-based medicine in the Cochrane Library, produced by the world-wide web virtual Cochrane Collection is available to libraries and via CD-ROM. Recently several universities in Texas have established evidence-based practice centers specifically for nursing. The Academic Center for Evidence-Based Practice (ACE) at the University of San Antonio School of Nursing was established in 2000. The Texas Tech University Health Sciences School of Nursing and the Medical Center Hospital in Odessa, Texas are establishing an evidence-based practice center in 2007. These are encouraging developments that need to make massive moves forward to provide the needed resources for nursing.

A critical need exists in nursing informatics for an updated, current practice, public health/community health terminology and classification (taxonomy). The mission of this chapter is to promote nursings' role in preventative and predictive care delivery systems which are primarily public health nursing and community health. The means to accomplish this is vis-à-vis classification research in public health nursing and evidence based care research. The American Nurses Association (ANA) has endorsed the inclusion of two classification systems related to home care, e.g., The Omaha Community Health Problems and Interventions Classification System (Omaha System) (Martin & Scheet, 1992) and the Clinical Care Classification (CCC), (Saba, 2007) (revised from Home Health Classification System (HHCC) of Nursing Diagnoses & Interventions, Saba, 1991). Both of these systems are outdated and do not reflect the current practice of public health/community health care. They are two of the eleven classification systems recognized by ANA. The Unified Medical Language System (UMLS) also includes the Omaha System and the CCC (formerly HHCC) system. Public health nursing and community health care require sophisticated cognitive knowledge and skills in socio-economic structures, diverse cultures and communication and these requirements are not included in the two classification systems currently fronted. These classification systems are not suited for urban or rural community health. A most glaring omission is the lack of attention to socio-economic and cultural variables for rural populations and poverty areas of a community. Increasingly the evidence demonstrates the pervasiveness of an early, sustained impoverished social status on poverty encased, disenfranchised individuals and their perception of their health (Marmot, 2000; Sapolsky, 2005). The attempt to limit nursing services to bedside-type functions, in both of these systems is outdated and outmoded.

The International Classification for Nursing Practice (ICNP®) Version 1 (2005) has the greatest potential for becoming a nursing language system. However this document has succumbed to the designation of "Nursing Diagnoses". Nursing diagnosis is too limiting and contradictory for public and community health care. Use of the terms 'Nursing Statement' or 'Nursing Emphasis' would be more inclusive of public health and community activities. Public health nursing is focused on population-based care. And the language is about primary prevention of illness and disease. Primary prevention is about wellness, health promotion and healthy lifestyles. Health and wellness do not require a 'diagnosis' or 'problem' to define their status. Therefore, the North American Nursing Diagnosis Association International (NANDA I) nursing diagnosis approach is not applicable. A new taxonomy is needed, to address wellness terminology and the education needed to sustain a healthy lifestyle. The controversy over NANDA I relates to its focus on physiological conditions and acute care, and exclusion of 'wellness' states, prevention, and client preference. It is possible to contend that wellness education topics may start with identification of the major causes (i.e., problems) of chronic disease, but this is albeit to making the foot-fit-the shoe.

IMPACT ON RURAL PUBLIC HEALTH NURSING

The impact of new care delivery patterns with predictive and preventative models, i.e., distance monitoring, patient/client controlled information registries and nursing case management are some of the future roles involving nursing informaticists. As the technological infrastructure continues to develop in the rural areas and care delivery expands, research is needed to design and develop solutions for nursing care delivery in sparsely populated areas with multiple socio-cultural differences. Rural care provision is complex and problematic (Williams, A, & Cutchin, M, 2002). Rurality is best defined by locality.

Rurality is rife with socio-cultural differences, distance and access problems and the need for collaboration between disciplines (Institute of Medicine [IOM], 2005).

A set of research questions for the rural nursing informaticists include defining the role of technology in distance monitoring from rural locations to urban institutions and from clients homes to home health agencies. Distance monitoring includes both telemedicine and home physical assessment monitoring. Building an information and communication infrastructure in rural America begins with attention to the culture, education and financial assistance needed at the basic level of care delivery.

Improving healthcare in rural areas begins with understanding and incorporating the strengths of these environments. Loyalty to family and healthcare providers, concern for neighbors, hardiness and a drive to survive are socio-culture patterns more common in rural environments. Small hospitals, community clinics, physicians' offices, home health agencies and public health departments are the sources of healthcare in rural areas. Emergency care and transport to these facilities often depends on emergency medical services personnel who may be volunteers, hospital employees or low-wage minimally trained individuals. Communication devices are usually personal equipment, subject to interference from weather, low range capability and lack of consistent transmission towers or satellites. Travel distances and remote home locations with poor road access add to the problem. Small hospitals treat common, chronic conditions, normal labor and delivery situations and minor emergencies. Patients needing specialist care are stabilized and transferred to tertiary care facilities. Regional public health departments are the major source of preventative education, well-child care and infectious disease surveillance and immunization. The Institute of Medicine's quality chasm series directed to improving rural healthcare illustrates some significant differences in rural versus urban populations. Some of these differences in rural areas are (1) a higher rate of smoking in adolescents and adults; (2) higher rate of self-reported obesity in women; (3) less active; and (4) more threats of death from motor vehicle injuries, falls, poisoning, and suffocation (IOM, 2005). These gaps in health care need to be addressed by a system-wide approach.

Searches for advances in healthcare monitoring techniques are retrieved primarily from commercial and biotechnology web sites. A variety of 'services', programs and equipment are available. Some vendors focus on home health services, with home monitoring devices, such as 'Health Buddy' (McKesson, 2008) which transmit patient data to field offices. These field offices may be home health agencies or other service type agencies. These types of remote monitoring techniques are low-technology with wireless technology or plug-ins to power outlets and phones and do not require a computer or Internet access. They are sold to be used with or without home care nurses. The use of these devices has ballooned into an extensive system of remote monitoring. At the high-technology end is the package of telehealth advisor solutions. These include disease management programs, healthcare monitoring, educational programs on prevention and communication technology provisions for care-givers, friends, and family to pharmists, chaplains and others. These health management plans provide tiers of vendor products to be used, and require late-model computers, cameras, monitoring devices and a sophisticated user. These invasive-type telehealth systems are focused on the electronically versed individual, i.e., some of the 'baby boomers'. They also may include personal health records and healthcare financial management systems.

Questions that arise from remote, home monitoring are akin to the questions asked post-humus about expansive and expensive, telemedicine projects. Many are focused on rural participants and tout universal healthcare edicts for most diseases and illness, or focus on a select few chronic disease.

No consideration has been given to rural family values, cultural differences, socio-economic variables, and lack of an information infrastructure for delivery of the system. No consideration is given to the individual, client, patient, consumer, user, and recipient of 'healthcare services'. The major thrust of reform proposed by the Institute of Medicine is to make the healthcare delivery system *patient-focused*!

Therefore, nurse informatists' must be concerned with remote monitoring which does not require intervention by the professional best prepared to assess, monitor and evaluate homecare, i.e., the home-health nurse and the public health nurse. Where is the evidence-base of research which supports remote monitoring? Should comparative logic look at telemedicine projects for evidence? Should questions of acceptance of remote monitoring by rural cultures be addressed? Other questions needing answers from informatists' include the following:

1. Is a set of data, i.e., weight, pulse, respiration, temperature and possibly, blood pressure, peak flow measurement, and blood glucose monitoring, collected via a remote device compromised by the abilities of the data collector, the quality assurance monitoring of the device itself, and/or the dynamics of the household?
2. How much invasive technology promotes the health and welfare of the client? Is the client in charge? Are other persons assuming or demanding control for nefarious reasons?
3. Privacy issues become problematic: Do friends and neighbors need to know personnel information about an elder client? Does the client acquiesce from fear of abandonment or lack of care?
4. Is treatment delayed or unnecessary due to inappropriate referral?
5. Will third-party payors pay for all aspects of a disease management system, which may be duplicative and ill-conceived for rural patients?

Remote monitoring devices, including video, audio and physical assessment monitoring are valuable tools for the armamentarium for the rural public health/community health nurse. However, the cautions need to be in addressed prior to investment in technology which may be shelved and/or provide false assurance. These are fundamental areas of work requiring the skills of the nurse informatists.

The development of a rural health information infrastructure is a needed component of a reformed healthcare system in the United States. A surprising 75 per cent of the U.S. is rural; 80 per cent of some states are rural, e.g., Texas (ERS/USDA Research emphasis, 2007). Therefore a major force to improve and reform healthcare must traverse these rural miles to attain a connectivity desired for seamless healthcare delivery. In other words a rural-urban continuum must be formed (Ricketts, Savitz, Gesler, & Osborne, 1994). Private investors, grants and governmental funds are needed to finance the technology infrastructure for electronic connectivity (IOM, 2005).

Rural residents seeking healthcare face a number of unique obstacles. Some obstacles are personal challenges, while many are system wide, political obstacles. When the rural resident is also a member of an ethnolinguistic culture other than English-speaking, White and Anglo the obstacles begin to expand. For Hispanics, the personal obstacles lessen with acculturation and improved legality of status (Escarce & Kapur, 2006). The political obstacles remain as challenges for healthcare providers and healthcare systems in all rural areas. The non-English speaking rural resident is vulnerable to a lack of healthcare, plus Spanish speaking healthcare workers are minimal to absence in small rural hospitals. The Anglo rural resident is also vulnerable, but most commonly enters the healthcare system due to an acute illness or crisis, and is confronted with multiple bewildering choices. Some of the answers come with electronic connectivity.

PERSONAL HEALTH RECORDS

Rural areas are unique in composition, culture and use of the healthcare system. Loyalty to local healthcare providers is a component which abrogates some changes, such as 'brokered care' insurance management and change in community services. However, healthcare services are seldom self-sufficient in a rural place. Operating ties exist between urban tertiary care systems and rural practitioners. The use of personal health records would be a major improvement in continuity of care and patient-focused care. Personal health records are electronic repositories of a person's health history and health status. A reduction in over-medication, duplicative medications and repeat testing could be minimized. Patient involvement in their changing health needs would be available for scrutiny and timely engagement in new practices, such as changes in insulin dosage based on glucose monitoring, diet and activity. The Robert Wood Johnson Foundation, a private philanthropic organization, established *Project Health Design* "to promote the development of interoperable personal health care record systems that will provide a range of flexible tools that support an individuals' needs and preferences." (Robert Wood Johnson Foundation, 2007, pg. 1). This project is directed by Patricia F. Brennan, PhD, R.N. The development of personal health records will give back control of information to the clients, allow correction of inaccuracies, and should be developed with client privacy as a major concern.

Another major movement for personal health records is in a major private industry development which will significantly impact the healthcare system in the USA. Dossia, an independent, secure Wed-based system of personal health care records will empower individuals to gather their own medical data from multiple sources and to create and utilize their own personal, private and portable electronic health record (Dossia, 2007). Major U.S. employers are partnering with Dossia. These include Applied Materials, BP America, Inc., Cardinal Health, Intel Corporation, Pitney Bowes, AT&T, and Wal Mart (Dossia, 2007). This is one of several movements to empower the clients and consumers.

Patients want to know about their health status which means more transparency, less physician-dominated language, timelier test results directly to the individual and a portable health history record. Personal health records will be in place before electronic health records (EHRs) are available as a significance source of data. Leading technology experts point to recent closures and slow-downs in construction of Regional Health Information Organizations (RHIO), which are the prime vehicle for EMRs. The closure of the leading RHIO at Santa Barbara, California in 2006 portended an urgent look at health data sharing between physicians, hospitals, clinics, pharmacy and insurers (McGee, 2007). Reasons for folding of the project were ending of financial support and a lack of physician support to continue the projects. Predictions are for another decade or two before EHRs are ubiquitous.

FUTURE TRENDS

The changing face of healthcare delivery will evolve into a new dimension, with a germane interest in the pendants of socio-cultural and socio-economic structures. The practice of medicine and nursing will become individualized, personalized and genomic driven. The question of how to introduce genomic information to individuals, care providers, third-party payors and employers will be a major hurdle in re-defining the privacy laws. The care delivery platforms will change to electronic exchanges between patients, care providers and service providers. Nurse informaticists will become widely recognized as the knowledge workers with clinical expertise.

Population-based care will continue but on a more select scale with smaller aggregates as the intended clients. Genetic variations and genomic complexes in humans, animals and plants will become the basis for intervenability. Diets, medications and behaviors tailored to the individuals present and future requirements will be the norm.

A significant caution exists for global effectiveness of healthcare delivery. Will we evolve into a society with two tiers of healthcare? One level would be the electronically enabled middle and upper class with demands and capabilities to direct their health future, with the poor and vulnerable populations left to partake of health services as available.

CONCLUSION

Population-based research is available to interested and in-touch healthcare providers. We need more operational population-based research. The population-based care method focuses on broad categories of morbidity as the indicator of health resource use, rather than a few chronic diseases (Mullen, 2007). All players in the healthcare arena will continue to be involved, but hopefully with a more rational policy-making role.

REFERENCES

Agency for Healthcare Research and Quality. (2007). Retrieved May 25, 2008, from http://www.ahrq.gov/clinic/epcix.htm

American Medical Informatics Association. (2007). Retrieved October 26, 2007, from http://www.amia.org/

American Nurses Association (ANA) Recognized terminologies and data elements set (2006, May 11). *ANA nursing practice information infrastructure.* Retrieved May, 25, 2008, from http://www.nursingworld.org/npii/terminologies.htm

Basler, B. (2007, April). *Care in the express lane.* AARP (American Association of Retired Persons Publications) Bulletin, 48(4), 12-14. New York: American Association of Retired Persons Publications.

Berg, A., Fleischer, S., & Behrens, J. (2005). Development of two search strategies for literature in MEDLINE-PubMed: Nursing diagnoses in the context of evidence-based nursing. *International Journal of Nursing Terminologies and Classifications, 16(2)*, 26-32.

Bu, D., Pan, E., Johnston, D., Walker, J., Adler-Milstein, J., Kendrick, D., et.al. (2007). *The value of information technology-Enabled diabetes management.* Charlestown, MA: Healthcare Information and Management System Society.

Cimino, J. (2001). Delivery of just in time information. *American Medical Informatics Association, 2001 Spring Congress Final Program, Developing a National Agenda for Public Health Informatics.* (p.13). Bethesda, Maryland: American Medical Informatics Association.

Corrigan, J., Kohn, L., & Donaldson, M. (Eds.) (2000). *To err is human: Building a safer health system.* National Academies Press: Washington, D.C.

Dossia gains momentum toward providing employees with personal, private, portable and secure health records (2007, October 3). [Press release] Retrieved May 25, 2008, from http://www.dossia.org/home/Dossia_Gains_Momentum_Sept_07.pdf

Electronic Research Service/ United States Department of Agriculture (ERS/USDA) Research Emphasis (2007). *An enhanced quality of life for rural Americans.* Retrieved October 21, 2007, from http//www.ers.usda.gov/emphases/rural/

Escarce, J., & Kapur, K. (2006). Access to and quality of healthcare. In M. Tienda & F. Mitchell (Eds.), *Hispanics & the American Future (pp.*

410-446). Washington, D.C.: National Academies Press.

Evidence-based Practice Centers Overview (2007, July). *Agency for Healthcare Research and Quality*, Rockville, MD. Retrieved August 19, 2007 from, http://www.ahrq.gov/clinic/epc/

Healthcare Terminologies and Classification: An action agenda for the United States (2006). *American Medical Informatics Association and American Health Information Management Association*. Retrieved May, 2008 from, http://www.amia.org/inside/initatives/docs/terminologiesandclassifications.pdf

Institute of Medicine, Committee on Quality of Health Care in America (2001). *Crossing the quality chasm: A new health system for the 21st Century*. Washington, D.C.: National Academies Press.

Institute of Medicine (2003). *The future of the public's health in the 21st Century*. Washington, D.C.: National Academies Press. Institute of Medicine, Committee on the Future of Rural Healthcare. (2005). *Quality through collaboration: The future of rural health*. Washington, D.C.: National Academies Press.

Institute of Medicine (IOM) (2007). *Nutrigenomics and beyond: Informing the future*. Washington, DC: The National Academies Press.

International Council of Nurses (2005). *International Classification for Nursing Practice, Version 1*. Geneva, Switzerland: Author.

Khoury, M., & Mensah, G. (2005, April). Genomics and the prevention and control of common chronic diseases: Emerging priorities for public health action. *Preventing Chronic Disease: Public Health Research, Practice and Policy, 2(2)1- 11.* Retrieved June 8, 2005, from, http://www.cdc.gov/pcd/ issues/2005/apr/05_0011.htm

Kimball, B., & O'Neil, E. (2003). *Healthcare's human crisis: The American nursing shortage.* Robert Woods Johnson Foundation. Retrieved May 25, 2008, from, http://www.rwjf.org/files/publications/other/NursingReport.pdf

Marmot, M., & Wilkinson, R. (Eds.). (1999). *Social determinants of health*. Oxford OX2: Oxford University Press.

Martin, K., & Scheet, N. (1992). *The Omaha System: Applications for community health nursing and The Omaha System: A pocket guide for community health nursing*. Philadelphia: Saunders.

McGee, M. (2007, May 28). Urgent care. *Information Week, 140*(1), 40-50.

McKesson Corporate: Healthcare Providers (2008). Retrieved May 25, 2008, from http://www.mckesson.com/en_us/McKesson.com/For+Healthcare+Providers/Home+Care/Telehealth+Solutions/McKesson+Telehealth+Advisor+Components/Health+Buddy+Appliance.html

Mullen, P. (2007, June). A conservation with Jonathan Weiner, DrPH: Mixing population-based care with market controls. *Managed Care*, *16*(6), 1-7. Retrieved August 8, 2007, from http://www.managedcaremag.comarchives/0706/0706.qna_weiner.html

National Office of Public Health Genomics [CDC] (2007). Retrieved August 10, 2007, from http://www.cdc.gov/genomics/activities.htm

Netting the Evidence (2007). Retrieved August 19, 2007, from http://www.shef.ac.uk/=scharr/ir/netting/

North America Nursing Diagnosis Association-International (NANDA-I) (2007-2008).*Nursing diagnosis: Definitions and classifications*. Philadelphia: NANDA.

Public Health Informatics Institute (2006). *Taking care of business: A collaboration to define local health department business processes*. Decatur: GA: Public Health Institute.

Public Health Informatics Institute (2006). *Common ground: Transforming public health information systems* (2006, August 1). Retrieved September 10, 2007, from http://commonground-program.org/

Ricketts, S., Gesler, W. & Osborne, D. (Eds.). (1994). *Geographic methods for health services research. A focus on the rural-urban continuum.* Maryland: United Press of *America, Inc.*

Robbins, D. & Brill, J. (2005, May-June). *Blending ethics and empowerment with consumer-driven healthcare.* Patient Safety & Quality Healthcare. Retrieved August 4, 2007, from http://www.psqh.com/mayjun05/ethics.html

Robert Wood Johnson Foundation. (2007). *Improving the health & healthcare of all Americans Project.* Retreived from http://www.rwjf.org/programareas//resources/product.jsp?id=21131&pid=1140&gsa=pa1140

Saba, V. (2006). *Clinical care classification (CCC) system manual. A guide to nursing documentation.* New York: Springer Publishing.

Saba. V. (1991). *Home health care classification project.* Washington, D.C.: Georgetown University (NTIS Pub. #PB92-177013/AS).

Sapolsky, R. (2005). Sick of poverty. *Scientific American, 293(6)92-99.* NewYork: Scientific American, Inc.

Tilson, H., & Berkowitz, B. (2006, July/August). The public health enterprise: Examining our twenty-first century policy challenges. *Health Affairs, 25*(4), 900-910. Retrieved August 10, 2007, from http://content.healthaffairs.org/cgi/content.full/25/4/900

United States Department of Health and Human Services (USDHHS). (2007, June 20). *Medicare preventative services: A healthier US starts here.* Retrieved May 25, 2008, from http://www.medicare.gov/Health/Overview.asp

Veterans Evidence-Based Research Dissemination Implementation Center (VERDICT). (2007). Retrieved August 19, 2007, from http://verdict.uthscsa.edu/verdict/default.htm

Waton, K. (2007, June 11). Corporate Wellness. *Advance for nurses, 5*(13), 31-32. King of Prussia, PA: Merion Publications, Inc.

Work, Stress and Health: Findings from the Whitehall 11 study. (2004). Retrieved September 1, 2007, from http://www.workstress.net/downloads/whitehall_11_study.pdf

Williams, A., & Cutchin, M. (2002). The rural context of health care provision. *Journal of Interprofessional Care, 16(2),* 107-115.

KEY TERMS

Chronic Disease Genomics: Is the process of applying family history, gene variations and human genomic information to preventing chronic disease and promoting health in individuals, families and communities (Khoury, M. & Mensah. G., 2005).

Nutrigenomics: "Nutritional genomics or nutrigenomics is the application of high-throughput genomic tools in nutritional research. Applied wisely, it will promote an increased understanding of how nutrition influences metabolic pathways and how this regulation is disturbed in the early phase of diet-related disease and to what extent individual genotypes contribute to such disease." (Nature Review Genetics, 2003).

Predictive Modeling: A generally accepted definition is a term for statistical methodologies and support technologies using historical data to predict future behavior; a risk management model use in healthcare to lower cost, predict home health care needs, and assign case management strategies; predictive modeling in this document refers to genomic analysis of biological predictabilities that may be susceptible to clinical interventions.

Primary Prevention: Public health efforts to prevent disease and injury by education on healthy lifestyles and safe life practices.

Public Health Nursing: A unique field combining public health practice and nursing practice with the primary focus on population groups; the core functions are assessment, policy development and assurance.

Rurality: Rurality is the sum total of factors and experiences lived and archived by individuals living outside population-dense areas.

Vulnerable Populations: No consensus is available on who are vulnerable populations; in a medical sense 'vulnerable populations' are more susceptible to disease; vulnerable populations as subgroups frequently include the following: racial or ethnic minorities, uninsured, children, the elderly, the poor, the chronically ill, the physically disabled or handicapped, the terminally ill, the mentally ill, persons with acquired immunodeficiency disease, alcohol or substance abusers, homeless individuals, residents in rural area, individuals who do not speak English, the poorly educated or illiterate, incarcerated individuals.

Chapter II
Assessment in a Computer-Based Nursing Documentation

Elfriede Fritz
University of Health Sciences, Medical Informatics and Technology, Austria

Daniela Deufert
University of Health Sciences, Medical Informatics and Technology, Austria

Johannes Hilbe
University of Health Sciences, Medical Informatics and Technology, Austria

Christa Them
University of Health Sciences, Medical Informatics and Technology, Austria

ABSTRACT

Experience in nursing practice shows that, in Austria, there are still problems with ***assessment*** *in computer-based nursing documentation. Nursing documentation includes the various steps of the nursing process and the* ***nursing diagnosis****. In addition, an assessment instrument, which captures the needs for care, must also be integrated into it. This chapter describes different Nursing* ***Assessment*** *Instruments and the advantages of Computer-Based Nursing Process Documentation. Quality criteria for assessment instruments are validity,* ***sensitivity****,* ***specificity****,* ***reliability****,* ***practicability****, and the appropriateness of the instrument. Quality criteria for computer-based systems are basically software ergonomic aspects, which are not part of this study. Each country should choose for itself those specific* ***assessment*** *instruments that capture the needs for care of their clients. These data enable comparison of facilities and reliable cost estimates in connection with nursing.*

INTRODUCTION

Very few nurses in Austria are acquainted with the theme of **assessment** in nursing and the corresponding instruments. This can be explained by the fact that institutes and courses on nursing science have been established in Austria only in the last few years. **Assessment** instruments are employed and developed further in the course of scientific activity. In the following, **assessment** will be considered in the context of a computer-based nursing process documentation system. In Austria there are currently problems with **assessment** instruments due to lack of guidelines for **assessment** instruments that are integrated into computer-based nursing documentation. A problem that is caused thereby is that those who choose the documentation system have only limited knowledge of the quality criteria of **assessment** instruments. In addition, quality criteria for **assessment** instruments integrated in a computer-based nursing documentation system are often not scrutinized or the instrument is changed in an institution, and thereafter is not subjected to re-examination according to quality criteria. Further difficulties with **assessment** instruments in a computer-based nursing documentation are, that links from the **assessment** instruments to the care plan are partial incomplete or nonexistent. E.g. an instrument which assesses the risk of skin ulcers is not linked to the relevant **nursing diagnosis**. Other problems are e.g. an instrument is developed for **assessment** of patients in an acute hospital but is employed in assessing clients in nursing homes or home care. Some of the instruments used for assessing the needs of clients comprise very few items; with these, not all needs of care of clients can be captured. Another problem of **assessment** instruments in the area of nursing care is that some of the instruments currently in use are not nursing care-specific since e.g. they were developed by physicians. Examples of such instruments are the Mini Nutritional Assessment (Guigoz, Vellas & Garry, 1994) for estimating the nutritional status or the Tinetti Performance-Oriented Mobility Scale (Tinetti, 1986). These instruments cover primarily medicine-relevant areas, and nursing-relevant parts are partially missing.

In the past, a paper-based nursing documentation system was frequently introduced in nursing homes for the elderly. Ammenwerth, Eichstädter, Haux, Pohl, Rebel & Ziegler (2001, p. 66) point out the following advantages of computer-based nursing documentation: "time saving during care planning and a clear improvement in legibility and completeness of the documentation". A further result of the investigation was that physicians and nurses reported improved communication. According to Ammenwerth et al. (2002), computer-based nursing documentation increases the completeness of documentation and improves transparency of nursing services. From nursing documentation, data can be generated for management, and professionalism of nursing care can be enhanced. Presumably, a computer-based nursing documentation system has also advantages in the **assessment** of clients.

BACKGROUND

According to Gottschalck (2003), **assessments** are carried out by nurses in order to gather basic data such as at admission of a patient to a hospital or a client to a nursing home or home care. **Assessment** serves the purpose of establishing the individual nursing needs of clients. **Assessments** simplify nursing documentation, help avoid unnecessary measures in relation to patients, enable estimation of individual reactions of clients to nursing care and facilitate monitoring of effectiveness of nursing (Gottschalck, 2003).

Before **assessment** instruments are employed in nursing practice, they should be examined for their test-theoretical quality criteria. Quality criteria for **assessment** instruments are validity, **sensitivity**, **specificity**, **reliability**, **practicability** and the appropriateness of the instrument (Isfort & Weidner, 2001). The minimum requirement in relation to **reliability** is **interrater reliability**, since without it, no statements can be made about the **reliability** of the instrument (Bartholomeyczik, 2006). Assessing **interrater reliability** consists in establishing if there is agreement and the extent of agreement between two independent investigators; Cohens's Kappa value is determined (Mayer, Nonn, Osterbrink & Evers, 2004). With regard to **sensitivity** and **specificity**, over 80% values must be reached, which, however, is not the case with some of the instruments currently in use in nursing practice. (Bartholomeyczik, 2006). An instrument is particularly useful when a client is changing his institution and both institutions employ the same instrument. The **assessment** instrument can be used in the process of transferring a client to his new institution or it can be used in a disease management programme for evaluation (Bartholomeyczik, 2004). If the same **assessment** instruments in computer-based nursing documentation in all Austrian nursing homes and home care are used, they will facilitate transfer of clients and enable comparability of nursing care facilities. A further advantage of a standardized instrument is that it allows nursing-relevant data on clients to be collected in the same fashion throughout the country and thus enables comprehensibility for other disciplines, keeping in mind that interdisciplinary cooperation is a goal to be aimed at in the future. Standardization of **assessment** instruments is necessary not only for nursing practice but also for research purposes. Without standardization, no reliable data can be gathered in research projects. According to Isfort & Weidner (2001), an **assessment** instrument is practicable if it is simple and comprehensible to work with, easy to implement and helpful in the presentation of results. In addition, the instrument must be formulated in simple language, keeping in mind the qualification levels of the user. The quality criteria mentioned above are also applicable to instruments in a computer-based nursing documentation system.

In the present article, **assessment** in a computer-based nursing documentation for nursing homes and home care is discussed. In Austria and Germany, often no standardized instrument is used in computer-based nursing documentation. The question arises as to why such a standardized instrument for **assessment** purposes is needed. In all areas, standardization is necessary whenever comparisons need to be made. A standardized instrument enables collection of data on nursing care a client has received and these data can then be used in evaluating and planning discharge of the client (Bartholomeyczik, 2004).

Beside information for the nursing personnel involved, **assessment** tools could be used for appropriate reimbursement of institutions and for nursing in the home care setting. However, integrating **assessment** tools into the care plans for quality assurance in nursing treatment continues to present some major challenges. Intensive work with diagnosticians, data entry persons, coders, economists, reimbursement specialists, on the one hand, and identified quality of life markers as well as patients, their care providers and families, on the other, will have to be carried out before any attempts can be made to decide on the suitable combination of instruments.

THE NURSING PROCESS

Some relevant concepts associated with computer-based nursing documentation system will be discussed in some detail below. The nursing process is a procedure that nurses use in problem solving, in which nursing needs are first determined, nursing measures are then planned and the effect of these measures evaluated (Sauter, Abderhalden, Needham & Wolff, 2006). Thus, the nursing process comprises the following steps: nursing **assessment**, **nursing diagnosis**, nursing care planning, implementation of nursing measures, and nursing care evaluation (Brobst et al., 2007). **Assessment** data serve initially in making a **nursing diagnosis** and thereafter in planning and implementation of nursing measures, the final step in this process being evaluation.

The first step of **assessment** in the nursing process is important, since if this is not carried out properly, it will have a negative effect on all subsequent steps of the nursing process. Thus, **assessment** can be defined as the basis of nursing process or nursing documentation. If, for instance, only partial patient-relevant data are collected, it will affect **nursing diagnosis** and the corresponding nursing interventions. The goal of **assessment** is to gather all relevant information. **Assessment** is a precise, comprehensible estimate, evaluation or judgement on nursing care (Fritz, Müller & Them, 2007). Sauter, Abderhalden, Needham & Wolff (2006) define **assessment** as follows: "**assessment** implies collection, classification, analysis, interpretation and documentation of information about patients, their health condition, health behaviour and subjective experience". Thus, during **assessment**, both subjective and objective data are collected. Subjective data include clients' statements about their pain such as, for instance, their description of the kind, severity, frequency and localisation of pain (Brobst et al., 2007). Objective data include measurable entities such as blood pressure, pulse or the size of a wound. **Assessment** in the context of nursing process is oriented to the current situation of the client and is carried out in different ways. Sauter, Abderhalden, Needham & Wolff (2006) distinguish between emergency **assessment** an initial estimate of a client, focus **assessment** for a specific **nursing diagnosis** and the screening **assessment**. During emergency **assessment**, only the most important information is gathered for an initial estimate of a client after admission to a nursing home, which is followed by a more comprehensive **assessment**. The screening **assessment** is a short estimate in the sense of a search test (Sauter, Abderhalden, Needham & Wolff, 2006). This test is followed, if necessary, by a more extensive **assessment**.

The aim of **assessment** of clients in the context of nursing process is making a nursing care-relevant **nursing diagnosis**. In the future, **nursing diagnosis** of the North American Nurses Diagnosis Association (NANDA) will be integrated into a computer-based nursing documentation in nursing homes or home care. According to Müller-Staub, Abderhalden, Needham, Odenbreit, Lavin & van Achterberg (2007), implementation of NANDA **nursing diagnosis**, the nursing intervention classification (NIC) and the nursing outcome classification (NOC) lead to a higher quality in nursing documentation. Making a **nursing diagnosis** and the carrying out of the nursing process as a whole are dependent on the qualification of the nursing personnel. Nursing diagnoses have been in use in Austrian nursing practice since about ten years, and it can be assumed that there are problems to this day in formulating such diagnoses. It must be pointed out that **nursing diagnosis** is not an **assessment** instrument, not can it replace an **assessment** instrument, but is established on the basis of precise **assessment** of clients (Bartholomeyczik, 2004).

ASSESSMENT INSTRUMENTS IN A COMPUTER-BASED NURSING DOCUMENTATION SYSTEM

Nursing Minimum Data Set (NMDS)

A core part of some **assessment** instruments is the **Nursing Minimum Data Set** (NMDS). In many countries, **assessment** instruments for estimating the needs for care of patients in hospitals and of clients in nursing homes and home care contain such NMDS. Werley, Devine, Zorn, Ryan & Westra (1991, p. 422) define NMDS as follows: "a minimum data set of items of information with uniform definitions and categories concerning the specific dimension of nursing, which meets the information needs of multiple data users in the health care system". The goals of **assessment** with NMDS, according to Werley, Devine, Zorn, Ryan & Westra (1991`, p. 422-423) are to:

- Establish comparability of nursing data across clinical populations, settings, geographic areas, and time;
- Describe the nursing care of clients and their families in a variety of settings;
- Demonstrate or project trends regarding nursing care provided and allocation of nursing resources to individuals or populations according to their health problems, or **nursing diagnosis**;
- Stimulate nursing research [...] and
- Provide data about nursing care to influence and facilitate health policy decision making.

Some or all of the following ADL and IADL scales can be found in newer instruments.

Activities of Daily Living (ADL) and Instrumental Activities of Daily Living (IADL)

The ADL index (Katz, Ford, Moskowitz, Jackson, & Jaffe, 1963), the Barthel index (Mahoney & Barthel, 1965) and the IADL scale of Lawton & Brody (1969) are the most well known instruments for assessing independence and functional ability of people. Developed decades ago, these instruments continue to this day to be part of some of the more comprehensive **assessment** instruments for estimating need for nursing care.

In 1963 Katz, Ford, Moskowitz, Jackson & Jaffe developed the ADL-Index in the context of an epidemiological investigation of orthopaedic patients with reference to their activities after fracture of the femoral neck (Halek, 2003). Developed on the basis of this investigation, the aim of the ADL index was to facilitate information gathering, not only on orthopaedic patients, but also geriatric patients, patients with chronic illnesses, hospitalized patients and those in nursing homes. Using the ADL index, information on the following domains can be gathered: body care (washing oneself, bathing), getting dressed, going to the toilet, transfer, continence and eating (Halek, 2003). In gathering data on these domains, observations of the past two weeks are included.

Very few studies so far have investigated the validity and **reliability** of Katz's ADL index (Halek, 2003). The instrument covers only six activities and consequently cannot make a comprehensive **assessment** of the needs for care of clients requiring nursing.

The Barthel index is another instrument with an ADL scale. This was developed by Mahoney & Barthel (1965) as index of independence in a hospital for the chronically ill. The client is assessed with this instrument on admission and thereafter at set intervals. A score of 100 points, the maximum that can be scored under this **assessment**, would mean that the client is independent in all domains of activity (Halek, 2003). Using the German version of the Barthel index in stroke patients, Heuschmann et al. (2005) showed it to have good **interrater reliability**. The Barthel index has been used in various studies with different population cohorts with partially modified versions so that no generalisations can be validly made on the quality criteria of the instrument. According to Halek (2003), the Barthel index is a standardized instrument that assesses the physical aspects of a client, but the individual factors are not taken into consideration, so that it can be used in assessing needs for care of clients only with some reservations.

The IADL index, with its items specially intended for persons in home care, is a further **assessment** instrument. The items in this index are: using the telephone, shopping, preparing food, housekeeping, doing laundry, travelling away from home, taking medications, and handling personal finances. Studies on the IADL scales show that some items such as preparing food, housekeeping and doing laundry are sex-specific and are also culturally influenced (Halek, 2003). The items of the IADL index show that this instrument should be used only in combination with the ADL scales.

One can distinguish between nursing measurement instruments that are condition-related and those that are effort-related. In the following sections, condition-related instruments are presented that can be integrated in a computer-based nursing documentation of elderly people.

Resident Assessment Instrument (RAI)

Resident Assessment Instrument (RAI) is a more comprehensive **assessment** instrument compared to the ADL and IADL scales described above. RAI was developed in the USA in 1987 with the goal of having an instrument that should be adequate for drawing up a nursing plan, measuring nursing quality and financing long-term care (Garms-Homolovà, Gilgen, 2000). RAI contains indicators of quality for assessing the quality of nursing results. Indicators of quality are "markers" that help determine the presence or absence of good quality (Brandenburg, 2004). RAI was developed for assessing clients needing care for more than 14 days and has been translated into a German version for clients in nursing homes and home care (Isfort, Weidner, 2001). Specialists in the USA have developed a minimum data set (MDS) for the **assessment** of clients. The MDS is the core functional **assessment** instrument in the RAI and covers such domains as physical functioning in the activities of daily living (ADLs), cognition, continence, mood, behaviour, nutritional status, vision and communication, activities, and psychosocial wellbeing (Hawes et al., 1997). Objective, standardized information on the condition of clients can be gathered with the MDS which is used for making nursing diagnoses. This forms the basis for measurement of quality and nursing outcomes (Garms-Homolovà, 2005, Brandenburg, 2004). In the literature, there are varying reports about the time needed for administering RAI-MDS. On average, 129 minutes seem to be required for the RAI-assessment (Isfort, Weidner, 2001). After training and after having administered the RAI about 18 times, the required time dropped to 80 minutes. Although RAI has been in use since many years in many countries for nursing **assessment** of clients in nursing homes or home care, in Austria only the RAI-Home Care is used in one province. The results of a survey of nursing personnel in this Austrian province working with the RAI-HC revealed that 30.4% of those surveyed required 61-90 minutes for completing the MDS, 27.8 % required 91-120 minutes and 24.8% needed more than 121 minutes for completing the MDS (Feuerstein, Fritz, 2007). These time differences may be due to differing experience of the survey participants with the use of RAI. Nursing personnel have often criticized the length of time needed for administering such a wide-ranging **assessment** instrument.

Numerous studies have been carried out in the USA on the **reliability**, acceptance and effectiveness of RAI. They have demonstrated high **interrater reliability** for RAI (Brandenburg, 2004). According to a majority of nurses who participated in an investigation (Hansebo et al., 1998), introduction of RAI led to improved nursing documentation and nursing planning. The RAI is used in many countries and has been tested for quality criteria. The **reliability** and validity of the German version of the RAI for use in German-speaking countries should be investigated in further studies.

Functional Independence Measure (FIM)

The Functional Independence Measure (FIM) was developed in 1986 at the Center for Functional Assessment Research (CFARF), State University of New York, USA and published for the first time by Granger, Hamilton, Linacre, Heinemann & Wright in 1993. FIM is a further development of the frequently used Barthel-Index and is employed primarily in rehabilitation as well as geriatrics (Isfort, Klug, Weidner, 2002). FIM enables **assessment** of physical and cognitive abilities in terms of independent functioning of a client and thus monitoring and evaluation of success of rehabilitation (Halek, 2003).

The German version of the FIM comprises 18 items with a seven-point rating scale (Isfort, Klug & Weidner, 2002). Level 7 of the FIM indicates complete independence (timely, safely) and level 1 indicates total assist (perform less than 25% of task) (Brain Injury Resource Foundation, 2008). The English version of the FIM from the Brain Injury Foundation has been expanded by 12 items and comprises 30 items in the domains of: self-care, sphincter control, mobility, locomotion, communication, psychosocial adjustment und cognitive function (Brain Injury Resource Foundation, 2008).

Haas, Mayer & Evers (2002) have shown good **interrater reliability** for the German version of the FIM in head and brain injuries. FIM is easy to use and data can be gathered within 20 to 30 minutes (Halek, 2003). In the USA, it is mandatory to use this instrument in rehabilitation facilities. In Switzerland, the use of this instrument in the area of rehabilitation is recommended (Isfort, Klug & Weidner, 2002). It is not suitable for comprehensive **assessment** of clients on admission to a nursing home or home care since it does not enable adequate collection of relevant data. According to Isfort & Weidner (2001), from the point of view of nursing theory, the categories of the FIM are not adequate for setting up individually-tailored and structured nursing plans.

Care Dependency Scale (CDS)

The Care Dependency Scale (CDS) was developed in the Netherlands in 1996 by Dijkstra for assessing the care needs of people with dementia and the mentally handicapped (Lohrmann, Dijkstra & Dassen, 2003). In nursing practice, it can be used as an **assessment** instrument or as a research instrument. According to Halek (2003), the CDS measures psychological and physical functioning, independence, treatment needs and need for nursing care of geriatric patients.

The CDS comprises 15 Items, and is based on Virginia Henderson's concept of 15 basic needs. The 15-item scale measures a person's care dependency with regard to eating and drinking, continence, body posture, mobility, day and night patterns, getting dressed and undressed, body temperature, hygiene, danger avoidance, communication, contact with others, sense of rules and values, daily activities, recreational activities, and learning abilities (Lohrmann, Dijkstra & Dassen, 2003, p. 41).

Assessment with the CDS yields a total score of 15 to 75 points. The smaller the score, the greater is the dependence of the client on nursing (Lohrmann, 2004). The CDS has been internationally tested several times, and its **reliability** and validity have been established in studies (Halek, 2003). The CDS is an instrument easy to use since client **assessment** can be completed in about eight minutes (Lohrmann, 2004). According to Halek (2003), the CDS is not suitable for assessing clients in a nursing home or home care since it does not permit collection of adequately differentiated information. The CDS can only be used as a screening instrument (Halek, 2003).

CONCLUSION

Computer-based nursing documentation systems will be increasingly employed in the future in assessing clients' needs for care in a nursing home or in a home care setting. The nursing process represents the procedure for problem solving. Special attention should be paid to nursing **assessment**, the very first step in this procedure. Failure to collect all relevant information about the client during nursing **assessment** will have negative effects on the entire nursing process and nursing documentation. All nurses in nursing homes or working in home care settings will have to concern themselves in the future with **assessment** instruments. This is required for high quality nursing, for documented proof of nursing measures implemented and financing for the nursing activities carried out.

Assessment instruments in a computer-based nursing documentation system should be checked for validity, **reliability, sensitivity, specificity** and **practicability** before being put into operation in nursing practice.

The Barthel-Index and the IADL-Index are frequently used to this day. The IADL-Index is relevant for **assessment** of clients in home care.

More comprehensive nursing instruments can be used to assess the condition of clients or nursing efforts. One of these comprehensive nursing instruments is the RAI used in nursing homes and home care in many countries. An MDS is integrated within the RAI which enables comprehensive **assessment** of clients. These data are the basis for making a **nursing diagnosis** and for the entire nursing documentation. Apart from this, the MDS data can be used for quality management, benchmarking, financing of nursing and rendering prognoses.

A further **assessment** instrument used worldwide in rehabilitation and geriatrics is FIM. This instrument is a developed version of the Barthel-Index that has been in use for years. FIM can also be used as a screening instrument; for a comprehensive estimation of clients' needs for care in nursing homes or home care, FIM is rather unsuitable.

An **assessment** instrument developed in Europe for estimating clients' needs for care is the CDS. The CDS takes into consideration the basic needs according to Henderson. Only 15 items can be captured with the CDS so that it is not suitable for the **assessment** of clients' needs for care in nursing homes or home care. The CDS can only be used as a screening instrument for nursing **assessment**.

NMDS data required for a given country must be defined for nursing **assessment** in a computer-based documentation system. Only with the correct data can comparisons of facilities and reliable calculations of nursing prognosis can be made. NMDS data will enable nursing measures and activities carried out both comprehensible and capable of being demonstrated.

REFERENCES

Ammenwerth, E., Eichstädter, R., Happek, T., Hoppe, B., Iller, C,, Kandert, M., Kutscha, A., Kutscha, U., Mansmann, U., Luther, G., & Mahler, C. (2002). Auswirkungen EDV-gestützter Pflegedokumentation – Ergebnisse von Studien am Universitätsklinikum Heidelberg. PrInternet, 11/02, 85-92.

Ammenwerth, E., Eichstädter, R., Haux, R., Pohl, U., Rebel, S., & Ziegler, S. (2001). A Randomized Evaluation of a Computer-based Nursing Documentation System. Method Inform Med. *40*, 61-68.

Bartholomeyczik, S. (2004). Operationalisierung von Pflegebedürftigkeit – Assessments und ihre Möglichkeiten. In: Bartholomeyczik, S., Halek, S. (Hrsg.) (2004). *Assessmentinstrumente in der Pflege*. Hannover: Schlütersche, 11-20.

Bartholomeyczik, S. (2006). *Pflegediagnostik, Assessment und Klassifikationen: Funktionen und Grenzen. PrInternet*, 9/06, 453-458.

Brandenburg, H. (2004). Das Resident Assessment Instrument (RAI) Eine Chance für die Pflege in Deutschland. In: Bartholomeyczik S., Halek S. (2004), *Assessmentinstrumente in der Pflege. Hannover: Schlütersche*, 69-89

Brain Injury Resource Foundation (2008). *Functional Independence Measure™ and Functional Assessment Measure Brain Injury*. Retrieved from http://www.birf.info/pdf/tools/-famform.pdf (18.03.2008)

Brobst, R., Clarke Coughlin, A. M., Cunningham, D., Feldman J. M. Hess, R. G., Mason J. E., Fenner McBride, L. A., Romano C. A., Warren, J. J., & Wright, W. (2007). *Der Pflegeprozess in der*

Praxis, 2. aktualisierte Auflage. Bern: Verlag Hans Huber.

Feuerstein, I., & Fritz, E. (2007). *Die Anwendung des RAI-HC 2.0 in der Steiermark – Ergebnisse einer Befragung von diplomierten Pflegepersonen.* Vortrag am 24.10.2007 beim Amt der Steiermärkischen Landesregierung FA 8 B - Gesundheitswesen (Sanitätsdirektion) Graz.

Fritz, E., Müller, G., & Them, C. (2007). Assessment für die Pflege? *Österreichische Pflegezeitschrift, 5*(7), 8-12.

Garms-Homolovà, V., & Gilgen, R. (Hrsg.) (2000). RAI 2.0 Resident Assessment Instrument. Bern, Verlag Hans Huber

Garms-Homolovà V (2005). *RAI-System als Voraussetzung der Erfüllung zeitgemäßer Qualitäts und Planungserfordernisse.* Retrieved from http://www.igk-forschung.de/RAI-GERMANY/rai-germany.html (15/12/2005).

Gottschalck, T. (2003). Assessmentinstrumente zur pflegerischen Beurteilung des Mundes. *Pflege, 16*, 273–282.

Granger, C. V., Hamilton, B. B., Linacre, J. M., Heinemann, A. W., & Wright, B. D. (1993). Performance profiles of the functional independence measure. *Am.J Phys Med Rehabil, 72*(2), 84-89.

Guigoz, Y., Vellas B. J., & Garry, P. J. (1994). Mini Nutrional Assessment: A practical assessment tool for grading the nutritional state of elderly patients. *Facts and research in gerontology, Supplement on Nutrition an Aging, 2*, 15-59. New York: Springer Publishing Co.

Haas, U., Mayer, H., & Evers, G. C. M. (2002). Die Interrater Reliabiliät des. Functional Independence Measure. (FIM) bei Patienten mit Schädel-Hirn-Verletzungen. In: *Pflege 2002, 15*, 191-197.

Hansebo, G., Kihlgren, M., Ljunggren, G., & Winblad, B. (1998). Staff views on the Resident Assessment Instrument, RAI/MDS, in nursing homes, and the use of the Cognitive Performance Scale, CPS, in different levels of care in Stockholm, Sweden. *Journal of Advanced Nursing, 28*(3), 642-653.

Hawes, C., Mor, V., Phillips, C. D., Fries, B. E., Morris, J. N., Steele-Friedlob, E., Greene, A. M., & Nennstiel, N. (1997). The OBRA-87 Nursing Home Regulations and Implementation of the Resident Assessment Instrument: Effects on Process Quality. *JAGS, 45*, 977-985.

Halek, M. (2003). *Wie misst man Pflegebedürftigkeit?* Hannover: Schlütersche.

Heuschmann, P.U., Kolominsky-Rabas, P.L., Nolte, C.H., Hünermund, G., Ruf, H.U., Laumeir, I., Meyrer, R., Alberti, T., Rahmann, A., Kurth, T., & Berger, K. (2005). Untersuchung der Reliabilität der deutschen Version des Barthel-Index sowie der Entwicklung einer postalischen und telefonischen Fassung für den Einsatz bei Schlaganfall-Patienten. *Fortschr Neurol Psychiat, 73*, 74-82.

Isfort, M., & Weidner, F. (2001). Pflegequalität und Pflegeleistungen I. Zwischenbericht zur ersten Phase des Projektes. *Entwicklung und Erprobung eines Modells zur Planung und Darstellung von Pflegequalität und Pflegeleistungen. Deutsches Institut für angewandte Pflegeforschung* (dip), Köln. http://www.dip-home.de/material /downloads/bericht-pflegeleistung1.pdf (18.03.2008).

Isfort, M., Klug, E., & Weidner, F. (2002). Pflegequalität und Pflegeleistungen II Zwischenbericht zur zweiten Phase des Projektes. *Entwicklung und Erprobung eines Modells zur Planung und Darstellung von Pflegequalität und Pflegeleistungen.* Deutsches Institut für angewandte Pflegeforschung (dip), Köln. http://www.dip-home.de/material/downloads/bericht-pflegeleistung2.pdf (18.03.2008).

Katz, S., Ford, A.B., Moskowitz, R. W., Jackson, B.A., & Jaffe, M. W. (1963, September). Studies of Ilness in the Aged. The Index of ADL: Standardized Measure of Biological and Psychosocial Function. *JAMA, 21*, 185, 914-9.

Lawton, M. P., & Brody, E. M. (1969). Assessment of older people: self-maintaining and instrumental activities of daily living. *Gerontologist, 9*(3), 179-86.

Lohrmann, C. (2004). Die Pflegeabhängigkeitsskala. In: Bartholomeyczik S., Halek S. (2004): Assessmentinstrumente in der Pflege. *Hannover, Schlütersche*, 55-60.

Lohrmann, C., & Dijkstra, D. T. (2003). The Care Dependency Scale An Assessment Instrument for Elderly Patients in German Hospitals. *Geriatr Nurs, 24*, 40-3.

Mahoney, F. I., & Barthel, D. W. (1965). Functional Evaluation. The Barthel Index. *MD State Med J, 14*, 61-65.

Mayer H., Nonn C., Osterbrink J., & Evers G. (2004). Qualitätskriterien von Assessmentinstrumenten – Cohen's Kappa als Maß der Interrater – Reliabilität (Teil 1). *Pflege, 17*, 36-46.

Müller-Staub, M., Needham, I., Odenbreit, M., Lavin, M.A., & van Achterberg, T. (2007). Improved Quality of Nursing Documentation: Results of a Nursing Diagnosis, Interventions, an Outcomes Implementation Study. International *Journal of Nursing Technologies and Classifications, 18*, 1, 5-17.

North American Nursing Diagnosis Association (NANDA) (1990). *Definition of Nursing Diagnosis*. http://www.enotes.com/nursing-encyclopedia/nursing-diagnosis (28.05.2008).

Sauter, D., Abderhalden, C., Needham, I., & Wolff, S. (2006). *Lehrbuch psychiatrische Pflege*. Bern: Verlag Hans Huber.

Tinetti, M. E. (1986). Performance-oriented assessment of mobility problems in elderly patients. *J Am Geriatr. Soc, 34*, 119-126.

Werley, H. H., Devine, E. C., Zorn, C. R., Ryan, P., & Westra, B. (1991). The nursing minimum data set: abstraction tool for standardized, comparable, essential data. *American Journal of Public Health, 81*, 421-426.

KEY TERMS

Computer-Based Nursing Documentation: Computer-based nursing documentation comprises assessment, nursing diagnosis, planning of nursing interventions and evaluation.

Nursing Assessment: This is a process during which information on clients in hospitals, nursing homes or home care is collected, classified, analysed, interpreted and documented.

Nursing Diagnosis: In 1990, the North American Nursing Diagnosis Association (NANDA) defined nursing diagnosis as "a clinical judgement about individual, family, or community responses to actual or potential health problems/life processes. Nursing diagnoses provide the basis for selection of nursing interventions to achieve outcomes for which the nurse is accountable".

Nursing Documentation: This consists of precise documentation of all nursing processes and can be carried out in a paper-or computer-based fashion.

Nursing Minimum Data Set (NMDS): Werley, Devine, Zorn, Ryan & Westra (1991, p. 422) define NMDS as follows: "a minimum data set of items of information with uniform definitions and categories concerning the specific dimension of nursing, which meets the information needs of multiple data users in the health care system".

Nursing Process: The nursing process is a procedure consisting of five or six steps and is employed by nurses for problem solving.

Chapter III
Clinical Decision Support Systems in Nursing

Dawn Dowding
University of York, UK

Rebecca Foster
University of Southampton, UK

Rebecca Randell
City University, UK

Valerie Lattimer
University of Southampton, UK

Natasha Mitchell
University of York, UK

Carl Thompson
University of York, UK

ABSTRACT

Increasingly, new and extended roles and responsibilities for nurses are being supported through the introduction of clinical decision support systems (CDSS). This chapter provides an overview of research on nurses' use of CDSS, considers the impact of CDSS on nurse decision making and patient outcomes, and explores the socio-technical factors that impact the use of CDSS. In addition to summarising previous research, both on nurses' use of CDSS and on use of CDSS more generally, the chapter presents the results of a multi-site case study that explored how CDSS are used by nurses in practice in a range of contexts. The chapter takes a socio-technical approach, exploring the barriers and facilitators to effective CDSS use at a level of the technology itself, the ways people work, and the organisations in which they operate.

INTRODUCTION

In high income countries, nurses are taking on increasing decision making responsibility, a trend that looks set to continue (Bryant-Lukosius, DiCenso, Browne, & Pinelli, 2004; Furlong & Smith, 2005). Clinical decision support systems (CDSS) have been introduced as one way of supporting nurses who are taking on such extended roles (e.g. (Fitzmaurice et al., 2000; O'Cathain, Sampson, Munro, Thomas, & Nicholl, 2004). However, despite the evidence for the potential benefits of using CDSS in health care (Garg et al., 2005), and the adoption of such systems by nurses, there is little evidence examining how nurses as a specific professional group use CDSS to support their practice.

In this chapter we provide an overview of research on nurses' use of CDSS, considering the impact of CDSS on nurse decision making and patient outcomes, while also exploring the socio-technical factors that impact the use of CDSS. The background section of this chapter first provides some essential terminology, before summarising previous research on doctors' use of CDSS and then considering previous research on nurses' use of CDSS. The main part of the chapter presents the results of a multi-site case study that explored nurses' use of CDSS in a range of contexts. This case study was conducted as part of a recently completed project, funded by the Policy Research Programme, Department of Health (England), which examined how nurses use new technologies (such as CDSS) to inform their clinical decision making. Possible future trends in CDSS use are then considered and the chapter concludes by summarising the research on this topic. In each section, we take a socio-technical approach, exploring barriers and facilitators (factors that may affect the impact of CDSS use on clinician performance and/or patient outcomes and/or encourage or discourage the use of CDSS) to effective CDSS use at the level of the technology and its interface with human operators, the work process level, and the organisational level.

BACKGROUND

Definitions

Clinicians have a range of decision tools available to them to support their decision making (Liu, Wyatt, & Altman, 2006). Examples of decision tools include nomograms (charts that simplify complex information such as Body Mass Index (BMI)), templates incorporated into electronic patient records (EPRs), predictive scores (such as early warning scoring systems for clinical event risk), formularies to support prescribing, and patient information leaflets. CDSS are a computer-based form of decision tool, integrating information (ideally from high-quality research studies) with the characteristics of individual patients, to provide advice to clinicians (Dowding, 2007). As such, CDSS are seen as a potential way of improving the quality, safety and effectiveness of clinical decisions, leading to improvement in clinician performance and patient outcomes (Garg et al., 2005). CDSS vary in their functionality, from 'passive' systems that only provide information to a clinician when they request it, through to 'active' systems that provide patient specific recommendations to a clinician automatically (Hajioff, 1998). For example, computerised clinical reminders (CRs) are an example of an active system, typically being integrated with an electronic patient record (EPR) and presenting reminders to the clinician regarding potentially appropriate interventions, based on an evaluation of the available patient data (Patterson, Nguyen, Halloran, & Asch, 2004; Saleem et al., 2005). Computerised provider order entry (CPOE), which enables computer-based ordering of medication, can also be a form of active CDSS, when decision support alerts the user to the risk of a dangerous drug interaction or advises the user of appropriate dosages (Aarts, Doorewaard, & Berg, 2004). Passive CDSS include electronic information tools that provide clinicians with access to online clinical practice guidelines and research evidence (Randell, Mitchell, Thompson, McCaughan, & Dowding, In press-a).

CDSS have a long history; a systematic review of the impact of CDSS contained 5 studies that were published in the 1970s (Garg et al., 2005). The review identified 100 studies, covering the activities of diagnosis, disease management and drug dosing and prescribing, and a range of clinical areas, including both primary and secondary care.

Previous Research on the use of CDSS

Previous research on the use of CDSS has highlighted the socio-technical nature of these systems. At the most basic level the effectiveness of the CDSS will be impacted by the quality of the knowledge base that underlies it. Thus, the failure of a CPOE system to detect significant drug interactions will most likely lead to a negative impact on patient outcomes (Coiera, Westbrook, & Wyatt, 2006).

However, there are also a range of other factors at the computer-interface level that can impact the success of a CDSS. Effective use is impacted by the usability (Fung, Woods, Asch, Glassman, & Doebbeling, 2004; Saleem et al., 2005), speed (Saleem et al., 2005) and flexibility of the CDSS (Ash, Berg, & Coiera, 2004; Saleem et al., 2005). Associated with this, interfaces that do not allow 'interruptive use' are seen as barriers, as are processes for information entry or retrieval that require the information to be overly structured or insist on completeness (Ash et al., 2004). Decision support overload (such as systems providing large numbers of unnecessary reminders, alerts or warnings) is seen as a barrier to effective CDSS use (Liu et al., 2006; Saleem et al., 2005). Therefore limiting the number of reminders that are presented to the user is seen as a positive strategy (Saleem et al., 2005). The provision of recommendations for action, rather than simple assessments of the patient's condition, is associated with improvements in clinical practice (Kawamoto, Houlihan, Balas, & Lobach, 2005).

At the work process level, the fit of the CDSS with the workflow has been shown, in both clinical trials and qualitative studies, to be of fundamental importance. One systematic review of the impact of CDSS found that automatic provision of decision support at the time and location of decision making was linked to improvements in clinical practice (Kawamoto et al., 2005). Barriers to effective CDSS use at the work process level include: the CDSS not being part of the standard workflow (Kawamoto et al., 2005; Saleem et al., 2005); additional work being created by use of the CDSS; and lack of time (especially when combined with additional work) (Patterson et al., 2004; Saleem et al., 2005). The level of distraction experienced by the clinician is considered to impact the use of the CDSS (Coiera et al., 2006), with high levels of distraction potentially leading to data entry errors and so to inappropriate recommendations. The perceived impact on provider-patient interaction (Patterson et al., 2004) and the perceived appropriateness of the recommendations provided by CDSS (Patterson et al., 2004; Saleem et al., 2005) are also thought to impact CDSS use, leading to decreased CDSS use when perceptions are negative. One systematic review examining the potential benefits of CDSS found better performance in studies in which the trial authors had developed the CDSS (Garg et al., 2005); while this may be the result of biases in assessing outcomes, it could also be the result of having a local champion or having more usable and locally appropriate software.

Additionally, the effectiveness of CDSS appears to depend on the type of decision they support. Systems that provide reminders to clinicians for preventive health care (such as screening and vaccination), assist clinicians with disease management, or provide drug dosing or prescribing advice all appear to improve practitioner behaviour (Garg et al., 2005). However, the evidence is not as strong for systems that are designed to support medical diagnosis (Garg et al., 2005), suggesting that there may be differences in the nature of such decisions that need to be considered (Randell, Mitchell, Thompson, McCaughan, & Dowding, In press-b).

At the organisational level, barriers to effective CDSS use include lack of clarity about responsibilities in relation to decision support, the perception amongst practitioners that CDSS use is a non-core activity (Saleem et al., 2005), and lack of training (Patterson et al., 2004). CDSS use can be encouraged by linking decision support with the audit and feedback of performance data (Fung et al., 2004), the documentation of system problems, and providing prompt feedback. Finally, it has been suggested that the amount of time the CDSS is in place affects its use, with effectiveness decreasing over time (Demakis et al., 2000).

These factors are summarised in Table 1. Considered as a whole, what these studies highlight is that the impact of CDSS use on clinician performance and patient outcomes is the result not just of the CDSS itself but the socio-technical system of which it is a part. While the usability of the interface and the quality of the knowledge base are of fundamental importance, for effective CDSS use we must also consider factors at the organisation level and, perhaps most significantly, the ways in which people work.

Table 1.

Computer interface level
Quality of underlying knowledge base Usability Speed Flexibility Number of reminders Provision of recommendation
Work process level
Part of standard workflow Provision of automatic decision support at time and location of decision making Time available Amount of additional work resulting from CDSS use, including documentation Level of distraction Perceived impact on provider-patient interaction Applicability of recommendations to situation
Organisational level
Clarity of responsibilities Training Perception of importance of decision support Link with audit and feedback of performance data Organisational support, in the form of ability to document problems and receive feedback Time in place

CDSS use by Nurses

CDSS are increasingly being used by nurses and there is a significant push in high income countries for the use of CDSS by nurses to be extended. In part, this is because recent changes in the way health care is being delivered in high income countries have led to nurses taking on extended roles that were previously carried out by junior doctors. For example, in the UK a number of specialist nurses now have responsibility for the management of care of patients with heart failure and diabetes (Horrocks, Anderson, & Salisbury, 2002). Nurses are also able to prescribe medication (Jones, 1999), and often run clinics within primary care and outpatient hospital settings (Rosen & Mountford, 2002).

The provision of CDSS has been identified as a way of supporting nurses within their extended roles, to work more autonomously and as a way of improving patient safety (Department of Health, 2000; Van de Castle et al., 2004). Examples of areas where nurses use decision support to help them with the decision making about patient care include the management of asthma (Eccles, McColl et al., 2002), diabetes (Eccles, Hawthorne et al., 2002) and angina (Eccles, McColl et al., 2002) and triage of patients in first contact care (Lattimer et al., 1998; Salisbury, Chalder, Scott, Pope, & Moore, 2002). However, until recently, little was known about the extent to which these systems are available to and used by nurses. As a starting point into our study of nurses' use of new technologies, we conducted a survey of the availability of CDSS to nurses working in England (Dowding et al., 2007). We found that approximately two thirds of NHS Trusts (providers) that responded had at least one CDSS that was used by nurses. Nurses who worked in Acute Hospital Trusts or Ambulance Trusts were more likely to have CDSS available to them than nurses who worked in other settings. The most frequently reported category of CDSS used by nurses were EPRs, followed by knowledge management systems, triage systems, assessment systems, test ordering and results systems and prescribing systems. The features that systems possessed varied according to their category, with EPR unlikely to provide automatic decision support or recommendations for action. In contrast, triage and prescribing systems were more likely to provide recommendations automatically, and be integrated within the clinical environment.

Previous Research on Nurses' use of CDSS

Despite the increasing use of CDSS by nurses, the design and evaluation of CDSS has largely focused on doctors as users; 92% of studies in the systematic review by Garg et al. (2005) enrolled doctors as primary users. Very few studies have looked at the use of CDSS by nurses. As part of our study of nurses' use of new technologies, we carried out a systematic review of clinical trials that evaluate the impact of CDSS on nurse decision making and patient outcomes (Randell, Mitchell, Dowding, Cullum, & Thompson, 2007). The review identified only eight studies, carried out in three clinical areas; anticoagulation management, telephone triage in first contact care, and glucose regulation in the intensive care unit. The effect of CDSS use on nurse performance and patient outcomes was inconsistent, suggesting the need for further studies to establish the context in which CDSS use by nurses is most effective. The CDSS used by nurses in the studies included in the review had many of the features that previous reviews have suggested are linked to improved outcomes, such as automatic provision of a recommendation at the time and location of decision making. However, these features did not appear to have the same association with better outcomes in this review. Unfortunately, a lack of detail in the reporting of the studies included in the review makes it difficult to determine whether the lack of impact was the result of computer-interface, work process or organisational level issues. For one of the studies the results suggest that the limitations were the result of the protocols on which the CDSS was based (Rood, Bosnan, van der Spoel, Taylor, & Zandstra, 2005), while for another study the objectives of the control group and the intervention group were possible in conflict (Richards et al., 2004).

There are few studies that have explored how nurses use CDSS in practice. However, there are a number of qualitative studies that explore nurses' use of CDSS within NHS Direct, the telephone triage and advice service for England. What is emphasised in these studies is the impact of issues at the work process level on how the nurses used the CDSS. Nurses adapted the questions recommended by the CDSS both to overcome the problem of not being able to see the patient, relying on detailed questions that are not suggested by the CDSS (Johnson Pettinari & Jessopp, 2001) and to suit the situation of individual callers (Greatbatch et al., 2005; Hanlon et al., 2005). Similarly they were prepared to override the CDSS in order to fit the recommendation with a range of factors, such as whether the patient had already received medical assistance, the patient's level of anxiety, and the nurse's knowledge of how local NHS services operate in practice (Greatbatch et al., 2005; Hanlon et al., 2005). Nurses reported that they were more likely to override the software recommendation, in either direction, if they had clinical knowledge and experience of the health problem under consideration. Nurses welcomed having a varied team around them, drawing on colleagues' knowledge and experience when considering triage decisions (Hanlon et al., 2005; O'Cathain et al., 2004) suggesting that the presence of the CDSS did not replace their previous sources of support for decision making.

A MULTI-SITE CASE STUDY

With heterogeneity in terms of the CDSS examined and the outcomes assessed in studies that evaluate the impact of CDSS on nurse decision making (Randell et al., 2007), there is a need to understand the barriers and facilitators to effective CDSS use in nursing. Qualitative studies of nurses' use of CDSS have predominantly focused on telephone triage. We wanted to explore how nurses use CDSS in other contexts and in support of other types of decisions. In order to examine in detail *how* nurses use CDSS in clinical practice to inform their decision making we carried out a multiple case site study, with different levels of analysis (clinician, unit, organisation). Further details of the case site study have also been published elsewhere (Dowding et al., In press).

Methods

Settings and Participants

Data from the survey study noted above (Dowding et al., 2007) were used to purposively select case sites according to the following criteria:

- The nursing staff within sites varied in terms of their experience and expertise using the systems
- There was variation in the types of CDSS supported decisions
- The CDSS could be compared across dimensions such as flexibility of use, type of interface
- Different contexts and implementation strategies could be compared.

While previous studies on the use of CDSS tend to highlight the failures of CDSS to be used effectively (e.g. (Hajioff, 1998; Patterson et al., 2004; Saleem et al., 2005), it should be pointed out that we intentionally sought case sites that appeared to be successfully using CDSS to support nurse decision making, so as to understand the factors associated with successful CDSS use.

Case Site 1: An Anticoagulation Management Clinic

This case site was an Anticoagulation Team based in a Primary Care Trust (PCT), which provided near patient testing to approximately 1700 patients. It offered a 'one-stop service' approach for patients registered with local GPs, enabling patients to attend clinics near to their home in order to undertake International Normalised Ratio (INR) monitoring and receive appropriate anticoagulant dosages. The team had used CDSS to support nurse decision making since their inception in 2001 and had been using the current CDSS since April 2005. The CDSS the team used was a stand-alone PC-based system that nurses accessed through either a desktop PC or a laptop whilst interacting with the patient. Nurses measured the patient's INR and entered this into the CDSS which calculated the patient's anticoagulant dosage (to which we will refer as the "dose recommendation") and the date of their next clinic visit (to which we will refer as the "date recommendation").

Case Site 2: A Spinal Assessment Clinic

This case site was based in the Spinal Assessment Clinic, a nurse led clinic, of a District General Hospital. The primary caseload for the clinic was patients suffering from back pain and referred leg pain. Patients were seen both within the hospital-based clinic and in clinics based in the community, for either initial assessment or review of their condition. On average the clinic saw 118 patients a month. Patients were referred by their GP to the clinic for assessment, and then given appointments to return for review if appropriate. Before each consultation, the patient answered a series of questions using the CDSS. The CDSS then calculated a range of quality of life scores (including pain and depression scores) for the patient. The CDSS was locally developed and had been in place, in various versions, for approximately 10 years.

Case Site 3: A Walk-In Centre

This case site was a Walk-in Centre based within a Community Hospital. It was managed by nurse practitioners, who diagnosed and treated a wide range of minor injuries and minor illnesses. Where necessary the nurse practitioners could refer patients to other health and social care providers. Patients did not need an appointment to attend the Walk-in Centre. The CDSS was based on algorithms that are logically structured, ordered, symptom-based questions, which lead to an end-point (disposition), which advised the appropriate level of care required. The CDSS had been in use since April 2000.

Case Site 4: A Respiratory Centre

This case site was a Respiratory Centre of a District General Hospital, which provided respiratory medical services to adults. Nurses in the Centre treated patients within the hospital, at health clinics and in patients' homes. Seven nurses in the Respiratory Centre used a CDSS to monitor patients with chronic obstructive pulmonary disease (COPD) who were living at home, with the aim of preventing their readmission to hospital. Patients used a Data Collection and Interaction (DCI) unit twice daily to answer a series of questions, so providing information about their own health and well being, such as level of breathlessness and amount of medication used. Collected data was sent to a secure database via the patient's telephone line. The database could be accessed by nurses in the Respiratory Centre and trends in patient responses monitored over time. The CDSS displayed warning alerts when patient responses exceeded a certain level, previously determined by the nurses in the Respiratory Centre. The CDSS had been in use since March 2006. Use of the CDSS was part of a pilot study, funded by the European Union via the INTERREG IIIC Telemedicine Project, which was managed by the local Primary Care Trust.

Data Collection

We collected data at three levels within each case site; practitioner/patient, clinical unit and Trust (organisational) level. At practitioner/patient level we observed consultations between nurses and patients, interviewed both nurses and patients immediately after their consultation and interviewed nurses about their use of CDSS. At clinical unit and Trust level we interviewed key staff. All consultations and interviews were digitally audio recorded and subsequently transcribed. We obtained both NHS ethical approval and research governance approval from each NHS Trust to carry out the study. Data were collected between June 2006 and March 2007.

We observed a total of 124 consultations, interviewed 38 patients and 36 nurses after their consultation and carried out in-depth interviews with 19 nurses working with the CDSS in the case sites. We also carried out 9 unit level and 9 Trust level interviews.

Analysis

The majority of the data collected in the case study were qualitative and analysed using thematic content analysis. The data was managed using the computer package Atlas-ti. Data were coded and classified according to themes that were developed inductively from the observation and interview data. The analysis presented below considers the influences on the use of the CDSS at three levels: the computer-interface level; the work processes level; and the organisational level. In this analysis, we are drawing primarily on the observations of the CDSS in use and the data collected in the nurse interviews to understand actual and perceived facilitators and barriers to the use of CDSS.

Findings

The Computer-Interface Level

In all case sites, use of the technology was largely quick and unproblematic. However, in some of the case sites the availability and design of the technology affected how nurses and patients interacted with the CDSS. In case site 2 (spinal assessment) and case site 4 (remote monitoring) there were issues associated with the equipment available to nurses and patients. In case site 2 there was a light pen attached to the computer for patient use, which had not worked for some time. This caused patients some difficulties when answering the questions on the computer, as four questions specifically asked them to use the light pen, rather than the mouse, to indicate where their pain was on a diagram. Availability of computers was also a problem in this case site, with only one reliable computer in the hospital clinic and one laptop (which was in the consultation room) for community clinics. Therefore if the clinic was running late or a patient turned up early they could not answer the questions on the CDSS. In case site 4 (remote monitoring) the nurses reported some problems due to the failure of some patient DCI units, the resulting gaps in patient data caused problems with patient monitoring.

In case site 3 (Walk-in centre) and case site 4 (remote monitoring) there were also issues with the CDSS software, which affected how nurses interacted with the system. In case site 3, nurses' experiences of using the algorithms inherent within the CDSS appeared to have left them with negative impressions of its capabilities. In particular, nurses appeared to find the structure of the algorithms inflexible. Issues such as having to work through an algorithm from start to finish, beginning with very basic questions, not being able to easily exit an algorithm and not being able to input all the information gleaned by examination of the patient, meant that they did not use the algorithms during consultations with patients. Nurses also commented on the lack of suitable algorithms for the variety of conditions with which they were presented.

In case site 4 (remote monitoring) most nurses found the software easy to use, however they did describe some problems with data interpretation because of the way in which data was presented by the CDSS. The graphical displays of patient data did not use a standard scale for each patient, causing some confusion, while the direction of some of the scales were described as 'counter-intuitive' (in that a higher score reflected a worsening of patient symptoms). The patients interviewed in case site 4 were very positive about using the CDSS, however some forgot to do so from time to time, resulting in missing data for the nurses. In cases where there was significant missing data, nurses found it difficult to build up a picture of a patient's symptoms and general health. Due to the flexibility of the CDSS software, the questions which patients had to answer and the levels at which alerts were triggered could be tailored to each individual patient. Patients commented that they liked the tailoring of questions to their own requirements which made the system more user-friendly. There were some nurse comments that the alert triggering mechanism could be over sensitive.

The Work Process Level

In several of the case sites, observation of the technology in use and interviews with the nurses highlighted a lack of fit between how nurses worked and the understanding of that work process inscribed within the technology. In case site 1 (anticoagulation), in only 6 of the 26 routine consultations we observed was the nurse recorded as accepting both the dose recommendation and the date recommendation made by the CDSS. Most commonly, the nurse accepted the dose recommendation but overrode the date recommendation. Reasons for overriding included a lack of 'fit' between the case site's routine practice and the

CDSS; the software would only allow a maximum gap between appointments of six weeks, whereas the anticoagulation team routinely saw stable patients only every eight weeks; and the inability of the CDSS to take into account patient factors (such as what they had eaten, whether or not they had drunk alcohol, the patient's medication had been changed) which nurses felt were important to inform their decisions.

In case site 3 (Walk-in centre) we rarely observed nurses using the CDSS to support the actual decision they made. They would instead fill out the decision algorithm related to a specific patient *after* the consultation. The nurses gave several reasons for this. Firstly, they felt that the support was unnecessary. They had often seen similar cases many times before and felt confident in their ability to ask the appropriate questions, perform the required examinations and make the necessary decisions about patient care. Secondly, nurses did not feel happy with many of the recommendations of the CDSS. They also commented that they felt the content of the algorithms was not always appropriate, in particular dispositions were seen as being too risk averse. However, although the nurses rarely used the CDSS in the consultations, this does not necessarily mean that the CDSS had no impact. Most nurses reported being very familiar with the content of the algorithms, knowing exactly what questions would be asked and the pathways down which they would be taken.

In case sites 1 (anticoagulation) and 3 (Walk-in centre), there was a conflict between nurses need to interact with the technology and a perceived responsibility to pay attention to the patient. The CDSS in both of these case sites was designed to be used during the consultation with the patient. To minimise the effect using the CDSS would have on their interactions with patients, in case site 1 often the nurse would have already brought up the patient's record and moved to the patient dosing screen before the patient entered the consulting room. Generally, the software was not discussed within the consultation. However, the nurse would sometimes make reference to the computer if it was slow in calculating the dose. In case site 3, the nurses felt that if they had to focus on the computer to enter data and read algorithms the quality and flow of their interaction with the patient would deteriorate and slow down, with the nurse potentially missing non-verbal cues. The majority of consultations required the nurse to interact physically with the patient, for example by feeling, bandaging or cleaning an injury, making interaction with the computer difficult.

The Organisational Level

In case sites 1 (anticoagulation) and 3 (Walk-in centre), the supportive nature of the team within which the nurse worked was identified as an important factor for both using the CDSS and for making decisions more generally. In case site 1, although the nurses worked across different locations, there was a sense that there was always someone at the end of the phone. Similarly in case site 3 a number of nurses commented on the supportive nature of the nursing team working in the Walk-in centre. It was reported that nurses were happy to ask for, or to give, a second opinion or advice in cases when there was uncertainty as to the best decision to make. In 4 of the 40 observed consultations in this study the nurse involved asked a colleague to give a second opinion. In case site 4 (remote monitoring) the nurse who had taken a leading role in the introduction of the CDSS was very supportive of the other nurses using the system, giving them help, advice and training. This was an important factor in the successful use of the CDSS in this case site.

All of the nurses were asked about the amount of education and training they had received both for general IT and also for the CDSS they were using. In general the nurses interviewed were confident in using computers and used computers outside of the work place. However, most of the nurses reported they had had very little formal training in IT skills, with most of them learning skills during their current or previous posts. Some of the nurses described their fears at having to use CDSS, describing learning to use the computer as "frightening" and a "steep learning curve".

There were variations in how nurses had been trained to use the CDSS across case sites, with nurses who were using commercially developed packages more likely to have received some form of formal education or training. In case site 1 (anticoagulation), before the CDSS was introduced, a number of team members went on a two-day practical training course with the system providers. The nurses who went on these training days were positive about it, although felt that you really only learn to use the system when you start using it in practice. They then taught the other team members how to use the system. Nurses who have subsequently joined the team have gone through an induction period, working in a supernumerary role, enabling them to gradually learn to use the software with the support and guidance of another nurse.

Similarly in case site 3 (Walk-in centre), those who had been working there when the CDSS was introduced had attended a five-day, off-site training course provided by an outside company. Those who had subsequently joined had been trained on-site with the help of on-screen training, booklets and support from supervisors and mentors. Nurses who had attended the five day training course made a variety of comments on their experiences with descriptions varying from 'excellent' to 'disastrous'. Of the four nurses who had attended, three described problems with the training relating to the use of the algorithms. Problems arose as the trainers, used to training nurses in how to use CDSS for telephone triage, stressed the importance of using the algorithms during the consultation, while the nurses were used to a face-to-face working environment and to making patient care decisions without a computerised aid. It was reported that the five day training course did not successfully teach some nurses how to use the CDSS. However, those nurses soon gained confidence and competence in using the CDSS use after returning to the Walk-in centre and using it in a real life situation. One of the nurses involved in training at the Walk-in centre mentioned that lack of time for update training led to nurses using the system in different ways and not always getting the most out of the system.

In case site 2 (spinal assessment), where the nurses used a locally developed system, none of the nurses had received any training on the use of the CDSS. However, they found the CDSS easy to use and did not feel the training was necessary.

In case site 4 (remote monitoring), training also varied amongst the nurses. Some nurses were trained on the system for a few hours whilst others were simply shown how to use the system in about 20 minutes. All the nurses felt able to speak to the nurse leading the pilot study to clarify how to use the system.

Discussion

The findings highlight not only how factors at the computer-interface level, work process level and organisational level impacted the use of the CDSS, but also how the nurses adapted their work practice in order to incorporate the CDSS into their practice, such as finding ways to limit the impact of the CDSS on their interaction with the patient (case site 1) and developing strategies to resolve alerts raised by the CDSS (case site 4). Many of the factors were the same as those previously identified in studies of doctors' use of CDSS (e.g. (Patterson et al., 2004; Saleem et al., 2005). At the computer-interface level, there were concerns over the flexibility of the CDSS (case sites 3 and 4), the quality of the underlying knowledge base (case site 3), the number of reminders (case site 4), and the ease of use (case site 4).

When considering how nurses used the CDSS within their work processes, there were concerns over the impact on interaction with the patient (case sites 1 and 3) and the applicability of the recommendations (case sites 1, 3, and 4). Nurses who used more 'active' CDSS were more likely to use or follow information provided by the system (case site 1) than nurses who used more 'passive' systems (such as case site 2 where it was unclear how nurses actually used the information provided by the system in their decision making). In case site 3 the CDSS did not easily fit with the workflow of the nurse, leading nurses to use the technology *after* the consultation for record keeping rather than decision support.

At the organisational level, there were fewer similarities with previous studies. The findings suggest an alternative form of organisational support that can be a facilitator of CDSS use, which is the supportive nature of the team in which the nurse works. This may be of particular relevance to nursing, where nurses are often using CDSS to take on extended roles. The nature of the training provided did not appear to have a significant impact on how the CDSS was used. Fitting with previous research (Demakis et al., 2000) the length of time over which the CDSS had been used did seem to have an impact on the use of the CDSS. However, while in case site 3 the nurses' increased confidence in their decision making led to them not using the CDSS, in case site 1 they continued to use the CDSS but were more confident in their ability to adapt the recommendations in light of additional information gathered from the patient. In case site 2, the nurses were motivated to use the CDSS as they considered it to support research, similar to the finding that the provision of audit data through a CDSS can encourage use.

The case study highlights the way in which flexibility is not only a computer-interface level issue but also an organisational level issue. In case site 1, the failure of the CDSS to fit with local practice in terms of the frequency with which patients needed to return to the clinic (a work process level issue) was balanced by the ease with which the nurse could override the recommendation (a computer-interface level issue) and support at the organisational level in terms of allowing nurses to override the recommendation where they felt it was appropriate. In case site 3, failure of the CDSS to fit with local practice was unfortunately matched with a lack of flexibility at the computer-interface level. However, there was again flexibility at the organisational level, allowing the nurses freedom to choose when to use the decision support. Such an approach meant that the technology was still used successfully for recording patient details and could still be accessed by the nurses when they felt it was appropriate, rather than abandoning the CDSS altogether.

This ties in with a more general issue that the results of the case study point to, which is that the success of a CDSS is not dependent on a set list of factors but rather is the result of a combination of factors. All of the CDSS in this case study could be considered to be 'successful' in the sense that nurses continued to use them, even if not in the way originally envisaged by the developers of the CDSS but in a way which they felt was beneficial to their practice. In all case sites, nurses found reasons to persist with the CDSS, despite a range of concerns at both the computer-interface and the work process level.

FUTURE TRENDS

Forecasting what is likely to happen in the future is an inexact science. However, we feel that on the basis of the current directions of health care policy both in the UK and other countries with developed health care systems, we can suggest what we consider to be likely future developments in nurses' use of CDSS. With the nationwide introduction of IT systems to support health care practice in the UK, and similar initiatives in other countries (e.g.(McMurray et al., 2007; Moo & Fletcher, 2007) the use of technology within health care practice is likely to expand. There is continuing investment within health care in specific types of systems, such as CPOE and EPRs. Similarly, it is likely that in more developed countries, for both political and economic reasons, nurses will continue to take on extended roles, often supported by some form of decision support. Both of these trends mean that it is likely that there will be an increase in the use of CDSS within nursing, either as stand alone systems or incorporated into existing technology such as EPRs. It is therefore important that the implementation of such systems is subject to robust evaluation of the likely impact both on patient outcomes and broader work practices for both nurses and the health care systems within which they work.

What is apparent from our project is the current lack of robust evidence to support the wide scale use of CDSS in nursing practice. The trials in this area that we identified in the systematic review were focused on two main areas of clinical practice (telephone triage for first contact care and anti-coagulation management) (Randell et al., 2007), whereas nurses have been reported to be using CDSS for a wide range of decision tasks, including chronic disease management (e.g.(Eccles, McColl et al., 2002). The survey data highlighted that the majority of nurses in England will be using EPR systems or knowledge management systems to support their practice; at present there appear to be no studies that have evaluated whether or not such systems have the potential to help improve nurse decision making or patient care, or what the likely effects on the broader health care system of using such technology may be. There is a need for robustly conducted trials that evaluate the use of CDSS within nursing, which also explore the ways in which CDSS are used in practice by nurses, using qualitative techniques. Through a combination of such methods it may be possibly to identify in more detail which CDSS work for nurses, and *why* the systems produce either positive or negative benefits to either professional practice and/or patient outcomes.

As discussed in the background to this chapter, CDSS can be classified according to whether they are 'passive' systems through to more 'active' systems that can provide nurses with guidance for action (Hajioff, 1998). The majority of CDSS currently available to nurses in England are passive systems, for which there is very little research evidence to suggest that their use will have a positive impact on either patient care or practitioner behaviour. However, as the presence of EPRs increases, there will hopefully be an increase in decision support that is integrated within such systems, making available relevant research information to health professionals at the point of the decision (Richards et al., 2004). For example, 'infobuttons' can be integrated into EPRs to provide patient-specific and context-sensitive links to research evidence (Hanlon et al., 2005). Unfortunately, as with much research in this area, the design and evaluation of such forms of CDSS have focused on doctors as users, not nurses. What is needed now is research that evaluates the impact that such systems have on nurse decision making.

SUMMARY

Nurses use CDSS as part of a wider socio-technical system. As CDSS to support nurse decision making increases, policy makers and clinicians require evidence of the effectiveness of such systems. Our study reveals that even in environments where CDSS use is considered to be successful, exactly *how* a system is used may vary considerably from the original intentions of the system designer. Evaluations of CDSS need to take into account the influence of the technology itself, how the system is incorporated into broader work practices and the organisations within which work is organised.

REFERENCES

Aarts, J., Doorewaard, H., & Berg, M. (2004). Understanding implementation: The case of a computerized physician order system in a large

Dutch university. *Journal of the American Informatics Association, 11*, 207-216.

Ash, J. S., Berg, M., & Coiera, E. (2004). Some Unintended Consequences of Information Technology in Health Care: The Nature of Patient Care Information System-related Errors. *J Am Med Inform Assoc, 11*, 104-112.

Bryant-Lukosius, D., DiCenso, A., Browne, G., & Pinelli, J. (2004). Advanced practice nursing roles: development, implementation and evaluation. *J Adv Nurs, 48*(5), 519-529.

Coiera, E., Westbrook, J. I., & Wyatt, J. (2006). The Safety and Quality of Decision Support Systems. *Methods Inf Med, 45*(Suppl 1), S20-25.

Demakis, J. G., Beauchamp, C., Cull, W. L., Denwood, R., Eisen, S. A., Lofgren, R., et al. (2000). Improving Residents' Compliance With Standards of Ambulatory Care: Results From the VA Cooperative Study on Computerized Reminders. *JAMA: the journal of the American Medical Association, 284*(11), 1411-1416.

Department of Health. (2000). *The NHS Plan: A plan for investment, a plan for reform*. London: The Stationary Office.

Dowding, D. (2007). Computerized decision support systems in nursing. In N. Cullum, D. Ciliska, B. Haynes & S. Marks (Eds.), *Evidence-based nursing: an introduction*. Oxford: Blackwell.

Dowding, D., Lattimer, V., Randell, R., Mitchell, N., Foster, B., Thompson, C., et al. (2007). How do nurses use new technologies to inform their decision making? Final Report, University of York, York.

Dowding D, Mitchell N, Randell R, Foster R, Lattimer V, Thompson C. Nurses' use of computerised clinical decision support systems: A case site analysis. *Journal of Clinical Nursing*. In press

Eccles, M., Hawthorne, G., Whitty, P., Steen, N., Vanoli, A., Grimshaw, J., et al. (2002). A randomised controlled trial of a patient based Diabetes Recall and Management system: The DREAM trial: a study protocol. *BMC Health Services Research, 2*(1), 5.

Eccles, M., McColl, E., Steen, N., Rousseau, N., Grimshaw, J., Parkin, D., et al. (2002). Effect of computerized evidence based guidelines on management of asthma and angina in adults in primary care: cluster randomised controlled trial. *British Medical Journal, 325*, 941.

Fitzmaurice, D., Hobbs, R., Murray, E., Holder, R., Allan, T., & Rose, P. (2000). Oral anticoagulation management in primary care with the use of computerized decision support and near-patient testing. *Archives of Internal Medicine, 160*, 2343-2348.

Fung, C. H., Woods, J. N., Asch, S. M., Glassman, P., & Doebbeling, B. N. (2004). Variation in Implementation and Use of Computerized Clinical Reminders in an Integrated Healthcare System. *American Journal of Managed Care, 10*(2), 878-885.

Furlong, E., & Smith, R. (2005). Advanced nursing practice: Policy, education and role development. *J Clin Nurs, 14*, 1059-1066.

Garg, A. X., Adhikari, N. K. J., McDonald, H., Rosas-Arellano, M. P., Devereaux, P. J., Beyene, J., et al. (2005). Effects of computerized clinical decision support systems on practitioner performance and patient outcomes: A systematic review. *JAMA: The journal of the American Medical Association, 293*(10), 1223-1238.

Greatbatch, D., Hanlon, G., Goode, J., O'Cathain, A., Strangleman, T., & Luff, D. (2005). Telephone triage, expert systems and clinical expertise. *Sociology of Health & Illness, 27*(6), 802-830.

Hajioff, S. (1998). Computerized decision support systems: an overview. *Health Informatics Journal, 4*, 23-28.

Hanlon, G., Strangleman, T., Goode, J., Luff, D., O'Cathain, A., & Greatbatch, D. (2005). Knowledge, technology and nursing: The case of NHS Direct. *Human Relations, 58*(2), 147-171.

Horrocks, S., Anderson, E., & Salisbury, C. (2002). Systematic review of whether nurse practitioners working in primary care can provide equivalent care to doctors. *BMJ, 324*, 819-823.

Johnson Pettinari, C., & Jessopp, L. (2001). Your ears become your eyes: Managing the absence of visibility in NHS Direct. *Journal of Advanced Nursing, 36*(5), 668-675.

Jones, M. (Ed.). (1999). *Nurse Prescribing: Politics to Practice*. London: Harcourt Publishers.

Kawamoto, K., Houlihan, C. A., Balas, E. A., & Lobach, D. F. (2005). Improving clinical practice using clinical decision support systems: A systematic review of trials to identify features critical to success. *BMJ, 330*(7494), 765-772.

Lattimer, V., George, S., Thompson, F., Thomas, E., Mullee, M., Turnbull, J., et al. (1998). Safety and effectiveness of nurse telephone consultation in out of hours primary care: randomised controlled trial. *British Medical Journal, 317*, 1054-1059.

Liu, J., Wyatt, J., & Altman, D. G. (2006). Decision tools in health care: Focus on the problem, not the solution. *BMC Medical Informatics and Decision Making, 6*(4).

McMurray, A., Gilbert, C., Reis, B., Chueh, H., Kohane, I., & Mandl, K. (2007). A self-scaling, distributed information architecture for public health, research and clinical care. *Journal of the American Informatics Association, 14*(4), 527-533.

Moo, S., & Fletcher, J. (2007). Northern Territory HealthConnect: Shared electronic health record service implementation experiences and benefits realised in indigenous health. *Medinfo, 12*(1), 297-301.

O'Cathain, A., Sampson, F. C., Munro, J. F., Thomas, K. J., & Nicholl, J. P. (2004). Nurses' views of using computerized decision support software in NHS Direct. *Journal of Advanced Nursing, 45*(3), 280-286.

Patterson, E. S., Nguyen, A. D., Halloran, J. P., & Asch, S. M. (2004). Human Factors Barriers to the Effective Use of Ten HIV Clinical Reminders. *J Am Med Inform Assoc, 11*, 50-59.

Randell, R., Mitchell, N., Dowding, D., Cullum, N., & Thompson, C. (2007). Effects of computerized decision support systems on nursing performance and patient outcomes. *Journal of Health Services Research and Policy, 12*(4), 242-249.

Randell, R., Mitchell, N., Thompson, C., McCaughan, D., & Dowding, D. (In press-a). From pull to push: Understanding nurses' information needs *Health Informatics Journal.*

Randell, R., Mitchell, N., Thompson, C., McCaughan, D., & Dowding, D. (In press-b). Supporting nurse decision making in primary care: exploring use of and attitude to decision tools *Health Informatics Journal.*

Richards, D., Godfrey, L., Tawfik, J., Ryan, M., Meakins, J., Dutton, E., et al. (2004). Direct versus general practice based triage for same day appointments in primary care: Cluster randomised controlled trial. *British Medical Journal, 329*, 774.

Rood, E., Bosnan, R., van der Spoel, J., Taylor, P., & Zandstra, D. (2005). Use of a computerized guideline for glucose regulation in the intensive care unit improved both guideline adherence and glucose regulation. *Journal of the American Informatics Association, 12*(2), 172-180.

Rosen, R., & Mountford, L. (2002). Developing and supporting extended nursing roles: the challenges of NHS walk-in centres. *Journal of Advanced Nursing, 39*(3), 241-248.

Saleem, J. J., Patterson, E. S., Militello, L., Render, M. L., Orshansky, G., & Asch, S. M. (2005). Exploring Barriers and Facilitators to the Use of Computerized Clinical Reminders. *JAMIA, 12*, 438-447.

Salisbury, C., Chalder, M., Scott, T. M., Pope, C., & Moore, L. (2002). What is the role of walk-in centres in the NHS? *BMJ, 324*, 399-402.

Van de Castle, B., Kim, J., Pedreira, M. L. G., Paiva, A., Goossen, W., & Bates, D. W. (2004). Information technology and patient safety in nursing practice: an international perspective. *International Journal of Medical Informatics, 73*, 607-614.

KEY TERMS

Active CDSS: CDSS that provide patient-specific recommendations to clinicians automatically as part of workflow.

Clinical Decision Support System (CDSS): Computer-based systems that integrate information, ideally from high-quality research studies, with patient characteristics to provide advice to clinicians.

Computerised Clinical Reminder (CR): A form of active CDSS, typically being integrated with an electronic patient record (EPR) and presenting reminders to the clinician regarding potentially appropriate interventions, based on an evaluation of the available patient data.

Computerised Provider Order Entry (CPOE): Computer-based systems that enable ordering of medication, often also providing decision support by alerting to the user to the risk of a dangerous drug interaction or by advising the user of appropriate dosages.

Decision Tool: Refers to a wide range of tools used by clinicians to support their decision making, including not only CDSS but also their paper-based counterparts, such as clinical practice guidelines, predictive scores (such as early warning scoring systems for clinical event risk), formularies to support prescribing, and patient information leaflets.

Passive CDSS: CDSS that provide clinicians with access to guidance but which do not provide support automatically.

Chapter IV
Culturally Sensitive Healthcare for Newcomer Immigrants

Jerono P. Rotich
North Carolina A & T State University, USA

ABSTRACT

This chapter will give an overview of the healthcare-related challenges that most newcomer immigrants and refugees encounter as they acculturate into their new environments in Western countries. It will highlight practical tips that can: enhance the caregiver and patient relationships across cultures and across continents; enhance culturally sensitive healthcare services; and help to create culturally inviting healthcare environments. Current demographics indicate that most developed countries continue to experience a growing influx of cross culturally diverse immigrants and refugees that represent the world's 210 nations. It is also evident that, although these newcomers enrich their new nations with their diverse backgrounds, language, and cultural differences continues to pose formidable obstacles to their health, healthcare providers and health system in general. While the patients and providers realize the effects of immigration on the quality and access to healthcare, they seem to be overwhelmed by the barriers.

INTRODUCTION

Most Western countries have experienced a drastic increase in the number of immigrants and refugees (Coppel, Dumont & Visco, 2001; Leininger & McFarland, 2006; & Westberg, Bumgardner, Melissa, Lind, & Patricia, 2005). Specific findings by Westberg et al (2006), indicated that immigrants made up 11.5% of the United States population and that approximately 1.5 million immigrants arrived each year. Noteworthy is the fact that, though the highest numbers of immigrants in the United States come from Mexico and other Hispanic-speaking regions, the first group of immigrants were from the Northern continent of Europe. Other regions of the world that are represented by the immigrants and refugees in America and many Western countries include: Africa, Southeast Asia, South America, Eastern Europe, and the former Soviet Union.

Despite the fact that most immigrants and refugees leave their home countries in good health (Fowler, 1998), and with myriad hopes and expectation (Bailey, 2002), it is unfortunate because their health seems to deteriorate over time. They seem to encounter numerous health access barriers, mental and emotional health related challenges as they acculturate and integrate into their new culture and environment (Bailey, 2002). Their acculturation and their ability to access health care has remained complex due to cultural and language related challenges. Unfortunately, this insurgent increase in health access barriers has been linked to the lack of cross culturally competent and sensitive front line workers, health care providers, policies and health care environments. Though the solutions to these problems may be complex, long –term, and multifaceted, it is believed that health care providers who are knowledgeable in cross cultural competency skills as well as health care systems that have designed culturally sensitive policies and environments will optimize the ability to help alleviate these disparities. Unlike other professionals, cross culturally competent health care providers have the unique ability to eliminate health access disparities and to improve the quality of care among cross-culturally diverse immigrant and refugee populations.

The purpose of this chapter is to highlight the health care access barriers that immigrants and refugees encounter as they acculturate into their new Western cultures and environments. It will also offer suggestions of cultural competency approaches and tips that can enhance the patient-provider and the system –community relationships across cultures. The specific objectives of this chapter are to:(1) provide an overview of the influx of immigrants and refugees into Western Countries ; (2) raise awareness of the health care access barriers that immigrants and refugees encounter upon arrival ; (3) provide information that can help providers become better acquainted with the health seeking behaviors, practices and perceptions of the diverse immigrants and refugees; and, (4) offer practical and cost –effective cross cultural competency suggestions and tips that can help health care providers and health care systems deliver culturally appropriate services and design cultural sensitive environments.

Background

The 2006 Census data indicated that the total number of immigrants and refugees in the United States of America had reached an all-time high of 37.5 million. It was also evident that although the numbers of immigrants and refugees in most Western countries continued to increase, the United States of America had the fastest-growing numbers in the world (Active Voice, 2003; Bailey, 2002; Macdonald, 2003; & Portes & Rumbaut, 1996). Specific reports from Active Voice (2003), indicated that in 2000, the United States of America was home to 56 million foreign born residents and children of immigrants, compared to 34 million that was reported three decades earlier. According to Frey (2006), the immigrant population in the United States represented more than 5 percent of the population in 29 states, and more than 10 percent in 15 other States. Active Voices also pointed out that these immigrants were from diverse cultures, ethnicities, nationalities, and socio-economic status and were settling and making new homes in large and small cities across the country.

Similar trends were reported in other western countries (Coppel, Dumont & Visco, 2001). According to the 2007 reports(2007, Biggest-invasion-since-1066), Government projections from the United Kingdom indicated that immigration will result in **an increase in the population of the UK of 6 million in the 27 years from 2004** that is 6 times the population of Birmingham. It is anticipated that immigration will account for 83% of future population growth in the UK.

Regardless of their reasons for emigrating into America, United Kingdom or any other Western country, it is evident that, all of them are searching for better standards of living. They are fleeing poverty and persecution, economic hardships, pursuing athletic or educational glory, and are seeking better and healthier ways of life (Bailey, 2002; Coppel, Dumont & Visco, 2001). According to Gavagan & Brodyaga (1998), the categories of immigrants and refugees who arrived to most Western countries included: legal immigrants, official refugees, asylum seekers, and undocumented residents among others. The refugees and asylees for example are a special category of immigrants who are admitted into other countries because they are fleeing religious, political or race persecution, or natural disaster (Bailey, 2002, Balgopal, 2000). Immigrants on the other hand enter Western countries voluntarily in search better ways of life. They arrive as students, or guest workers.

Although all immigrants and refugees perceive their new environment to be a beacon of hope and although most of them arrive in good health, they tend to become unhealthy over time. According to Gavagan & Brodyaga (1998), the physical and psychological effects of acculturation and integration into their new environment largely depend on their reasons for emigration. Several studies (Gellert, 1993; & MacPherson, 1993) have attested to this. Their findings indicated that anemia, dental problems, intestinal parasites, nutritional deficiencies and immunization irregularities were very prevalent among newly arrived refugees especially those from developing countries. Mental and emotional health problems on the other hand were prevalent among all immigrants and refugees. Most immigrants and refugees experience post-traumatic stress, due to past experiences and on-going acculturation challenges. Those who have reported stress have linked it to separation from loved ones, cultural shock, different environment, shift in or change in family roles and norms, financial difficulties and language and communication barriers. Similar findings (Bailey, 2002; Kaleidoscope, 2003; & Portes & Rumbant, 1996) indicated that a confluence of communication, cultural and socio-economic barriers have contributed to their acculturation challenges. Of paramount importance are the social determinants of health (Bailey, 2002; Fowler, 1998; & Kaleidoscope, 2003). Some of the specific determinants that they outlined include: communication due to verbal and written language barriers, cultural differences, age, social isolation, financial hardships, immigration status vulnerabilities, eligibility restrictions, limited information on available health care resources, discriminating workforce, and educational systems that do not respond to their diverse needs. Bailey also mentioned the fact that most theorists recognize that the western concept of the "melting pot," was not a reality, but it was a myth. He illustrated this by pointing out the fact that most immigrants and their traditions, identities, values and practices are not swallowed up by their new mainstream culture, but they continue to remain over time. Specific research findings on immigrant health (Angell & Cetron, 2005; Bailey, 2002; Kaleidoscope, 2003; & Portes & Rumbant, 1996*)*, alluded to the fact that healthcare barriers for immigrants and refugees existed at the following levels: (1) *systems level* due to no insurance, or low insurance coverage and culturally uninviting health care systems or environments; (2) *patient level* due to cultural beliefs or values , linguistic obstacles or lack of transportation; and (3) *provider level* due to culturally insensitive staff and providers.

Findings from a study that was done in Denmark **(Norredam.M; Mygind, A; Nielsen' S.N; Bagger, J & Krasnik. A, 2007)** attributed the high volumes of visits to the emergency room by more immigrants to the lack of access to health care and the convenience. The study indicated that most immigrants preferred to seek health care from the emergency room because they either did not have a physician, health insurance, or did not know how to explain their problem over the phone. These findings therefore reaffirm the need for cross cultural competent health care providers, culturally sensitive health care policies and culturally inviting health care systems and environments.

OBSTACLES IN ACCESSING PRIMARY HEALTH CARE AMONG IMMIGRANTS AND REFUGEES IN WESTERN COUNTRIES

Unable to Communicate: Language has played a pivotal and instrumental role in determining the level and quality of health care access that immigrants and refugees receive. Their inability to communicate well in English or their host country's official language appears to be the most significant health access barrier. It makes it difficult for health care personnel to provide adequate health care services. Immigrants and refugees who are less proficient in the official language (i.e. English) find it extremely difficult to navigate the formal health care system. And as a result most of them end up going to the emergency room as a last resort. Those who have attempted to seek services outside of the emergency room have indicated that, it takes forever to make appointments. Given the above barriers, recent findings (**Norredam.M; Mygind, A; Nielsen·S.N; Bagger, J & Krasnik. A, 2007; &** Kaleidoscope, 2003), indicated that most immigrants and refugees are less likely to: seek routine preventive health care, return for follow up appointments, finish their prescribed medications or follow up with their medication instructions. Findings from a study that was conducted in Ontario, Canada (Fowler, 1998), indicated that immigrants who did not speak English at home were less likely to classify their health as either very good or excellent.

Although efforts have been made to translate health care materials such as forms, side effects of medications, eligibility guidelines among many others, they are mainly in Spanish. It is therefore evident that, the current available translated materials may not reflective of all the diverse languages and communities (i.e. Arabic, jarai, B'nong, Swahili, loas, Cambodian, Vietnamese and etc).

The literature on access barriers also indicates that some immigrants and refugees are illiterate in their own language. According to Kaleidoscope (2003), the number of immigrants and refugees who are illiterate in their own languages is increasingly high.

Underinsured/uninsured: Income and health insurance are critical for entry into the formal health care system in most Western Countries (Leclere, Jensen & Biddlecom, 1994). Due to socioeconomic hardships, a vast majority of immigrants and refugees are underinsured or uninsured, thus face substantial financial barriers to medical access. Most of them come from large families that are inappropriately poor, and work in low paying manual jobs that provide minimal or no health insurance. Coupled with the lack of work insurance, most of them have limited access to publicly-funded programs such as Medicaid and Medicare. According to the provisions of the 1996 welfare reform law, undocumented immigrants are not eligible for normal benefits through Medicaid or the State Children's Health Insurance Program (SCHIP) and the normal Medicaid and SCHIP benefits for the first five years they reside in the United States. Others (mostly refugees) have to wait for a period of five years before they could become eligible for most public benefits. Due to lack of insurance most of them do not have a regular physician or health care provider thus making it difficult for them to obtain timely care.

Underrepresented: Most immigrants and refugees find it difficult to seek health care because they do not "see a health care provider who looks like them" in most of the health care agencies or systems. It is unfortunate that the racial and ethnic makeup of the current health care workforce in most Western Countries is not reflective of the nation's increasing cultural diversity. This makes it difficult for most immigrants to seek health care. For one, they may not trust the provider because they are afraid that they may not understand their cultural views as regards to treatment and prevention. Secondly, they realize that it takes longer to get treatment and services because they have to involve an interpreter. On the contrary, they are known to frequent immigrant and refugee owned clinics or those agencies that have a diverse workforce. They seem to prefer them because they do not need to worry about their cultural and language barriers.

Uninformed: Most immigrants and refugees do not utilize the formal health care system because they lack the knowledge on how to access available services. A vast majority of immigrants and refugees do not seek health care because they do not understand how to navigate the seemingly complex health care system. They are unfamiliar with the bureaucracy, protocols and procedures such as making appointments, insurance requirements, paper work, time concept , payments, follow up and referrals among others. And as result they do not receive timely and relevant information on prevention and treatment. A vast majority end up getting diagnosed late and are less likely to receive timely preventive care or treatment. Additionally, the on going individual mobility that is very prevalent among most immigrant and refugee communities makes it difficult for them to become knowledgeable and familiar with the services available in their respective community.

Under Resourced/ Underserved: The impact of the increase in income inequality on the health and well being of most immigrants and refugee continues to be significant. Due to low incomes, manual jobs, most of them are forced to settle in poorer and impoverished neighborhoods that do not offer health care resources and services. Because of the fear of the "unknown", most immigrants and refugees feel at ease living among their people. They therefore tend to gravitate towards areas and neighborhoods that have people who "look like them" and people who "speak like them. They form enclaves which over time help contribute to the ever occurring segregation. As a result of this, most of them find themselves in neighborhoods that have limited health care resources. Generally, the more underserved the area is, the greater the problems of access to health care due to geographic distances, and transportation problems.

Undocumented: Lack of legal documents makes it hard for most immigrants to seek for health care services. Families and individuals who are not documented do not seek health care because they are constantly living in fear of deportation. The undocumented immigrants particularly feel uncomfortable when they get overwhelmed with lots of paper work or questions. As a result some have chosen to stay away from such programs because of fear of immigration consequences. Others refrain from using public benefits because they are afraid that this may affect their chances of obtaining permanent residency or citizenship in the near future. This immigration related fears continue to be further compounded and complicated by the contentious politics that currently surround immigration.

Untrusting: It takes time to develop trust: Due to past experience, immigrants and refugees take time before they can discuss their problems openly with providers. They are particularly turned off by health care providers who ask too many questions or individuals who do not explain their procedures. According to Kaleidoscope (2003), the decisions of all family elders and community members as to when to seek healthcare takes precedence over follow up appointments. This process may deter individuals from follow up appointments or preventive health care measures.

WHAT HEALTH CARE PROVIDERS NEED TO KNOW ABOUT IMMIGRANTS AND REFUGEES

Did you know that most immigrants and refugees (Active Voice, 2003; Bailey, 2002; Kaleidoscope, 2003; Macdonald, 2003; Matt, 1997; Portes & Rumbaut, 1996; & Cultural Competency for Health Care Providers, 2006):

1. Are less likely to seek regular check ups, physical examination or routine screening;
2. Shy away from seeking health care because of culturally insensitive health care providers and health care systems;
3. Are more likely to report poorer emotional health compared with other English speakers;
4. More familiar with the informal health care system (prevalent in their countries of origin) than the formal care system (prevent in America or other Western nations);
5. Utilize the health care system at later stages of illness verse at earlier stages. Due to financial barriers most of them only go to the doctor or emergency room when they are very sick especially the male/men;
6. Relay on cultural brokers, community leaders and family members to facilitate their cognitive access to the health care system;
7. Do not understand the concept of making appointments. Most were used to walk in clinics and therefore find it cumbersome to make appointments. In any case most of them wait until the illness is so advance before they can attempt to make appointments and because of the urgent need for care, then they often end up at the emergencies rooms;
8. May not always comply with the treatment medications or instructions provider by providers or pharmacist;
9. Are very unfamiliar and uncomfortable with the bureaucracy in health care. They are not very familiar with medical protocols that are so detailed in western countries;
10. Do not always seek treatment for mental health or depression related illnesses;
11. Have conflicting beliefs on diseases and treatment. Medical need is determined by the presence of physical illness as well as the cultural perceptions;
12. Have health beliefs and taboos that may affect their health seeking behaviors especially issues that pertain to mental and reproductive health;
13. Are not overly keen with keeping time. It is not uncommon for them to show up late
14. Have large households. They Live with extended families members because they depend on pooled resources;
15. Came from countries that had few hospitals (if any) that were in poor condition, and lacked the necessary equipment and medications;
16. Have health problems that resulted from years of poverty, war, and inadequate health care services as well as lack of enough trained providers;
17. Are less likely to have documentation of vaccination records, birth dates or medical history. Most providers are forced to rely on verbal reports;
18. Will try home remedies before seeking health care. some communities such as the Hmong people sacrificed animals and bought expensive amulets to guide the return of a death soul's;
19. Women, are much less likely to smoke, seek routine check ups or screening for cervical or breast cancer;
20. Women do not receive formal reproductive, prenatal and postnatal health education;
21. Women are the last ones to learn English because of child bearing responsibilities;
22. Women are victims of domestic violence and may never report it to providers
23. Women tend to get jobs faster than their male counterparts;

24. Men/husbands make most of the family decisions including those that pertain to health care; and that ,
25. Men will not translate well for women because of cultural barriers.

*Did You Know that **some** Immigrants and Refugees Communities and Individuals(S):*

1. Still practice female genital mutilation (female circumcision);
2. Use traditional medicine and more serious illnesses are more likely to be associated with angry spirits within an ill person. In the event that this happens, healing ceremonies are often performed to abbess the spirits;
3. Are very sensitive to body language during their health care visits;
4. Consider hand shaking to be inappropriate especially with people from the opposite sex;
5. Belief in divine healing powers. Those who had no access to health care services would go to sit in churches and wait to be cured by God;
6. Belief that mental illness are a result of a curse;
7. Consider direct eye contact to be rude and therefore unacceptable; and ,
8. Prohibited physical contact between those of opposite sex in public unless it is a member of the same family.

Things to Remember About Immigrants and Refugees from Specific Regions

*Did You Know that **most** African Immigrant and Refugees* (Kaleidoscope, 2003; & Cultural Competency for Health Care Providers, 2006):

1. Feel very uncomfortable with long periods of silence;
2. Represent 51 different countries with diverse languages, values, perceptions and beliefs. Therefore do not assume or stereotype;
3. Mostly visit the doctors when they extremely sick especially the men. Most try home remedies first;
4. Consider direct eye contact to be rude therefore is not acceptable;
5. Prohibited physical contact between individuals of opposite sex. It is acceptable for members of the same family unless;
6. From some communities circumcise females at the age of 13-15 years. Though some communities do not circumcise their males/boys, most get circumcised between the ages of 13-15;
7. Have rates of individuals that are affected by HIV/AIDS. Despite this prevalence ,it is not freely or openly talked about;
8. Most have not conceptualized the importance of keeping time. It is not uncommon to find them missing appointment or not show up at all;
9. Though greetings vary, they appreciate greetings such as hand shake or hugs because they symbolize peace and harmony;
10. Women, especially Muslim are not permitted to keep direct eye contact with unknown or men who are perceived to be unholy;
11. Have encountered major ailments such as: malaria, tuberculosis, cholera, respiratory infections, and measles (infants);and ,
12. Do not acknowledge that mental health problems though it continuous to be prevalent. They associated mental health with from demonic possession.

*Did You Know that most Latinos/**Hispanics*** (Kaleidoscope, 2003; & Cultural Competency for Health Care Providers, 2006):

1. Use the terms Latino/Hispanics refers to an ethnic group and not a racial group. They include individuals from over 25 different countries. Out of these, Mexicans, Puerto Ricans and Cubans make up 75% of the total Hispanic/Latino population nationally;

2. Do not like to be addressed as Latinos if they are Hispanics and vice versa;
3. Latino/Hispanics comprise the largest immigrants in the United States of America
4. Indicate that Latino is the most commonly spoken language;
5. Are not literate in written Spanish. And that not all Hispanics are Spanish speakers;
6. Have more than two names which are often mistaken for cheating;
7. Are not overly keen with keeping time. It is not uncommon for them to show up late;
8. Acknowledge that family relationships take precedence over all other things such as money;
9. Women are stay home mothers and serve as care givers; and,
10. Fathers/men provide leadership, finances and make all decisions for the home such as healthcare.

Did You Know that Southeast ***Asian(s)*** (Kaleidoscope, 2003; & Cultural Competency for Health Care Providers, 2006):

1. Speak diverse languages are from different regions and represent diverse cultures i.e. Cambodians, Laotians, Vietnamese, Montagnards;
2. Are uncomfortable with direct eye contact and head touching. It is inappropriate to touch their heads;
3. Do not verbally express their dissatisfaction with care, but if they feel unhappy with the care they received, they may never return for care again;
4. Are very sensitive to body language. They find some forms of "leg crossing" and body postures to be very offensive;
5. Belief in their traditional medicine and may not always adhere to western medicine;
6. Relay on elders and church leaders for information on health. They often consult them whenever they are in doubt; and
7. Vietnamese and Montagnards do not always speak the same languages and have different cultures. A montagnard for example gets very offended if you refer to them as a Vietnamese and vice versa.

Did You Know that ***Eastern European(s)*** (Kaleidoscope, 2003; & Cultural Competency for Health Care Providers, 2006):

1. Had more access to advanced health care back in their home countries as compared to other immigrants from Africa or other regions. Bosnians for example had free access to health care in their country;
2. Are racially categorized as white or Caucasians;
3. Are very diverse and are mainly from Bosnia, Croatia, Macedonian, Russia, and Ukraine among others;
4. Grew up in industrialized advanced community similar to that in America;
5. Are not offended by direct eye contact or hand shaking;
6. Highly respect their elders and are charged with making all important family decisions; and
7. Some are resistant to the health care system in the United States i.e. it is not uncommon for older Meskhetian Turks to ask their family members and friends to send medications from Russia.

TIPS TO IMPROVE HEALTH CARE ACCESS FOR IMMIGRANTS AND REFUGEES

Cultural Competency Tips for the Health Care Providers

Given all the health related barriers that immigrants and refugees face, it evident that a comprehensive multi-system strategies are needed in order to address the disparities that immigrants and refugees face. It is imperative that health care providers and agencies provide quality health care and equal access to health care while attending to the language, cultural and acculturation barriers (Kaleidoscope, 2003; Bailey, 2002; & Ponce et al, 2006). The following are suggested approaches and tips for health care providers:

1. *Use trained interpreters and not family members or friends.* Research findings indicated that good communication between patients and health care providers has contributed to better health, consistency with seeking health care and adherence to treatment and greater patient satisfaction. Family members or friends are known to add or omit information based on their comfort level and experience with the patient.
2. *Allow time.* Allow more appointment time for individuals who need or will be using interpreters. Speak slowly, listen carefully and be patient with clients who need language help. Most of them feel uncomfortable when they are rushed especially after waiting for long hours in the waiting room.
3. *Translate written materials into all needed languages.* Translated materials ensure that informational is available to all diverse individuals. Provide easily understood patient related materials. It is also important to have a profession member of the community double check terminologies in all translated materials because language terminologies differ even if individuals are from the same country.
4. *Be Patient.* Recognize the potential difference in culture and help seeking behaviors. Allow them time to open up and to get comfortable. This will help create a rapport with your client.
5. *Empathize with your patient.* Learn to be sensitive to their feelings and acknowledge their fears and perception. Women in particular can get very uncomfortable with male providers.
6. *Become educated on other cultures.* Learn about other cultures appropriate communication skills. Asks questions about the cultural beliefs and values that may influence the care (cause of disease, perceptions of care, and their prior history). This will include information such as body language, personal space and voice projection etc. Learn to listen carefully and pay close attention to the verbal and non-verbal communication signs.
7. *Know your patient* .Take time to talk to the patient and try to identify and discover as much information through their conversations and observation (i.e. country of origin, name preference, language spoken at home, help seeking behaviors, age, marital status, as well as education and reading level. Ask them questions about traditional beliefs that may affect the health care and follow up.
8. *Help them learn the system.* Emphasis the importance of keeping time, following procedures, protocol, compliance with medication and follow up with appointments.
9. *Home Remedies.* Find out about home remedies that they client may be taking or using. Most immigrants and refugees use home remedies, but may never report unless they are prompted. For example some communities such as the Hmong people sacrificed animals and bought expensive amulets to guide the return of death souls. Incorporate beliefs, home remedies and traditional practices into treatment plans when possible and whenever they do not contradict with modern medications.
10. *Recognize and respect the diverse cultures and beliefs.* Show respect and value for the patient's cultural beliefs and perceptions. Respect and show dignity for all their patients regardless of their age, gender, religion, class, sexual orientation, ethnic, country of

origin or cultural group. Respects the rights of patients to receive or follow up with care. Some communities find some practices and questions offensive, so take time to understand and use cultural brokers as needed.

11. *Involve the whole family* or entire community when providing health care services or prevention interventions. Most health care decisions are made by the entire family because of pooled resources.
12. *Utilize community resources.* Become familiar with available resources such as interpreters, cultural brokers, and translators as much as you can. Collaborate with community leaders and their faith based organizations or churches.

Tips for Working with Interpreters

Chevalier, (2003); Kaleidoscope, (2003); Refugee & Immigrant Service Center, (1995); Gerrish et al (2004); and Karliner et al., (2007), suggested that health care providers these guidelines when working with interpreters:

1. Create a culturally inviting environment for both interpreter and patient. Greet the patient and interpreter in their own language and introduce yourself and the session.
2. Ensure that the exam room or office is conducive i.e. quiet and free of distraction
3. Allow more time for appointment. Most languages require 25% more words in order to express or interpret the English words. Remember that the interpreter has an ethical responsibility and cannot omit, add or edit any information.
4. Set guidelines and expectations with the interpreter and give background information before entering the exam room. This will ensure that everybody is on the same page.
5. Keep control of the interaction and use short sentence.
6. Address the patient, not the interpreter. Maintain eye contact with the patient at all times and only use the interpreter as a voice.
7. Be patient and allow plenty of time the patient and interpreter.
8. Speak slowly and avoid using medical jargon and idiomatic expressions that make it difficult for the interpreter.
9. Provide all of the information about diagnosis, testing, and treatment
10. Allow time for patient to ask questions. Always encourage them to give explanations.
11. Interpreter to clarify concepts he/she might not understand.
12. Confirm understanding and agreement. Ensuring that the patient understands what is being said is critical to their compliance.
13. Use the interpreter as YOUR resource. Do not ask interpreter for his opinions about patients.
14. Do not raise you voice when speaking English.
15. Do not allow interpreter to engage in side conversations. This can be destructive to the patient and the provider.
16. Do not assume anything. Get clarifications when in doubt.

TIPS TO IMPROVE HEALTH CARE ACCESS FOR IMMIGRANTS AND REFUGEES

Cultural Competency Tips for the Health Care Systems

It is also paramount that health care systems create culturally sensitive environments. Specific information from the Michigan Physicians Mutual

Liability Company attests to this. They underwrote malpractice policies so that doctors receive a 2-5% premium reduction for doctors who attend or participate in cultural diversity seminars or conference. Another example is the Pennsylvania Health Law Project. Its tireless efforts to ensure stronger linguistic and cultural standards in federally funded health programs show it's commitment to cultural diversity. Health care industry ought to embrace the needs for diversity by integrating cultural competence into their existing programs i.e. Staff development and on-going educational programs. It is therefore paramount that all health care system provides:

- *Cross cultural competency trainings.* Provide trainings on cultural competency for all staff (top to low level). Conduct workshops that highlight the needs, cultures, values and challenges of specific immigrants and refugee groups. Where possible invite cultural brokers, community and agency leaders. Opportunities and support for exchange programs or travel abroad for cultural and language emersion could particularly helpful for providers.
- *Trained interpreters.* Use trained interpreters at all times. Face-to-face trained interpreters are preferred by most patients. Telephone interpreters should be used during emergencies or in cases where an interpreter that speaks the patients' language cannot be accessed. Identify an agency that can provide the system with a pool of trained interpreters. It is important to train all providers and all personnel on how to effectively use interpreters.
- *Translated materials.* Provide written material (i.e. application forms, consent forms, medical treatment instructions among other vital documents) in all represented languages. Make sure the level of language used in documents is basic. If possible post signage in the languages of the commonly encountered groups if not all in all service areas.
- *Diverse workforce.* Hire and recruit diverse workforce (Front line workers, nurses, certified nurse assistants, doctors, cleaning etc). Recruit and train minority populations. Encourage minority to enroll in health care careers. Provide education advancement opportunities for immigrants i.e. those who are CNA'S or LPN'S. Reports indicate that minorities who pursue health care careers especially in areas with few professionals are more likely to come back and work for their communities after graduation.
- *Collaborations.* Collaborate with community leaders and cultural brokers to provide outreach to the diverse communities. Involve community leaders from the various immigrant and refugee communities. They will guide and provide a road map of how to appropriate, reach and serve the diverse immigrant and refugee communities. They will also help them to identify immigrant-owned businesses and agencies within the respective communities. *This* will ensure that quality and culturally sensitive health care is provided for diverse communities and individual (Hispanics, Latinos, Vietnamese, Montagnards, Africans, Muslims etc).
- *Verbal translation.* Make accommodations for individuals who cannot read their own native language. Though most patients are fluent in their languages, not all of them can read and comprehend the written language.
- *Inviting Environment.* Create culturally inviting and sensitive health care environment (i.e. directions and signs in different languages, use of pictures and signs, posters, the "I speak "flash cards and culturally competent front line workers etc).
- *Information.* Provide a road map of available services that should include: list of

resources with some contact information, detailed information on eligibility as well as expectations, services that are available to uninsured, payment plans as well as the consequences and detailed information on billing of services.

- *Utilize Media.* Use local and ethnic media channels such as television, newspapers and radios to reach out to more immigrant and refugee communities.
- *Transportation.* Provide a one stop clinic or services (i.e. physician, specialists, lab work etc should be at one place) or Provide transportation where possible and necessary.
- *Forums with immigrant and refugees. Provide* on going forums and education for the immigrant and refugees in their communities. This will help to develop trust and rapport with the health care providers as well as the system in general.
- *Take services to immigrant and refugee neighborhoods.* Provide mobile clinics, and health fairs in their neighborhoods or churches
- *Incentive.* Provide economic incentives for practices and strategies that can improve the patient-provider communication, rapport and trust.
- *Lay Health advisors* .Use community health workers or Lay Health Advisors who will serve as cultural brokers. Word of mouth is very powerful among immigrants and refugees.

FUTURE TRENDS

Given the increase in the influx of diverse immigrants and refugees into the United States of America and many other Western countries, it is evident that interventions to serve cross culturally and linguistically diverse populations are inevitable. Though some progress has been made at the individual and at the systems levels; there is room for more improvements. The increase in the diversity of the immigrant and refugee patients attests to the complexity and the lifelong commitment that is required from all the stakeholders. It is thus evident that cross culturally competent health care providers, cross cultural sensitive environments, culturally appropriate training materials, a representative workforce and partnerships with the immigrant and refugee communities should remain the focus of future efforts to provide quality health care to diverse immigrant and refugee populations.

To ensure continuity and long term results of these efforts, young practitioners and institutions can seek the mentorship and guidance from health care providers who have expertise in cross cultural competency. Additionally training institutions should integrate cross-cultural competency content in the curriculum training for future health care providers and administrator. Training toolkits and modules on how to access the health care systems could be developed by health care providers and health care systems. Explore and evaluate the effectiveness of trained peers such as women with women.

CONCLUSION

It is evident that immigrants and refugees encounter numerous health access barriers that suggest an urgent need for cross cultural competency. As indicated above, their disparities could be reduced by training or hiring cross culturally competent health care providers and by creating cross culturally sensitive health care policies and environments. Attention to cultural biases, cultural differences, perceptions and values of health, home remedies, immigration status, linguistic differences and health seeking behaviors are recommended for all providers and agencies that serve diverse immigrant and refugee patients. Networking and collaborating with immigrant and refugee communities will also help to uncover some of the information that may help providers and systems design quality cross culturally appropriate intervention services and programs.

REFERENCES

Active Voice (2003). *The New Americans.* {Information posted on the website}. Retrieved November 18, 2007 from the web: http://www.activevoice.net.

Angell Y. S, & Cetron, M. S (2005). Health Disparities among Travelers Visiting Friends and Relatives Abroad. *Ann Intern Med. January 4, 2005; 142*(1) 67-72.

Bailey, R. (2002). *Demographics of Immigrants in Guilford County, NC.* {Report posted on the Web}.Retrieved December, 2007 from the CNNC web.

The Biggest –Invasion –Since 1066 (2007). Retrieved on May 22, 2008, from http://bookwormroom.wordpress.com/2007/11/15/biggest-invasion-since-1066/.

Berlin, E., & Fowkes, W. (1983). Teaching Framework for Cross Cultural Care. An Application in Family Practice. *West J.Med.,139*(6), 934-938.

Chevalier (2003). *Tips for Working Effectively with Interpreters.* Center for New North Carolinians.

Coppel, J., Dumont, J., & Visco, I. (2001). Trends in Immigration and Economic Consequences. *OECD Economics Department Working Papers*, No. 284, OECD Publishing. Doi: 10.1787/553515678780.

Cultural Competency for Health Care Providers (2007). Champlain Valley Area Health Education Center, 2007.

Dipietro, L., & Caspersen, C. (1991). National Estimates of Physical Activity among White and Black Americans. *Journal of Med Science Sports Exercise*, (23).

Fowler (1998). Providing Primary to Health Care Immigrants and Refugees: The North Hamilton Experience. *Canadian Medical Association, 159*(4), 388-391.

Frey, H. (2006). *Charticle: The Milken Institute Review.*

Gavagan, T., & Brodyaga, J. (1998). Medical Care for Immigrants and Refugee. *American Family Physicians, 57*(5).

Gellert, G. A. (1993). International migration and control of communicable diseases. Soc Sci Med 1993, 37(12), 1489-99.

Gerrish, K., Chau, R., Sobowale, A., & Birks, E. (2004). Bridging the language barrier: the use of interpreters in primary care nursing. *Health & Social Care in the Community* 12 (5), 407–413.

Kaleidoscope (2003). Cultural Diversity in Guilford County. *A training handbook for Health and human service providers.*

Karliner, L. S., Jacobs, E. A., Chen, A. H., & Mutha, S. (2007). Do Professional Interpreters Improve Clinical Care for Patients with Limited English Proficiency. *A Systematic Review of the Literature Health Services Research, 42*(2), 727–754.

Lacere, F., Jensen, L., & Biddlecom, A. (1994). Healthcare Utilization, Family Context, and Adaptation among Immigrants to the United States. *Journal of Health & Social Behavior, 35*(4), 370-384.

Leininger, M., & McFarland, M. M. (2006). Culture Care Diversity and Universality: A Worldwide Nursing Theory. Sudbury: Jones and Barlett publishers.

Maat, M. B. (1997). A group Art Therapy Experience for Immigrant Adolescents. *American Journal of Arts Therapy, 36*, 11-19.

Macdonald, I. J. (2003). Immigrant and Refugee Community Organization: Project interwoven tapestry. *Paper presented at the Annual meeting of the Society for Applied Anthropology*, Portland Oregon.

Macpherson, D. W. (1993). Immigrant health issues: assessment guidelines for the Physician. *Can J Contin Med Education,* (5) 59-66.

Norredam, M., Mygind, A., Nielsen, S. N, Bagger, J., & Krasnik, A. (2007). Motivation and relevance of emergency room visits among immigrants and patients of Danish origin. *The European Journal of Public Health* 2007, *17*(5), 497-502.

OECD (1999). *Trends in International Migration*, Australian Department of Immigration and Multicultural Affairs (DIMA), Citizenship and Immigration Canada, New Zealand Immigration Service, U.S. Immigration and Naturalization Service, European Migration Centre (EMZ).

Ponce, N. A., Hays, R. D., & Cunningham, E. W. (2006). Linguistic Disparities in Health Care Access and Health Status among Older Adults. *Journal of General Internal Medicine, 21*(7), 786–791.

Population Estimates Program, Bureau of the Census, Department of Commerce, Washington, DC, May 2006

Portes, A., & Rumbaut, R. G. (1996). Immigrant America, Berkeley, CA: University of California –Press.

Rafnsson, S. B., & Bhopal, R. J. (2008, May). *Public Health, 122(5), 532-534.*

Refugee and Immigrant Service Center (1995). *Working Effectively with Interpreters: A Guide for Service Providers.* Olympia, W.A.

Westberg, S., Bumgardner, M., & Lind, P. (2005) Enhancing Cultural Competency in a College of Pharmacy Curriculum. *American Journal of Pharmaceutical Education* 2005 (6) 211-222.

KEY TERMS

Asylees: This refers to a group of individuals who enter the United States by different methods (I.e. including student visas, as tourists, or even illegally using false documents), But file for refugee status upon arrival.

Cross-Cultural: Individuals from many diverse cultures (i.e. region, language etc).

Cultural Competence: The ability of the health care systems and providers to interact, communicate and provide culturally sensitive services and environments to patients from cross-culturally diverse communities. It calls for providers to make a conscious effort to understand and appreciate difference among and between groups and individuals.

Culture: It refers to an integrated pattern of human behavior that includes thoughts, communications, actions, customs, beliefs, values and institutions of a racial, ethnic, religious or social group.

Cross-Cultural Competence: The ability of the health care providers to demonstrate actions, behaviors and feelings that acknowledge and show respect to individuals from other cultures, nationalities and those who speak other languages.

Immigrants: Refers to a group of individuals who come to America voluntarily. They come in search of better opportunities i.e. education, economic. They have limitations in accessing health care services.

Interpreter: Interprets/translate orally conversations.

Refugees: This refers to a special category of immigrants who are admitted into the United

States because they are fleeing their country because of extreme fear of persecution due to war, race or politics among others (Bailey, 2001, 2002, Balgopal, 2000). Unlike Immigrants, they are eligible for work, school, housing, health care services.

Title VI Obligations: These are guidelines that regulate health and human service providers to remove barriers to immigrant access to public benefits and service.

Translator: Individual who interprets written text only.

Chapter V
Mobile Technology in a Developing Context:
Impacts and Directions for Nursing

Pammla Petrucka
University of Saskatchewan, Canada

Sandra Bassendowski
University of Saskatchewan, Canada

Thomas F. James
Apogia Networks, Ltd., Canada

Hazel Roberts
Government of St. Kitts-Nevis, Ministry of Health, St. Kitts-Nevis

June Anonson
University of Saskatchewan, Canada

ABSTRACT

This chapter presents the imperatives of mobile technologies in healthcare as these impact (or potentially) impact on development. It presents the contextual overview in development of the diffusion, penetration, and uptake of health-related mobile technologies. A consideration of the roles and responsibilities of the diaspora in the embracing of information and communication technologies is emphasized. The emphasis is on the impact of technologies, generally, and mobile technologies, specifically, in the global health context. The authors provide key exemplars of mobile technologies in development to increase understanding and demonstrate promising practices in this emergent field.

CHAPTER OVERVIEW

The goal of the chapter is to highlight the need for increased emphasis on nursing informatics as integral to quality of care and quality of work life in developing countries. The chapter will focus on the social and socio-technical considerations as these relate to the appropriation and utilization of information and communication technologies ICTs by nurses in select developing contexts. The topics will be framed within the relevant content on the current state in developing nations on technologies, generally, and mobile technologies (i.e., cellular phones, personal digital assistants), specifically. The issues, challenges, and opportunities related to technical capacities, human resources, and systemic limitations within the developing context will be presented. Further, the chapter will present critical issues on the social, cultural, and gender considerations as these pertain to nursing informatics in furthering the development agenda. Special attention will be given to the role of nursing informatics in achieving, monitoring, and evaluating the Millennium Goal agenda (World Health Organization [WHO], 2003). The chapter will include examples and promising practices of nursing informatics from developing countries' perspectives, including a case study of the "Linkage for Education and Research for Nurses (LeaRN): A Caribbean Exemplar". The final elements of the chapter will include a vision for future direction, research, and globalization of nursing informatics.

In accordance with the definition of the Nursing Informatics Special Interest Group:

Nursing informatics is the integration of nursing, its information, and information management with information processing and communication technology, to support the health of people world wide. International Medical Informatics Association-Nursing Informatics[2] definition, adopted August 1998, Seoul, Korea

This definition reminds us that there is an imperative for nurses to consider information and communication technologies (ICTs) and informatics as critical aspects of the global health care environment. Hence, this chapter is committed to a consideration of nursing informatics in an international context, generally, and a developing context, specifically. As health related ICTs and informatics are being increasingly integrated and supported in the Western world, there is an imperative to understand the implications and potentials within the developing context.

TECHNOLOGIES IN THE GLOBAL CONTEXT

Technology is said to be at the heart of progress. It is important to understand the role which technologies play within development and within health care. However, this understanding is only possible, if we understand the role and function of technologies globally.

According to Alan Gelb, Chief Economist of the World Bank, technology is a critical determinant of sustainable growth and poverty reduction, as much of the socio-economic progress of recent years has been due to technology (World Bank, 2008). Despite this rapid technological progress in the developing context, there still remains a significant technology gap (a.k.a. digital divide). So where are the inequities? And what has contributed to perpetuation of these inequities?

Penetration of Technical Achievement Correlates with Income Level...to a Point

In general, the level of technological achievement observed in a country is positively correlated with income levels (see Table 1). However, considerable variation is apparent within income groups, geography, and the nature of the technology. According to the World Bank (2008), "the (technological) penetration of older technologies, such as fixed-line telephones, transportation, and health care services—many of which were originally provided by governments— is only weakly correlated with income" (p. 4), such that almost regardless of income there is high penetration of these older technologies.

The issue of how long it takes for technology to be embraced or gain presence in developing countries is one part of the challenge; however, the more serious impediment is technological diffusion or technological uptake (see Table 2). In the past, it would take almost 100 years for a developing country to significantly exploit a new technological innovation; today, this has been reduced to about 20 years (World Bank, 2008, p. 6). For example, developing countries are only now approaching the level of penetration of mobile phones that has been enjoyed in the Western world since the mid-nineties. Another consideration is the issue of equitable diffusion of the technology within a country, which tends to favor urban centres and under-penetrate rural, remote, and slum areas.

Furthering the Technological Penetration...

Government policy, enabling trade agreements, and investment in human capital can markedly increase technological penetration and technological diffusion. Although there are a number of contributing factors as to whether a technological innovation is adopted, such as the overall macroeconomic, private sector, and governance environments, basic technological literacy and skills in the population significantly influence the rate of technological penetration (World Bank, 2008). Technological progress requires additional improvements in the quality of the labor force beyond strengthening educational systems. One such impact on technology penetration is international migration and diasporic involvement in

Table 1. Technological achievement in developing countries relative to that in high income countries (percent of level in high income countries)

Income Group	Penetration of Older technologies	Penetration of recent technologies
High	100.0	100.0
Upper Middle	58.4	49.6
Lower Middle	41.6	31.8
Low	23.7	22.7

Source: World Bank. (2008)

Table 2. Diffusion of recent technologies (2005) (per 1000 users)

Income Group	Internet Users	Personal Computers	Cellular Subscribers
High	527	579	77
Upper Middle	196	113	48
Lower Middle	95	45	24
Low	44	11	4

Source. World Bank. (2008)

developing countries (Petrucka, Bassendowski, & James, 2007). For example, the diaspora may contribute to the penetration of technologies through investments, networking, and remittances (World Bank, 2008).

Although challenges in human capital have, at times, impeded technological penetration, business and government tend to bring more significant impediments. For example, regulations and labour mobility can significantly impact the technological uptake and technological diffusion. In addition, national economic trends, civil stability, and governance strategies variously strengthen or weaken the penetration of any given technology.

The World Bank (2008) stated that "most developing countries lack the ability to generate innovations at the technological frontier" which is operationalized as the adoption and adaptation of pre-existing technologies rather than research and development in these countries (p. 3). Hence, what appears to be necessary to further technological penetration in development are policies which enable infrastructure and human resource capacity building rather than innovation and research and development.

Further, one should not underestimate the nature of the technology itself as a barrier (or facilitator) of penetration. For example, some emerging technologies (i.e., mobile phones) require less complex and less expensive infrastructure, human capital investment, and policy frameworks for successful technology penetration.

Making the Impacts Far-Reaching...

Silberglitt, Anton, Howell, & Wong (2006) described a list of emerging technologies expected by 2020, which focus on the front-runners being health services applications (i.e., improved diagnostic and surgical methods), access to information (i.e., wireless), and environmental sustainability (i.e., water purification). Many important technological innovations have been health related, such as clean drinking water and sanitation, yet the diffusion of technology was unequal and slow. For example, between one in three and one in five people in developing countries lack access to clean water and as many as one in two lack access to proper sanitation.

According to Primo Braga, Daly, and Sareen (2003), the falling costs of computing and wireless Internet have enabled some low income countries to show capacity for advanced level technologies but these potentials have been constrained due to lack of human capital and policy-enabling environments.

Technological innovations do not need to be complex or overly sophisticated to have important development impacts. In fact, affordability and simplicity tend to be better predictors of reach and sustainability of a technology in the developing context. The larger challenge appears to be equity (or inequity) in the experiencing of the benefits or impacts, and this is where future efforts must be directed to ensure benefits are shared across groups and sectors.

The Determinants of Technological Uptakein Development ...

The speed with which a country absorbs and adopts technology is not a linear process and not without challenges. An enabling environment with policies and regulatory frames to promote ICTs as a development catalyst is a critical determinant. Two key areas, which have not been addressed, are related to the human resources of the country – technological literacy and diasporic contributions.

Technological literacy. Technological progress is contingent upon the technological competencies of the people. The dirth of basic life and literacy skills in developing countries is a significant barrier to technological uptake. WHO (2008) states that the failure to control HIV/AIDS is an example of poor dissemination of technology and the ongoing technological literacy incompetencies of the next generation will perpetuate poor health outcomes (Bell, Devarajan, & Gersbach, 2004) and reduced opportunities for progress (World Bank, 2008).

According to Caselli and Coleman (2001), technological uptake is related to the educational attainment of the population which leaves the developing nations and certain subpopulations (i.e., women) in a deficit position. Literacy rates have consistently improved worldwide, but these are generally reserved for traditional reading, writing, and numeracy skills, without an indicator for technology literacy. Further, even these improvements have not been equally represented throughout developing populations with women often being left behind statistically (Rosenzweig and Wolpen, 1994; Behman et al., 1999).

Diaspora. Often associated with brain drain (in which there is a move of the well educated to developed countries), it is the opportunity for brain gain or repatriation that holds the greatest promise (Brinkerhoff, 2006; Petrucka, Bassendowski, & James, 2007). Not to be underrepresented, since 1990, the highly educated diaspora of developing countries has doubled in size. The members of the diaspora have a key role in introducing, promoting, and financing knowledge and technology transfers. According to Agrawal, Kapur, and McHale (2004), technological diffusion tends to adhere to cultural and national linkages. However, to date, it has not been made clear to what extent they have successfully influenced technological development and technological uptake in their home countries.

Current Trends... Going Mobile ...

Mobile phone ownership rates in developing countries—even in the poorest countries—are rising rapidly, having almost doubled in low income countries between 2000 and 2004 (World Bank, 2008). In slightly more than a quarter century, mobile phones have begun to displace older technologies in conducting economic, service, and knowledge transactions in virtually every country. As we move towards new infrastructure such as WiMax (wireless, broadband Internet standards) the potential for ongoing change to the accessibility of mobile technologies can be anticipated globally.

TECHNOLOGIES IN THE NURSING CONTEXT

"Technological developments make more effective health care a possibility; however, they do not make it a reality." (Burke & Weill (2005), p. 205)

The above quote invites us to a vision that it is health care providers, including nurses who can make technological diffusion and technological uptake in development a reality.

Nurses are the largest single group of health professionals who directly influence the quality of most health services provided and their outcomes (Laschinger, 2006). Scientific knowledge, generally, and nursing knowledge, specifically, is accumulating at an exponential rate. In light of the increasingly complex and diverse client groups, nurses have significant needs for timely, accurate, and appropriate information and must be prepared to consider ICTs and informatics in the provision of the best possible care for their clients (Pan American Health Organization [PAHO], 2004). Information is a central element in decision making and an essential requisite for the effective provision and management of health care. Access to information is recognized as a critical ingredient for health services and health program planning, operation, supervision, and control, and ICT are seen as indispensable tools for the evaluation of clinical and managerial interventions (WHO, 2003; PAHO, 2004).

Impacting the Global Health Agenda

According to WHO (2003), three critical challenges to nursing in the context of development are:

a. Addressing the impact of HIV/AIDS;
b. Addressing internal and international migration of nurses; and
c. Achieving effective health sector reform and reorganization.

Although these are all extremely important challenges, the latter two will be the focus, as the clinical and disease specific components are beyond this discussion.

Each of these challenges is rooted in ensuring adequacy (i.e., quantity and accessibility) of information and quality of nursing professionals to meet the health care needs and to address the Millennium Development Goals (MDGs). The eight MDGs – which range from halving extreme poverty to arresting the spread of HIV/AIDS to providing universal primary education, all by the target date of 2015 – form a blueprint agreed to by all the world's countries and leading development institutions.

Many of the causes of such challenges (i.e., quality and quantity) are chronic and inter-sectoral problems. For example, in terms of addressing the impact of HIV/AIDS, there is a need to consider the role of technologies in addressing the growing demands on the health care systems within many developing countries due to the prevalence of the disease among the healthcare workforce and extra demands the disease and its treatment impose on already overburdened health systems (WHO, 2003).

The mobile nurses' and technology's potential. In relation to the internal and international migration of nurses, there are significant concerns respecting the mal-distribution of staff and a lack of resources to recruit, train, and support health care workers. Underlying this discussion is the need to understand what human capacity in health care means. Human capacity development (HCD) is a comprehensive process of creating the political will, capabilities, and management systems to enable governments and organizations to respond effectively to the human resource crisis. According to WHO (2003), health human capacity is "the cumulative stock of all individuals engaged in promoting, protecting, or improving the health of populations." This means all those contributing to health services, both formal (doctors, nurses) and informal (traditional healers, volunteers).

One might query 'how significant is the human capacity issue and nursing in development?' WHO (2006) stated there is a shortage of more than 4 million health care workers in 57 developing countries. Commonwealth Deputy Secretary-General Winston Cox (2005) states that "recent studies estimate that for 1999-2000 the cost of nurses migrating from CARICOM countries was in the region of US$16.7 million". The impact of the nursing crisis is being felt throughout the Caribbean region. In Barbados, between 1999 and 2004, 229 registered nurses resigned, reaching a peak of 63 in the year 2000 (Walcott, 2005). Many of the most experienced, skilled and specialized nurses have left for greener and more professionally rewarding pastures, including higher remuneration, better working conditions, greater opportunities for professional development/ career opportunities (Walcott). About 35 percent of nursing posts in the Caribbean region's health sector are currently vacant. In sub-Saharan Africa, the situation is even more dramatic (or perhaps dismal) with only 3% of the global health care workforce (Kaiser Daily HIV/AIDS Report, 4/7). In 2006, there were 937 nurses for every 100,000 United States residents, Canada 995, Japan 779, compared with 114 in Kenya, 28 in Nigeria, and 21 in Ethiopia (WHO, 2006). The World Health Report (WHO, 2003) noted "the most critical issue facing health care systems is the shortage of people who make them work" (p. 110).

A nursing shortage is not just an organizational challenge or a topic for economic analysis; it has major negative impacts on health care in areas such as patient safety (Fischer, Stewart, Mehta, Wax, & Lapinsky (2003) and lack of sufficient expertise. Failure to deal with a nursing shortage – be it local, regional, national or global – is likely to lead to failure to maintain or improve health care (Buchan, 2004). The Honorable Dr. Jerome Walcott (2005), Minister of Health for Barbados stated that "there is a high correlation between the level of health care, the standard of nursing care, and the productivity of a country". Buchan (2004) stated that current research on health human resources highlights that single interventions are unlikely to achieve widespread or long-term benefits in workforce sustainability, but rather it requires a coordinated effort across the range of inter-dependent components. It is the potential of nursing informatics which holds the promise to assist developing countries to address challenges such as increasing productivity, reducing errors, improving patient care, and increasing worker retention (Davenport, 2004).

Achieving health sector reform. We must consider health information as an essential function of every health system (World Bank, 2001). Therefore, a key intervention aimed at strengthening health systems must necessarily include efforts to enhance national Health Information Management Systems (HIMS) or Health Information Systems (HISs).

Boned-Ombuena (2007) in a study for the World Bank released in September 2007 on Health Information Management Systems (HIMs) recommended:

- Integrating HIMS as essential components of health systems for purposes of quality, results-based health systems;
- Developing and retaining a skilled and motivated workforce as key in the development and sustaining of HIMS. Staff training must be complemented with other substantial investments to develop the necessary information infrastructure;
- Establishing HIMS tools and infrastructure to capture the necessary data in a timely and user appropriate manner;
- Strengthening HIMS in order to enhance monitoring and achieving progress toward the Millennium Development Goals;
- Developing partnerships between the different health information actors in order to coordinate the implementation of national HIMS because alliances ensure that all partners subscribe to common goals and complementary approaches.

Manfredi (1993) and PAHO (1999) suggested that health information management in developing countries is further challenged by:

- High demand for nursing care;
- Insufficient registered nurses;
- Predominance of non-professionally designated staff;
- Lack of standardized documentation;
- Lack of recognition of importance of documentation;
- Lack of an information and technology culture.

Technology Appropriation in Nursing...

Unfortunately, progress in improving the capacity of developing countries to absorb and make use of those technologies has been sub-optimal. As mentioned previously, the lack of equitable access to technologies, minimal technological competencies, and disabling policy/regulatory environments have been impediments to the technological uptake. According to the Kaul Report (2002), connectivity is a major concern which influences the ability of individuals to access online programs and resources, to gain skills necessary for computer literacy, and to adopt e-learning and e-health opportunities.

Anecdotal and experiential evidence suggests there is minimal ICT technological uptake within the health care sectors in developing countries – except in the administrative and management areas, as indicated in the Canadian Nurses Association's (2006) e-Nursing Strategy document. Despite nursing informatics' increased visibility and emphasis, the culture within the health care sector in developing countries tends towards traditional, paper-based, labour intensive mechanisms. Exposure, coupled with education, is seen as a critical and valuable catalyst to addressing this deficit.

Gender Implications in Technology Appropriation

Any discussion of technology and nursing would be remiss without consideration of gender impacts and implications. Generally, major ICT and science, technology, and innovation frameworks fail to address gender issues and inclusiveness in the knowledge society. Women's rate of Internet access and use do not naturally mirror national rates of technology penetration for the population as a whole. A range of socio-economic and political factors affect and frame this gender divide, including social and cultural barriers to technology use, education and skill levels, privacy and security, and location/mode of access to technology.

Nursing, more than most professions, is associated with a feminine dominant gender role due to the caring involved. Nurses are often seen in subordinate or service roles to other professions and this relationship is especially pronounced in the context of developing countries. Gideon (2006) argues that the division of labour in health care constitutes the most blatant form of the sexual division of labour between male (usually associated with medicine) and female (usually associated with nursing), despite the obvious emerging gender shifts within those professions. In addition, Barriteau's (2003) framework of material and ideological relations of gender would suggest that introduction of technology may not significantly impact the ideological relations.

Considering Mobile Technologies in Nursing and Development...

Nursing informatics has a significant role in addressing these challenges in innovative and responsive ways. Nurses are among the most skilled members in the health team when it comes to information management, routinely collecting and organizing data, seeking evidence, and researching treatments/interventions. However, most do so without the benefit of any ICT resources. According to Hebert, nursing culture does not encourage nurses to use information technology (IT) to manage information (The National Advisory Council on Nurse Education and Practice, 1997). In addition, computer anxiety may cause nurses to avoid using ICT (Orr, n.d.). Yet, nurses spend up to 1/3 of their time documenting with Lindsay (2001) and Houck (2001).

One potential mobile technology solution is the personal digital assistant (PDA), which according to Peterson (2004), is the newest tool in the academic and professional toolbox bringing powerful capabilities and portability to the pockets of nurses in a wide variety of settings. This device brings the potential for better information management that puts the answers in the nurses' hands, not at the nurses' station. It is also a strategic innovation which recognizes that nursing documentation is moving beyond inputting data into a paper format to that of collecting data and inputting it directly into a mobile system at the point of care delivery. These types of mobile technologies have been featured in a number of developing country exemplars in Africa and Asia where they have demonstrated improved practitioner capacity to treat patients effectively; increased level of job satisfaction and nurses' positive perceptions about quality of care; and enhanced cost and resource efficiencies. For the purpose of this discussion, the PDA will be the focus exemplar of mobile technologies. It is, however, recognized that other tools such as smart phones, tablets, cellphones, and other devices (ipods™) are equally as powerful.

PDAs - the Newest Tool in Nursing's Toolkit...

Imagine nurses having a reference library in the palm of their hand...drug formularies...laboratory and diagnostic manuals...textbooks...journal articles. All of these become possible through a simple tool – the PDA. Many researchers (Choia, Chun, Lee, Lee, Shin, Hyun, Kim, & Kim, 2004; Blair, 2006; Colevins, Bond & Clark, 2006) consider the potential for handheld mobile devices in the nursing arena.

Describing PDAs. According to Peterson (2004), the PDA is the newest tool in the academic and professional toolbox which brings powerful capabilities and portability to the pockets of nurses in a wide variety of settings. Personal digital assistants (PDAs) were introduced in the mid 1990s in their current format, however, as recently as 2003 Forrester's Consumers Technographics Study found that only 559,800 North American nurses were using PDAs in their practice (Davenport, 2004). This trend exists despite the potential for PDAs to give better information management in a light and mobile model that puts the answers in the nurses' hands, not at the nurses' station. In a 2001 survey of clinicians in Toronto 42% of general internists (mean age 46), 70% of house staff (mean age 25) and 32% of family physicians (mean age 45) used a PDA in practice (Strauss et al., 2001). It is noteworthy that in 2002, physician technological uptake of PDA technology was over 18% in the United States with nurses showing only about 1% technological uptake (Hunt, 2002). By 2003, the results from the Canadian Medical Association Physician Resource Questionnaire (Martin, 2003) indicated that a third of Canadian physicians were using some type of hand held device in their practice; and, by 2004, Solworthy indicated 47% of US physicians used PDAs in their practice with approximately 18% of nurses using PDAs.

According to Bryant (2002), "the (PDA) is able to respond to these needs in a way that no other form of ICT is able.... It provides portable, reliable access to up-to-date journals and texts, can maintain up-dated norms and standards and training materials, can be used with local content easily, provides the opportunity for easy sharing and consultation, and provides a unique opportunity to collect, analyze, and disseminate data for decision making". Further, a PDA offers the potential to profoundly change the functioning of health systems and yield improvements in both access to and quality of service delivery by:

- Ensuring that every provider has the most recent and up-to-date norms and standards of care available;
- Ensuring that every practitioner has access to relevant and current textbooks;
- Ensuring access to current treatment algorithms (i.e., HIV/AIDS care; IMCI);
- Permitting the recording, analysis of trends, and identify potential problem areas for client care;
- Allowing providers to access local and global discussion groups to maintain connection to the larger discussion of health issues; and
- Improving accuracy, minimizes errors and speeding information sharing (Bryant).

Miller (2003) summarized a survey conducted by Skyscape, a provider of PDA references, in which ninety percent of the 900 physicians reported better patient care, 85% had less medical errors, and 40% said they treated more patients each day. Descriptive analysis of 946 respondents revealed that the PDA drug database saved time during information retrieval, was easily incorporated into workflow, and improved decision-making. But, what is known about the specifics of uses of PDAs in international settings?

International PDA Experiences. PDAs are featured in a number of developing country exemplars in Africa and Asia. Of special note are projects in Kenya[1], Uganda[2], Ghana[3], and the Caribbean[4]. These projects focused on guidelines for critical diseases such as malaria, tuberculosis and HIV/AIDS, drug lists, medical references/texts, and medical calculators. Key findings, according to Satellife (2005), were:

- Improving practitioner capacity to treat patients effectively;
- Mastering of basic functions is less than 2 days;
- Reporting high degree of satisfaction and felt the technology helped them perform tasks better;
- Saving costs and resources in place of paper and pencil methods;
- Improving data collection accuracy and timeliness.

International trends indicate that nursing documentation is moving beyond inputting data into a stationary format to that of collecting data and inputting it directly into a mobile system at the point of care delivery. Hence, PDAs appear to be emerging as the platform of choice for this function worldwide (PDA Cortex, 2002). An international study from Germany (Stengel, Bauwens, Walter, Kopfer, & Ekkernkamp, 2004) compared the use of handheld computer-assisted documentation with traditional paper chart documentation. According to this study, documentation quality ratings improved significantly with the introduction of the handheld devices ($p < 0.01$) with respect to the correct assessment of a patient's progress and assessment of patient data. Similar projects are being conducted in India (i.e., India Health Care Project) where they have found health workers have experienced 40-60% reduction in time for processing data through PDAs (Sastry, 2003).

A major example of PDA use in health care for development occurred in Uganda with health care workers and physicians using PDAs to access, record, and transmit data. The study considered the technology's functionality, ease of user technological uptake in day-to-day workflow, and data quality (IDRC, 2004). It was noted that through this type of initiative, practitioners were "now able to access the latest treatment guidelines for tuberculosis and malaria and learn of the most effective approaches to fight HIV/AIDS" (PDA Cortex, 2004, p. 2). Other key findings that have relevance to the proposed project are that PDAs were seen to increase documentation accuracy, increase sharing of health information, and email utilization using PDAs. As a result of the Uganda project, the Uganda Red Cross has undertaken a similar project and, medical students at Makere University now receive and use PDAs in their studies and clinical experiences (Bridges.org, 2003).

Mobile Applications for PDAs. Two unique applications for PDAs are discussed to further demonstrate the utility and adaptability of the tool to local, regional, and international contexts.

In December 2005, the editors of the New Oxford Dictionary identified 'podcast' as the word of the year (Skiba, 2006). Podcasting is defined as a new audio medium that allows individuals to subscribe to, store, and consume audio content at their choice of time and place (Cochrane, 2005). Podcasts can be received and stored on computers as well as a variety of mobile devices such as iPods© and personal digital assistants (PDAs). Podcasting and vodcasting (video-based) are evolving rapidly and having significant impact on how communication is occurring as information is shifted between cell phones, computers, PDAs, cameras, and other mobile devices. Podcasting is tool for learning but not in the traditional way of thinking about how content is created, distributed, and owned by the user (Kankaanranta, 2005; Seitzinger, 2006). Generally, podcasts are between 3 to 8 minutes, and provide updates on the latest evidence-based practices, provide information on a specific issue, or stimulate critical thinking

(Kadel, 2006; Kaplan-Leiserson, 2005). This strategy has significant potential in the developing context in that it is relatively inexpensive to access and/or create, user-friendly, and directed messaging capable.

Secondly, rapid advances in low-cost, wireless personal area networks (i.e., Bluetooth) foreshadow the emergence of remote health monitoring as a crucial tool for affordable future healthcare delivery and management. A limited number of personal health monitoring products are already available in the market (Honeywell HomMed, Health Hero Network, American Telecare, AMD Telemedicine. While these products vary in sophistication and cost, they range from basic systems that collect data wirelessly from biomedical devices and store them for later access to more advanced solutions that collect the data, distribute it to a managed care team and proactively trigger alerts for care teams. The real power of such remote monitoring will be harnessed by permitting advances such as proactive detection of emerging medical conditions, individually customized treatments, and monitoring or connecting remotely located patients with clinicians.

The prevailing and most widely accepted architecture for such remote health care monitoring involves the use of a personal gateway device (such as a PDA or smart phone) interposed between the biomedical sensors and the remote server acting as the repository of biomedical data streams. As the sensors typically have no wide-area networking interface due to energy and form-factor limitations, they transmit their sensed data to the gateway device via a short-range technology such as Bluetooth. This gateway device is assumed to possess wide-area wireless connectivity, and is responsible for relaying such transmitted data back to the remote server for either real-time or offline analysis. Such a three-tiered architecture has been proposed and prototyped in several research initiatives (Chakravorty, 2006). Such a three-tiered architecture, especially one that leverages a simple device such as a PDA is especially attractive, as it allows remote monitoring to become simply a value-added application.

Challenges of PDAs. According to George and Davidson (2005), nurses rated barriers that were related to technical issues and literacy as modest. These results were also reflected in the research of Dee, Teolis, and Todd (n.d.) who surveyed 131 healthcare PDA users and found that users were limited by lack of software, PDA memory limits, not understanding the software, and not understanding how to download the software. Lusky (2002) felt that nurses' stumbling blocks for PDA utilization are that nurses aren't very technologically savvy and information technology (IT) resistant. pda.cortex (2003) stated that nurses had trouble adopting IT because they are an aging population with little or no IT training, nursing schools do not have enough IT training, and nurses feel that IT is dehumanizing. However, this lays in direct contrast to the outcomes of the Uganda and Kenya projects described earlier with other professional and para-professional groups.

The Future Roles and Trends For Mobile Technologies...

The future is fast and furious. The introduction and innovation of mobile technologies has continued to far surpass anyone's imagination and expectations. However, there is an imperative to remember that PDAs are no substitute for sound clinical knowledge, experience, and keen assessment skills (Baumgart, 2005).

There are some critical questions respecting the promise of ICT to improve health in the developing world, such as:

- Can develop processes that respect the workload of caregivers and get the data into the hands of those who can really use it to make a difference? (Satellife, 2005)
- Can ICT be used to stem the mass migration of healthcare providers from the South to the North and ameliorate the devastating

diminishment of medical and health care skills, knowledge, and experience in poor countries? And given the stress on existing personnel, can we manage the human resource challenges posed by introducing new technologies? (Satellife, 2005)

- What are the strategies and possibilities for interaction and collaboration with members of the diaspora through technologies (Levitt & Nyberg-Sorenson, 2004)
- How will the future nursing education models in developing countries allow them to meet the demands of the workplace with inclusion of mobile technologies as part of the foundational toolkit?
- Can we re-create the current health care context in developing countries to facilitate nursing's technological uptake and utilization of mobile technologies?

In looking at a number of promising practices, we might begin to envision the range and scope of the successes of mobile technologies in health care for developing countries.

Promising Practices

A community link. In Bangladesh, D-NET Pallitathay Help Line provided a link between information suppliers and the target beneficiaries. Essentially, the network has an 'info-mediary', a mobile operator who goes door to door with a mobile phone. Through the phone, queries are placed and responded to by Help Desk operators at the D-Net site who are supported by a database-driven software application. To date, the majority of queries are related to health (primarily from housewives) and agriculture (primarily from farmers). The queries have assisted with the creation of awareness raising campaigns (e.g., www.pallitathya.org.bd).

A national link. In Kenya, the AfriAfya – African Network for Health Knowledge Management and Communication – considers means to use ICT for community health primarily in rural Kenya (but some African continental involvement is included). There is a focus on locating information from the Ministry of Health, the National AIDS and STDs Control Program, Partner Agencies, NGOs, and the Internet and making the information usable by lay community members (http://www.afriafya.org)

A regional link. The Caribbean Knowledge and Learning Network (CKLN) is a multilateral project supported by the OAS, the World Bank, the European Union, and the Canadian International Development Agency (CIDA). The project involves the Caribbean Community (CARICOM) and the Organization of Eastern Caribbean States (OECS) in an effort "to enhance the competitiveness of Caribbean countries using ICTs to connect the Caribbean to the global pool of knowledge, developing human resources, and facilitating greater regional integration." This initiative enables e-learning, e-health, e-governance and other e-enabled activities to be undertaken (e.g., http://www.ckln.org).

An inter-regional link. Linkage for Education and Research for Nurses (LeaRN) is a four island initiative which advocates the use of a simple ICT infrastructure and toolkit (i.e., PDAs, wireless connectivity, health relevant software) to address the critical challenges and, ultimately, affecting health information system effectiveness. During the project, the emphasis was on having the nurses gain a working knowledge of the equipment and basic applications. There was significant variation in the technical skills of nurses across sites ranging from no experience to related competencies (i.e., text messaging). The nurses in the English speaking sites have a palette of nursing programs downloaded on their machines, whereas the Spanish site has a basic program health care available for download. Further, the nurse participants in each site have shown great enthusiasm and willingness to incorporate PDAs into their work environments and beyond. The creation of a video, funded by IDRC, to capture the intent and perceptions of the participants is both a testimonial to their technological uptake of the project and the potential for the project to contribute to the quality of their work life and care. Within the majority of participants, it was found that the selected ICT was easy to learn and implement in their respective environments. Ensuring Nurses Access to Care Quality Knowledge through Technology (ENACQKT) will continue the introduction of the technology through a training the trainer mechanism to both build capacity and to enhance the investment in the nurse participants in the study. During the LeaRN project, a number of key contacts and linkages to governments and regional agencies emerged that will further support the sustainability of the project. Meetings with government officials (most significantly in Dominican Republic, Dominica, and St. Kitts) and potential partnering agencies (i.e., UNDP) have continued to provide insights into the linkage of this project to health information systems and e-portals which are envisioned as imperative to the health and health care systems in the region. (http://www.usask.ca/nursing/leaRN).

REFERENCES

Agrawal, K., Kapur, D., & McHale, J. (2004). *Defying distance: examining the influence of the diaspora on scientific knowledge flows*. Queen's School of Business, Queen's University, ON. Presented at the Fourth Annual Roundtable for Engineering Entrepreneurship Research, Georgia Institute of Technology, College of Management, December 4, 2004.

Barriteau, E. (2003). *Confronting power, theorizing gender: Interdisciplinary perspectives in the Caribbean*. University of West Indies Press.

Baumgart, D. C. (2005). Personal digital assistants in health care: Experienced clinicians in the palm of your hand? *Lancet, 366(9492)*, 1210-1222.

Behrman, J. R., Foster, A. D., Rosenzweig, M. R., & Vashishtha, P. (1999). Women's schooling, home teaching, and economic growth. *Journal of Political Economy, 107(4)*, 632–714.

Bell, C., Devarajan, S., & Gersbach, H. (2004). Thinking about the long-run economic costs of AIDS. In *The Macroeconomics of HIV/AIDS*, M. Haacker, (Ed.). (pp. 96–133). Washington, DC: International Monetary Fund.

Blair, R. (2006). Take-along tech and the training of specialty nurses. *Health Management Technology, 27*(3).

Boned-Ombuena, A. (2007). *Development assistance to health information systems strengthening*. Washington, DC: Health, Nutrition and Population Unit in Human Development Network, World Bank.

bridges.org. (2003). *The Satellife PDA project*. Retrieved March 12, 2007 from http://www.bridges.org/case_studies/351

Brinkerhoff, J. M. (2006). Diasporas, mobilization factors, and policy options. In *Converting migration drains into gains: Harnessing the resources of overseas professionals*, C. Wescott and J. Brinkerhoff (Eds.). (pp. 127–53). Manila: Asian Development Bank.

Bryant, M. (2002). *The expanding role of ICTs in HIV/AIDS program design and implementation*. Retrieved November 13, 2005 from http://topics.developmentgateway.org/hiv/sdm/previewDocument.do~activeDocumentID

Buchan, J. (2004). What Difference Does ("Good") HRM make? *Human Resources for Health*, 2:6 (7 June 2004), World Health Organization, Geneva, Switzerland.

Burke, L., & Weill, B. (2005). *Information technology for the health professions. 2nd Ed.* Chicago, IL: Prentice Hall.

Canadian Nurses Association. (2006). *E-Nursing strategy for Canada.* Ottawa: Author.

Caselli, F., & Coleman, W. J. (2001).Cross-country technology diffusion: The case of computers. *American Economic Review Papers and Proceedings, 91(2)*, 328–35.

Chakravorty, R. (2006, March). MobiCare: A Programmable Service Architecture for Mobile Medical Care. *Proceedings of UbiCare 2006: The First Workshop on Ubiquitous and Pervasive Healthcare.*

Choia, J., Chun, J., Lee, K., Lee, S., Shin, D., Hyun, S., Kim, D., & Kim, D. (2004). MobileNurse: Handheld information system for point of nursing care. *Computer Methods and Programs in Biomedicine, 74(3)*, 245-254.

Cochrane, T. (2005). *Podcasting: Do it yourself guide.* Indianapolis, IND: Wiley Publishing Inc.

Colevins, H., Bond, D., & Clark, K. (2006). Nurse refresher students get a hand from handhelds. *Computers in Libraries, 26(4),* 6-8; 46-48.

Cox, W. (2005). Commonwealth Secretariat: Towards a trade and development approach in the Caribbean region. Retrieved March 12, 2007 from http://www.thecommonwealth.org/speech/34293/35178/152062/152049/143178/towards_a_trade_address_to_the_symposium.htm

Davenport, C.B. (2004). *What nurses need to know about personal digital assistants (PDAs).* Retrieved March 20, 2007 from http://eaa-knowledge.com/ojni/ni/8_3/davenport.htm

Dee, C. R., Teolis, M., & Todd, A. (n.d.). Multi-state study of health professionals' use of the personal digital assistant (PDA). Retrieved on October 22, 2005 from http://www.mc.vanderbuilt.edu/biblio/scmla/pres/dee.pdf

Fischer, S., Stewart, T. E., Mehta, S., Wax, R., & Lapinsky, S. E. (2003). Handheld computing in medicine. *Journal of the American Medical Informatics Association, 10*(2), 139-149.

George, L., & Davidson, L. (2005). PDA use in nursing education: Prepared for today, poised for tomorrow. *Online Journal of Nursing Informatics, 9(2).* Retrieved on February 19, 2007 from http://www.ojni.org/9_2/george.htm

Gideon, J. (2006). Integrated gender interests into health policy. *Development and Change, 37(2)*, 329-352.

Hebert, M. (n.d.) National nursing informatics project discussion paper [Electronic version]. Retrieved on December 8, 2003 from http://www.cna-nurses.ca/pages/resources/nni/nni_discussion_paper.doc

Houck, J. B. (2001). PDAs-Stat-for busy nurses. Retrieved October 22, 2005 from http://www.wirelessnewsfactor.com

Hunt, E.C. (2002). The value of a PDA to a nurse. Retrieved October 22, 2005 from http://www.unc.edu5/~dbailey1/CONI/nsgpdavalue.doc

International Development Research Centre. (2004). *Uganda Health Information Network.* Technical report – IDRC Grant No. 102136-001. Ottawa, ON: IDRC.

International Medical Informatics Association – Nursing Informatics. (2008). The Nursing Special Interest Group. Retrieved March 20, 2008 from http://www.imiani.org/

Kadel, R. (2006). Coursecasting: The wave of the future? ... Bit by bit: Podcasting with purpose. Retrieved May 20, 2008 from InfoTrac OneFile database.

Kaiser Daily. (2006). Short of health care workers in developing countries undermines essential services. Retrieved May 20, 2008 from http://www.kaisernetwork.org/daily_reports/rep_index.cfm?DR_ID=44073

Kankaanranta M (2005). International perspectives on the pedagogically innovative uses of technology. *Human Technology, 1(2),* 111–116.

Kaplan-Leiserson, E. (2005). Trend: Podcasting in academic and corporate learning. Retrieved May 20, 2007 from http://www.learningcircuits.org/2005/jun2005/0506_trends

Kaul, I. (2002). Kaul Report. Retrieved May 20, 2008 from www.undp.org/globalpublicgoods/globalization/pdfs/Kaul%20162-180.pdf

Laschinger, H. K. S. (2006). Effect of empowerment on professional practice environments, work satisfaction, and patient care quality: Further testing the nursing worklife model. *Journal of Nursing Care Quality, 20.*

Levitt, P., & Nyberg-Sorenson, N. (2004). *The transnational turn in migration studies.* Global Commission on International Migration: Global Migration Perspectives, No. 6.

Lindsay, C. (2001). PDAs give nurses more time. *Nurse Week*, August 8, 2001.

Lusky, K. (2002). *Is a personal digital assistant in your future?* Retrieved on February 15, 2004 from http://www.nurses.com

Manfredi, M. (1993). The development of nursing in Latin America: A strategic view. *Review Latin American Enfermagem, 1(1)*, 23-35.

Martin, S. (2003). News: Pulse. *Canadian Medical Association Journal, 169 (9).* Retrieved February 5, 2004 from http://www.cmaj.ca/cgi/content/full/169/9/952a

Miller, J. (2003). *Doctors say PDAs improves [sic] medical care.* Retrieved on October 22, 2005 from Rim Road: News at http://www.rimroad.com

National Advisory Council on Nurse Education and Practice. (1997). *A national informatics agenda for nursing education and practice: report to the secretary of health and human services.* Rockville, MD: U.S. Department of Health and Human Services, Health Resources and Services Administration, Bureau of Health Professions, Division of Nursing.

Orr, L. V. (n.d.) *Computer anxiety: University of Southern Main, Communication 499.* Retrieved on January 26, 2004 from http://www.usm.maine.edu/~com/lindap~1.htm

Pan American Health Organization. (2004). *Nursing and Midwifery Services Contributing to Equity, Access, Coverage, Quality, and Sustainability in the Health Services.* Washington, DC: Health Services Organization (OS) - Technology and Health Services Delivery (THS).

Pan American Health Organization. (1999). *Setting up healthcare services information systems: A guide for requirement analysis, application specification, and procurement.* Washington, DC: Essential Drugs and Technology Program, Division of Health systems and Services Development. PAHA/WHO.

PDA Cortex.com (2002). First hand intelligence. *Journal of Mobile Informatics.* Retrieved November 13, 2005 from http://www.pdacortex.com

PDA Cortex.com (2003). *Adopting mobile technology to enhance patient care.* Retrieved on October 22, 2005 from http://www.pdacortex.com/issues_and_attitudes.htm

PDA Cortex. (2004). *Analysis of PDAs in nursing: benefits and barriers.* Retrieved from May 14, 2005 from http://pdacortex.com/Analysis_PDAs_Nursing.htm

Peterson, M. (2004). PDA and its future in nursing. *Kansas Nurse*, October.

Petrucka, P., Bassendowski, S., & James, T. (2007). The role of ICTs in enhancing diasporic citizenry and connectedness: A Caribbean exemplar. *The International Journal of Technology, Knowledge and Society, 2(7)*, 43-48.

Primo Braga, C. A., Daly, J., and Sareen, B. (2003). The Future of Information and Communication

Technologies for Development. *Paper presented at the Information and Communications Technology Development Forum*, Petersburg, Germany, May 21.

Rosenzweig, M. R., & Wolpen, K. I. (1994). Are there increasing returns to the intergenerational production of human capital? Maternal schooling and child intellectual achievement. *Journal of Human Resources 29 (2),* 670–93.

Sastry, C.L.R. (2003). *India Health Care Project: An application of IT in rural health care at grass root level.* Retrieved March 12, 2007 from www.iimahd.ernet.in/egov/ifip/jun2003/article4.htm

Satellife. (2005). *Handhelds for health: Satellife's experience in Africa and Asia.* Ottawa, ON: IDRC.

Seitzinger, J. (2006). *Be constructive, blogs, podcasts, and wikis as constructivist learning tools.* Retrieved May 2, 2007 from http://www3.griffith.edu.au/03/ltn/docs/Design_Strategies.pdf

Silberglitt, R., Anton, P.S., Howell, D.R., & Wong, A. (2006). *The global technology revolution 2020.* Santa Monica, CA: RAND Corporation, National Security Research Division.

Skiba, D. (2006). The 2005 Word of the Year: Podcast. *Nursing Education Perspectives, 27* (1).

Stengel, D., Bauwens, K., Walter, M., Kopfer, T, & Ekkernkamp, A. (2004). Comparison of handheld computer-assisted and conventional paper chart documentation a randomized controlled trial. *Journal Bone and Joint Surgery of America, 86-A(3),* 553-560.

Stolworthy, Y. (2003). *RNs are mobilizing.* Retrieved on October 22, 2005 from http://www.rnpalm.com/RNs_are_Mobilizing.htm

Straus, S.E., Takeshita, H., Davis, D., & Rodrigues-Gianolli P. (2001). *Bringing evidence to the point of care.* Retrieved June 27, 2002 from http://www.cs.toronto.edu/~prg/

Walcott, J. (2005). Opening Address to Commonwealth Secretariat Seminar on managed migration of nurses. 30-31 March 2005. Sherbourne Conference Centre, Barbados.

World Bank. (2008). *Global Economic Perspectives: Technology Diffusion in Developing World.* Washington, DC: Office of the Publisher, World Bank.

World Bank. (2001). *World Development Indicators.* Washington, DC: Office of the Publisher, World Bank.

World Health Organization. (2003). *World Health Report.* Geneva: WHO.

World Health Organization. (2006). The World Health Report 2006 - working together for health. Retrieved May 20, 2007 from http://www.who.int/whr/2006/annex/06_annex4_en.pdf

KEY TERMS

Millennium Development Goals: Articulated goals by the United Nations in the effort to reduce (halve) global by the year 2015. The eight goals are:

- Eradiate extreme poverty and hunger;
- Achieve universal primary education;
- Promote gender equality and empower women;
- Reduce child mortality;
- Improve maternal health;
- Combat HIV/AIDS, malaria, and other diseases;
- Ensure environmental sustainability
- Develop a global partnership for development.

Mobile Technology: Portable technologies (such as laptops, personal digital assistants, cellphones) using connectivity strategies including

WiFI, bluetooth, dial up, and third generation technologies (i.e., GSM, GPRS)

Nursing Informatics: Integration of nursing, its information, and information management using information processing and communication technology (ICT) for the purposes of improving individual, community and global health

Personal Digital Assistant (PDA): Portable handheld or palmtop computer which have a range of functions such as email, word processing, bar coding, global positioning system, and telephone capabilities. PDAs may include Wi-Fi, bluetooth, and infra-red functionalities which enable sharing of information and resources

Podcasts: Series of digital media files (audio and video files) shared over the Internet for purposes of education, knowledge building, and sharing. Podcasts can refer either to the series of content itself or to the method (often called podcasting).

ENDNOTES

1. Medical students at Moi University used PDAs with content relevant resources in obstetrics/gynecology, internal medicine, and pediatrics.
2. Practicing physicians affiliated with Makerere University used handhelds with basic reference materials.
3. Red Cross Volunteers conducted surveys on a disease/immunization project using PDAs.
4. LeaRN described later in the promising practices section.

Chapter VI
Nursing Documentation in a Mature EHR System

Kenric W. Hammond
VA Puget Sound Health Care System, USA

Charlene R. Weir
George W. Allen VA Medical Center, USA

Efthimis N. Efthimiadis
University of Washington, USA

ABSTRACT

Computerized patient care documentation (CPD) is a vital part of a Patient Care Information System (PCIS). Studying CPD in a well-established PCIS is useful because problems of system adoption and startup do not interfere with observations. Factors interfering with optimal nursing use of CPD are particularly challenging and of great concern, given today's shortage of nursing manpower. We describe problems and advantages of CPD usage identified by nurses in a series of research interviews. The chief advantages of CPD for nurses found were better accessibility and reliability of patient care documentation. The main disadvantage was an awkward fit between current input technology and nursing workflow. A second disadvantage was difficulty in translating portrayal of the nursing process into readable documentation that is useful to all members of the clinical team. We interpret these findings to show that explicit consideration of nursing workflow constraints and communication processes is necessary for development of effective nursing documentation systems. Some findings point to a PCIS reconfiguration strategy that is feasible in the short term. Other findings suggest the value of considering mobile and team-oriented technologies in future versions of the PCIS.

INTRODUCTION

Patient care information systems do not exist in a vacuum. Inevitably, these systems articulate with the cognitive, social and practical dynamics of teams of information workers in a health care environment. To the extent that workers' tasks and the functionality of the information systems they use mesh well, these systems are accepted by their users and may demonstrate benefits measurable in terms of efficiency, safety and clinical effectiveness. Present computerized systems do not meet this challenge uniformly (Chaudhry et al., 2006) and are particularly poor at meeting the complex, multi-faceted information needs of nursing. Much of the nursing role in health care delivery is at the final delivery point of care. Nemeth, et al. (2005) call this aspect of health care delivery the "sharp end" of care. As these authors note " . . . sharp end knowledge is dense, complex, changes rapidly, and is embedded in a complex social setting that resists scrutiny by those who are considered to be outsiders."(2005, p. 19)

One important aspect of a patient care information system (PCIS) is input and retrieval of electronic text, which we refer to as computerized patient care documentation or CPD. In this chapter, we will review CPD as practiced by direct providers of health care, focusing on nursing documentation. We will report on an ongoing investigation of CPD as it exists in a mature, complete and widely-deployed patient care information system, the United States Department of Veterans Affairs (VA) Computerized Patient Record System, known as CPRS. We will offer a preliminary analysis of these findings, taking a cognitive work analysis perspective, and illustrate our points with excerpts from individual and group interviews conducted in VA settings. Our findings will show important advantages of CPD for nursing in the VA and important problems, especially with the "task-technology fit" (Goodhue & Thompson, 1995) of CPD and nursing practice.

We will review applicable medical informatics literature and present hypotheses about the origins of the current state of affairs. We will discuss the scope and purpose of nursing documentation activity, and make some short and long term suggestions for improving the "fit" of CPD with nursing work, especially in inpatient care. Improving the "fit" of the CPD system with inpatient nursing care is important. Patient safety has been shown to be highly correlated with nurse (especially RN) staffing intensity, as reviewed by Hinshaw (2008). It is generally accepted that availability to patients is important to safety. In addition, numerous studies of medical errors suggest that effective inter-staff communication is also crucial (Bhasale, Miller, Reid, & Britt, 1998; Coiera, 2000; Wilson, Harrison, Gibberd, & Hamilton, 1999). In hospitals, ward nurses play a critical role in both areas. The more time nurses spend being pulled away from patient and staff contact to work with CPD the less time is available for safety-promoting activities of communication and patient monitoring. Nurses' work with CPD should be as productive and relevant as possible. While our present scope is limited to examining nursing usage of the VA's CPD system in a single facility, many of our most important observations address fundamental cognitive and workflow issues that would apply to nursing documentation in any health care setting using a PCIS.

BACKGROUND

CPD and its Place in the PCIS

The term "Patient Care Information System" refers more or less to the generation of health care information systems that succeeded departmental information systems serving various operational sectors in health care settings, typically: patient registration, appointment scheduling, pharmacy, laboratory, radiology and finance. Three transitions characterized emergence of the PCIS from these systems: integrated data access, provider order entry, and computerized patient care documentation, or CPD.

Free-form narrative documentation is necessary informational "glue" that connects and coordinates health care work. Narrative, because it is immediately accessible to human thought, serves to supplement, integrate, interpret and communicate the structured data in an organization's information system. In the 1980s, when putting this narrative component on line was first contemplated, resistance from users, especially those reluctant to type, was anticipated. With time, increased computer skills in the population, and establishment of the norm that health care professionals type, resistance abated.

Full integration of structured data, narrative and order entry creates powerful synergy that brings the PCIS "to life". The impact of having all documentation rapidly accessible at workstations, simultaneously viewable by many users cannot be understated. An information system lacking access to clinical documentation cannot be considered a "complete" PCIS, and a PCIS lacking a high penetration of direct user CPD entry cannot be considered optimal.

The VA CPRS: A Mature PCIS

The VA CPRS system originated in the late 1970's, driven by small groups of users with special interests united in a vision of an integrated hospital-based system that supported business and clinical needs (Kolodner & Douglas, 1997, pp. 39-56). By the mid-1980's, this system, based on relatively inexpensive "mini-computers", written in the MUMPS (later M and Caché), and deployed with a standardized, portable data base management program, was established in over 160 VA hospitals across the United States. The initial "core" version served basic business functions: laboratory, patient registration and appointing, and the pharmacy. Extended "core" functionality addressed clinical needs in Medicine, Surgery, Mental Health and Nursing. The earliest implementation of CPD functionality was found in a "Progress Notes" section of the Mental Health package.

In the early 1990's it was recognized that order entry and general clinical access to a documentation system was needed, and a text integration utility was developed. Nursing package development included a Vital Signs utility and a Care Plan. At this stage, the CPRS was implemented on "dumb" ASCII terminals.

In the mid-1990's policy, fiscal, and technological forces converged to accelerate general clinical adoption of a paperless PCIS. In 1997, in exchange for complying with Medicare requirements, the VA was permitted to bill private insurance carriers and facilities were allowed to recoup some of these billings. This drove documentation to support billing, and track diagnoses and procedures. This was initially accomplished via paper forms. Soon, though, plain text terminals gave way to client-server architecture and workstations and a graphical user interface (GUI) version of the CPRS was deployed. The GUI allowed viewing multiple data sources together on the same screen and offered a friendlier text editor. By the late 1990's, billing and workload tracking policy had evolved to require documentation of all outpatient clinic visits. For inpatient care, the discharge summaries and procedure notes were the primary documents used for billing. By 2002, most VA Medical Centers and clinics had implemented paperless systems. A national data repository architecture allowed access to patient records at any VA facility in the country from any VA workstation. This system, with 180,000 clinical employees, including 61,000 nurses, provides care for approximately 4.5 million veterans annually.

This rapid summary glosses the challenge faced by all VA clinical staff changing over from paper to computer documentation, but the challenge was met. VA has a highly computer-literate workforce that uniformly values the satisfactions of delivering care with this powerful tool. The VA has received repeated recognition for its accomplishment, and regularly leads other large systems in indices of care quality (Perlin, Kolodner, & Roswell, 2004). It is recognized as a leader in deployment of patient care information systems, and may possess the world's largest PCIS network in a single organization.

Influenced by incentives in fiscal reimbursement policy and a corollary workload and resource allocation structure, the last 15 years of CPRS and CPD development evolved to provide system support for practitioners – *not* nurses. In the present arrangement, only practitioner services can be directly billed. Notwithstanding, nurses in clinics and wards adopted this CPD system as well, because it had enough flexibility to address basic documentation needs, and VA nurses mastered the computer skills to use the system regularly.

Background on CPD

CPD includes electronic progress notes, discharge summaries, consult reports and other text documents that until recently were on paper. In addition to direct clinical use, CPD serves important administrative functions, including billing, quality review and information exchange between institutions. Input methods for CPD vary and include dictation, input assistance through templates, direct typing of narrative, and insertion of stored patient data. In the VA system, dictated entry accounts for less than 1% of CPD. VA data bases currently store approximately 1 billion patient care documents nationwide.

Background on Nursing Documentation and the Nursing Process

Inpatient nursing documentation consists of assessments, treatment and response flow sheets, periodic interval notes (every shift, daily, etc) and care plans. In some settings, these documents resided in a nursing care section of the record, but in others, such as the VA, electronic nursing documents are mingled with the document from all authors. Outpatient nursing documentation includes patient screenings, telephone contacts and follow-up notes, and these are typically interspersed in the general "progress notes" record. Our focus will be on inpatient nursing documentation.

Since the 1980s, documentation of "the nursing process" has been influenced by nursing theory. Most recent efforts to systematize nursing documentation incorporate specialized language associated with nursing theory to describe identification of clinical problems, treatment goals and interventions managed by nurses. This effort has not been altogether popular with nurses or other health professions, and considerable difficulty implementing documentation based in nursing theory has ensued. Not the least of these is that the specialized language incorporated in the nursing documentation is difficult for other professionals to understand.

Nursing Document Creation Tasks

As noted in the introductory section, document creation tools used by nurses were the same as those developed to support office based practice. Documents in the VA system are stored as ASCII text. Customized nursing content is accomplished by using document templates to build blocks of text that are then inserted as *unstructured* text into a document data structure which can be edited before saving the note. The initial implementation of nursing documents (assessments, care plans and other charting) involved templates consisting of editable checklists and boilerplate presented to authors. Later versions of the template tool supported selecting items from a dialog box.

Nursing Assessment

Patient assessment documentation occurs with each inpatient episode. In the first 7 years of use, assessments consisted of checklists customized to each unit. The limitations of the checklist approach are evident: meeting the requirement to use a "complete" assessment with standardized problem-specific language faithful to nursing terminology required a lengthy checklist. Applicable items are marked with an "X", but unchecked inapplicable items often remain in the resulting documents, as shown in Figure 1(a).

A great disadvantage of the resulting documents was that the "dumped" checklists were unreadable and generally ignored. Documents met administrative and theoretical requirements, but were not perceived to improve nursing performance in rendering care. The most useful parts of these documents were the nurses' free text, which tended to be buried in the boilerplate, as shown below in an "Assessment" paragraph (Figure 2.) from the same patient.

Figure 1. Nursing assessment template

(a) ICU Nursing status checklist in record	**(b) ICU Nursing plan as seen in record**
[X] Oral Care ____X/Shift BATH Assistance [] Skin Care [x] Bed [] Sitz [X] Peri/Catheter Care [] Shower [] Tub [] HS Care Diet/Nutrition Intake [] Good [] Fair [] Poor [] Per Tube Feeding [X] NPO [] Patient Feeds Self [] Requires Some Assistance [] Requires Complete Assistance Nutritional Supplement: [] Snack [] High-Protein Liquid Nutrition [] Good [] Fair [] Poor Patient's response: Feeds [] Self [] Some Assistance [] Complete Assistance [] Dysphagia Precautions NPO [X] Slept WITH SEDATION. [] Awake at intervals [] Awake most of the shift [] Ambulatory, Independent ___X/Shift [] Activities, with Assist ___X/Shift [] Transfer to Chair, Dangle, BSC, WC [] Ambulates in Hall, BRP Assistive Devices: []Belt []Cane []Walker[]Crutches [X] Pt is on Bedrest [] Turns Self or [X] Turn/Position W/Assist ____X/Shift	PLAN:Risk for urinary infection related to indwelling catheter The Patient will: 1. have no evidence of urinary tract infection Nursing will: 1. assess for elevated temperature and cloudy, foul-smelling urine qshift 2. catheter care q shift 3. maintain closed system with catheter securely anchored to inner thigh 4. observe color and characteristics of urine Risk for violence related to withdrawal from alcohol and accompanying depression The patient will: 1. exhibit no self-destructive or violent behavior 2. maintain control over behavior 3. accept help as needed 4. use effective coping mechanisms to handle stress Nursing will: 1. assess level of risk as evidenced by feelings of fear, suicidal or homicidal thoughts, poor impulse control or panic. 2. provide a safe environment for the patient 3. use medications as ordered 4. communicate expectation of need to maintain control of behavior in a clear and simple manner 5. provide reassurance.

Figure 2. Nursing assessment free text

ASSESSMENT:Aroused and attempting to get out of bed,pulling at foley cath and iv tubing at 0150.Given Haldol 1 mg at 0153.temp at this time 101.4 tylenol supp per rectum.temp at 1420 100.2.Foley cath draining dark amber Urine had 300 in bag voided between 2400 and 0300.sump suctioning brownish Gray gastrick secretions via cont. Low suction.100cc out between 2300and 0400.iv d51/2 with MVI+thiamine infusing at 100cc hr and completed at 0445,d51/2 hung due to unavailability of MVI and thiamine. Wrist restrained At 2430 patient was attempting to pull out iv and foley cath in addition to attempting to get out of bed. Abd bowel sounds quiet., abd distented. On CM sr heart rate 100s.

Nursing Care Planning

Documentation of nursing care plans has evolved, and in the setting we studied, written care plans are a much less prominent part of nursing documentation. Efforts to develop support for a computerized structured nursing care plan in the 1990's were largely dropped because of difficult usability of the system. Figure 1(b) shows the intervention section of a care plan created in 2003. Our nurse informants told us that while care planning still occurs, its documentation is less formalized.

The diminished role of formal written nursing care plans is noteworthy. For at least a generation, in pursuit of a professional identity for nurses distinct from physicians, academic nursing has

Figure 3. January 2003 assessment document

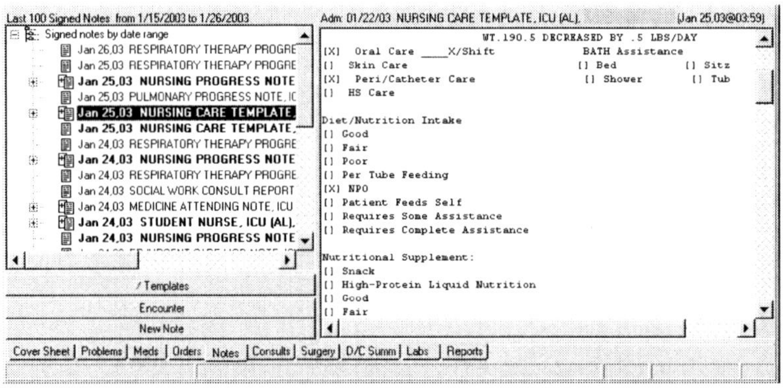

Figure 4. December, 2007 Version of assessment document

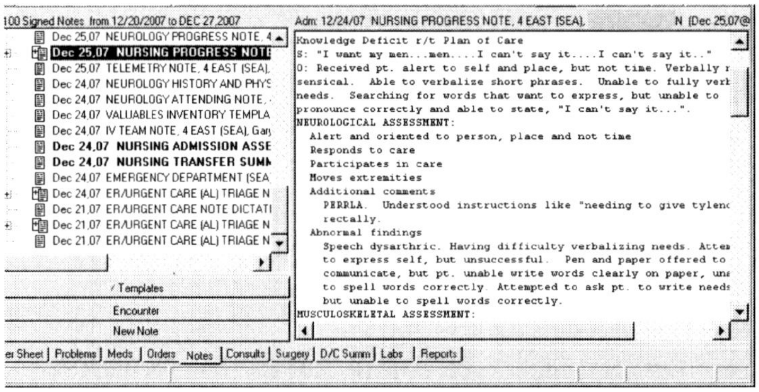

emphasized development of the "Nursing Process" and attendant terminology systems of nursing diagnoses, interventions and outcomes. Nursing classification systems have been prominent, if not predominant in the nursing informatics literature. Numerous computerized nursing care planning systems have been developed, including one for the VA that was largely abandoned a decade ago. The preceding figures illustrate the streamlining that has occurred in recent years. The more streamlined version contains more free text and less white space.

RESEARCH FINDINGS

Motivation

The goal of our ongoing research has been to increase understanding of computerized documentation in order to identify "valued" characteristics of patient care documents that might facilitate their retrieval for the benefit of users. A secondary goal is to use insights gained to shape recommendations for improving current and future versions of the VA's CPD system.

An important part of this research effort has been a qualitative investigation of CPD users' experiences using the VA CPRS system, specifically its practitioner, nursing and administrative stakeholders. We believed that determining document quality from an information theory perspective requires understanding what health care workers experience when creating and using CPD in their daily work. Accordingly, our investigation focused on users' experiences conducting typical work tasks. Our analytic perspective is that of cognitive work analysis. (Cam, Efthimiadis, & Hammond, 2008; Rasmussen, 1994; Weir et al., 2007). We are reporting initial findings from this work, focusing most on what we learned from nurses at the first of five VA sites we will study.

Methods

We began interviewing staff (practitioners, administrators and nurses) at the VA Puget Sound Health Care System individually and in separate focus groups in May, 2007. Nurse participants (described by role and location in Table 1) were recruited by asking for volunteers with the assistance of the chief nurse executive's office, and thus represented a non-random convenience sample. 24 nurses were interviewed individually or in focus groups. We also interviewed 25 practitioners and 12 administrative staff at the same site.

83% were inpatient nurses, a proportion similar to that found in the medical center. Compared to outpatient care, inpatient care is more document-intensive. Patients who only receive outpatient care typically accumulate ten to thirty documents per *year*. Inpatients usually accumulate more than 100 documents per *week*.

Our methodology was informed by the Cognitive Work Analysis (CWA) conceptual framework for work-centered evaluation and design (Rasmussen, 1994). This framework has been developed as a general approach to help information system designers analyze and understand the complex interaction between (a) the activities, organizational relationships and constraints of work domains, and (b) users' cognitive and social activities and their

Table 1. Roles and locations of nurses interviewed

	Inpatient	Outpatient	Direct care	Support	NP	RN	LPN
Focus Group	17	3	17	3	2	17	2
Individual	3	1	3	1	1	2	
	20	4	20	4	3	19	
	83%	18%	83%	18%	12.5%	80%	17%

subjective preferences during task performance (Vicente, 2003). The framework is the result of generalization of experiences from field studies that led to the design of support systems for a variety of modern work domains, such as process plants, manufacturing, hospitals, and libraries.

The CWA work-centered approach to the evaluation and design of information systems assumes that information interaction was determined by a number of dimensions. To facilitate an evaluation, a framework for cognitive work analysis is constructed. This analysis addresses dimensions such as: task situation in terms of work domain, decision making, and mental strategies that can be used; the organization in terms of division of work and social organization; user characteristics, resources and values. CWA in health care is not new. Over the past fifteen years the methodology has been used in the design of clinical displays, clinical information systems, medical equipment, and modeling intensive care unit patients (J. Effken, Loeb, Johnson, Johnson, & Reyna, 2001; J. A. Effken, 2002; Miller, 2004; Rasmussen, 1994; Vicente, 2003; Weir et al., 2007).

Procedures

We began interviewing VA staff (practitioners, administrators and nurses) individually and in focus groups in 2007 to learn about usage of computerized patient care documentation.

Subject recruitment was assisted by the chief nurse executive's office, and thus represented a non-random convenience sample. Of 19 nurse participants, 80% were inpatient nurses, a proportion similar to the nurse distribution in the medical center. Of the non-inpatient nurses, one worked in interventional radiology, two in a same day surgery unit and one provided administrative and clinical support to line nurses. Missing were the perspectives of outpatient, community care and telephone care nurses. The skewing of the sample toward inpatient care is also reflected in document statistics. In our document data set we found that patients who only receive outpatient care typically accumulate ten to thirty documents per *year*. When admitted to a ward, patient documents accumulate at a rate of over 100 documents per *week*.

All subjects gave informed consent to be interviewed. 30-minute individual interviews were conducted to pilot the focus group procedure. These interviews were recorded, transcribed and anonymized. From the individual inteviews, we developed a, semi-structured interview script for the focus groups which asked participants to identify key tasks associated with using CPD; to discuss benefits obtained and barriers encountered; and to describe the work strategies used to overcome the barriers. One-hour focus groups of 8-15 participants each were conducted, recorded, transcribed, anonymized and analyzed.

Analysis

Analysis consisted of reading transcripts to identify key nursing tasks and common themes emerging in the interviews. Preliminary theme identification was achieved by discussions held by the investigators.

Results

We found that the VA's CPD system was valued and accepted by all the stakeholder groups. Users were well-trained and had excellent computer and typing skills. Most had four or more years of experience using the system. Direct service providers reported using documentation functions between 30 and 40% of their total working day. A striking difference found was that practitioners and administrators found the CPD system to fit much better with their work flow than nurses, especially nurses providing inpatient care. Perhaps the most useful way to present these preliminary results is to tell a series of "stories" about the nursing experience with CPD.

Nursing CPD Tasks Identified

The topic and scripting method yielded rich and affectively open responses about nurses' use of CPD system. Eight sub-tasks in three categories emerged.

The first group of tasks concerned the creation of documents. Sub-tasks identified included *writing*: (1) Assessments, (2) Care Plans, (3) periodic progress notes and (4) summaries (discharge, transfer, and interval notes) documents, all of which corresponded closely to traditional Nursing Process Documentation.

The second group of responses involved processing information. Sub-tasks identified included (5) *reading* documents written by core members of the clinical team and peripheral sources (consultants and off-unit therapists) as patient care episodes unfolded, and (6) *reviewing*, as time permitted, documents from previous inpatient and outpatient care episodes.

The third task category identified involved sharing information: (7) *integrating* document information with other patient care process information and (8) *communicating* (primarily verbally, but occasionally as a written addendum to a note) processed document information with other members of the care team, especially, but not exclusively, with other nurses.

Nurses reported spending about 30% of their shift performing these tasks related to documentation. We estimated that they spent two thirds (20% overall) of this time *writing* documentation, and one-third (10% overall) *reading, reviewing, integrating* and *communicating* information in the continuously flowing narrative stream characteristic of an inpatient ward. Below we will describe details we learned about these tasks.

Care Planning

Care plan documentation followed a similar procedure, as shown above (b). Documents produced at the time care planning was mandated used standardized nursing language, but did not have an "individualized look and feel". Nurses, at the time we interviewed them, did not hesitate to criticize this:

Nurse: *There's been a bit of a controversy of what sort of notes nurses should use... There's been an informal expectation that nurses should all use the same format... But as practitioners, unless it's mandated (like you won't have your job), practitioners aren't going to do that. ...They find the part of the system that works best for them, with that individual patient...* ***So, you can't cookie-cut****: a patient that's first-day post-op, and a person who's tenth-day post-op, have very different needs, and different documentation needs as well...*

One unanticipated finding was that all members of the care team, including the nurses expressed lack of interest in reading nursing notes. Administrative personnel, such the coder below, also reported little use for nursing documentation.

Coder: *Typically, to look for procedures I won't initially click on a nursing note; mainly I'm going to go to – for example, here's a medicine attending note: I'll kind of want to glance at that, to see if there's anything there that I might want to note... Sometimes nursing notes do give me what I need – they'll insert a foley into a patient – and I will look for that from time to time, but for now I'm just going to click on the notes where I see the physicians for now – I might need to go back and look at nursing notes later, but for now I'm going to click on physicians and look at those...*

The awkwardness of the template approach to nursing documentation was eventually recognized. Notes containing checklists with empty items were especially difficult to read and users of all categories soon learned to ignore them. About six years after introduction of the paperless system a more compact and readable version of nursing notes and plans was implemented.

At the time of our investigation, the VA center we studied had used a paperless system for 10 years. One striking finding was that *written* nursing care planning, conventionally considered the core of the Nursing Process, played a diminished role in this "mature" system. The only units where formal written care plans persisted were psychiatric programs, where multidisciplinary treatment planning remained mandated by an accreditation agency. On medical and surgical units, nurse informants reported that formal written treatment plans were no longer the norm, but but created by exception, when necessary. The following remarks trace a nurse's perception of how written treatment planning became streamlined.

Interviewer: *Do you all do daily charting and treatment planning?*

Nurse 1: *Not so much treatment planning.*

Interviewer: *OK, so explain more about that.*

Nurse 1: *I think last year they actually had on one of the menus you could bring up 'care plan'.*

Nurse 2: *That's the way we did it three years ago.*

Nurse 1: *That sort of disappeared. And so they actually have one of the books... (laughter)*

Nurse 2: *They actually have one of the books in the references where we can pull it up, look at care plans and hopefully get to use that - copy and put it in if we need to - but we are basically just making it up.*

Interviewer: *So would that be part of your daily charting?*

Nurse 1: *It used to be, and in a lot of facilities it's still the standard that you do have an active care plan and you put these things in your notes saying 'this is what we're working on'.*

Nurse 2: *There used to be a nursing standard that you always had a care plan. Always. And then about 3 years ago we were going through and cleaning up the notes because there were thousands and thousands in there and they weren't being used and so at that point we had another little group get together and we went through the care plans and we said OK let's go and change the formatting and everything and so they took them away and* ***never put them back****. [Author emphasis].*

Interviewer: *But you're not doing that anymore?*

Nurse 1: *Occasionally, because I'll sit there and I'll type it out, but it's a lot of work to sit there and type these things out.*

Charting and Summaries

Nurse informants did not reject all standardized approaches to documentation. They valued the mnemonic properties of the checklist approach because it encouraged completeness in a variety of critical situations.

Nurse: *We have an admission/assessment template; we have a discharge template; we have a transfer template – those would all be considered when patients are changing not location as much as they're changing clinical status. So, if someone's being admitted, they're just starting they're pre-op work-up. But if they're being transferred out of the unit, their condition has changed – you've gone to surgery, gone to critical care, coming back to the ward; or they've had surgery, they've been here, and they're going into SICU – so, those three there's a definite template to use.*

Nurse: *As far as a patient who might be two-days post-operative, a nurse has a variety of notes she can choose from to document. She can document on a daily assessment, or a progress note*

– we're trying to standardize it, but nurses still have choices.

Despite the awkwardness of the Patient Assessment tool, they used it consistently for guidance, even if the notes created no longer resembled the structure of the parent template.

Interviewer: ... *All right, we've heard about the problems. How is it helpful?*

Nurse 1: *Well sometimes there are so many things we have to cover and so many details that it helps jog your mind on all the areas that you to cover. You can't forget anything. It won't let you. You can't sign it if you miss them.*

Nurse 2: *So, when you go into the nursing progress note, you can cancel out the SOAP format, and make it a narrative – all systems drop off. Which is a nurse's choice.*

They also found ways to bypass limitations of system design inherited from office practice, such as a twenty-minute time-out for completing a note.

Nurse: *Well, one thing that's not helpful, I mean the admission template. Once you start it you can't really pause – or you'll lose your information that you wrote... Lose the entire document....*

Interviewer: *So, if you're called away to do something or if you have to communicate with someone or something like that it...*

Nurse 3: *And even if you want to explore something further with the patient – say, for example, even in extended care admissions – part of admitting a patients ... is allowing the patient the opportunity to ... just be able to tell their story. And it's amazing the healing process occurs in just being able to get that out. And having someone hear them and listen to them. You don't have time. The computer will cut you off.*

Nurse 4: *It's very difficult with the admissions. The template kicks; it won't really let you out. You have to finish that. You have to finish any template to completion. You cannot stop and go do anything else. You must complete a template in one sitting.*

Nurse 4: ***That's why we have this copy in Extended Care Home. That we have this blank copy hooked up to a pseudopatient. And when you're done writing it down personally for a patient, you go back and now it's safe.*** *[Author emphasis].*

Interviewer: *Were there other shortcuts or ways that you- strategies you use so that you can try to get your work done?*

Nurse 5: *Well sometimes you can put, what I do, for admission assessments is open two CPRS sessions at the same time. You have to flip back and forth.*

Barriers: Document Creation Burden

The 20% of the day spent creating documents was universally addressed with feelings of frustration and even sorrow at having to spend time away from patients. One nurse remarked:

Nurse: *For us... being on the floor as the charge nurse you're all night – an octopus with lots of tentacles... Then you have only 8 hours ... and financially what the VA is saying 'you have too much overtime!' ... That's our problem also, we have to ... be at all the patients' bedside. We need to get all. But it's known, we have to put it on the computer.... And I didn't even learn how to type long time ago! It's really hard to put all those hours in that little table. Without going to overtime. Or we don't, really, and you feel* ***guilty*** *if you are not* *able to do, to put everything that is there. Because they will say 'ooh, that's only one patient, you put your 8 hours there?' Oh my God!*

Interviewer: *You feel guilty?*

Nurse: *You feel guilty because you didn't put everything in that you're supposed to. You* ***know*** *what you did at your patient's bedside.*

One consequence of the document burden is that it steals time from other traditional nursing tasks. In the VA we studied, one consequence of work reallocation was the disappearance of the nursing treatment record. The nurse below pleads for computer support integrating documentation of treatment with the treatment action plan found in the "Kardex", a capability yet unsupported in the VA computer system.

Interviewer: *Can you explain the Kardex...?*

Nurse 1: *Sure. The Kardex, first of all, is not part of the medical record. It's a pre-printed document that nurses write-on in pencil, about the daily changes in a person's care plan, driven by the order set. So, a person is coming to 3 east, and the nurse takes their order set, and pencils in categories of those orders onto the cardex. So, for example: diet, activity, respiratory treatment, IV fluids, consult, procedures, labs. All the stuff you see in the order set is transcribed via pencil onto the cardex, to be used as a guide and report guide...*

Nurse 1: *The other part is that there's no treatments that you can document – nursing treatments are still done on paper as well. Well, what happens is – I'm supposed to be telling the truth –* ***we don't put it on paper.*** *[Author emphasis] So, things that used to be documented, when there was no computer and we were a paper chart, we had a thing called treatment sheets, and things on there were foot care, wound care...* ***Well, we don't have anything for example that exists to document those things in the computer****. [Author emphasis]*
So, what's happened is those have all fallen-off, because everyone is doing everything in the computer, except the Kardex, ***the treatment sheets...the treatment sheets have fallen totally into a black hole****. [Author emphasis] I've given up – I've tried for a couple of years to get that on the top of the list, we need to get this in the computer so people are actually compliant, but now I take the energy that I had to divide through all these various duties and what I want people to continue doing on paper is the Kardex, because that's driving the report system.*

Reading and Processing Notes

One unexpected finding was strong voicing by nurses that the entire patient care documentation record was of immense value to pursuing their work, despite general readability challenges of boilerplate, inserted data and checklists. Nurses described the power of being able to access a large volume of patient documentation.

Nurse: *We do chart review; not just when the patient is being admitted. When they're being admitted to us, we go back on discharge summary, way back until, you know years later, or months later and then we see how long is the history of what's going on with the patient. And how you see his behavior when he comes to the ward. If he'd be dangerous. All those important details.*

Interviewer: *So, does that make you feel safer? More powerful to have this information?*

Nurse 1: *I think so (several voices agreeing). Yes. You know what to expect.*

Nurse 2: *The other thing is that we see something in there that doesn't look right in the note we're going to talk among the staff and discuss it with* *them and say "you know, in your note you said this patient blah blah this and we saw something totally different". So if you bring that around where everybody else can see to that there's two different things going on that everybody else can see. And your seeing one side and a lot of times you do. Because of the shifts – the time of day.*

Nurse 1: *[what] you read in the ER ... it's not the story they give us when they're on our unit. They want to come to our unit. So that what they said over there is not what they tell us when we sit down with them.*

Nurse 2: *And in the same thing, what they say to me, or to her can be completely different from what they say to the physician in order to buy more time to stay on the ward.*

Interviewer: *So is that useful that all that information makes it into the record?*

Several voices: *Yes.*

Nurse 3: *Because it creates more balance.*

Both nurses and physicians noted that authors' "original thoughts", often difficult to locate, were valuable. A nurse stated:

But what's interesting as you look at the record as a whole, even though some people have kind of an aversion to the narrative, the narrative often captures more of the data – all they say is what's happening; you don't have a lot of the miscellaneous stuff.

A physician nicely summarized the cognitive task of reading documentation:

Yeah, so going through the template, you're editing the template in your eyes and in your mind to get all the boilerplate out of the way and actually see the two or three lines that might be in the note. The boilerplate gets in the way. You'll find that some people have 98% boilerplate and 2% fresh thoughts... Searching a note for fresh input is very challenging.

Sharing Information

The above quotations begin to illustrate that with sufficient nurse-nurse and nurse-team contact, insights from readings of the documentation are eagerly shared. When we began our series of interviews our expectation was that the typical document-related tasks for nurses would consist of creating and reading documents. We soon heard repeatedly that *seeking, processing* and *sharing* the information in documents were equally important.

Interviewer: *Do you use the documentation system for preparing for rounds? How do you prepare for rounds?*

Nurse 1: *Basically, by the time the teams are making rounds you know your patients. When we first come in at the start of the shift we'll review almost all of the patients records. We'll review the last note or so, we'll review our medication, we'll look at their orders and get to know it that way. Plus we do a face to face handoff when we do our reports. We sit there, we talk and we tell: "this is what's going on. This is the history" and that kind of thing. Because for a lot of the patients in the Intensive Care Unit they have a huge number of notes for their stay. That for us to sit there and read through everything in order to get the patient we'd never get the patient. So we do a really brief face to face handoff we don't use CPRS for that. We use it when we admit a patient. We get a call saying somebody's coming in. We pull up usually the most recent history/physical notes by the surgical team - why this patient's coming in - that type of a thing.*

Interviewer: *How would you describe that activity?*

Nurse 1: *Most of us work 12 hr shifts. So by the end of your 12 hr shift you know your patient fairly well, and so we don't refer back to CPRS during the course of the shift. We'll go in and we'll read patient history, to understand how long has this been happening....*

Nurse 2: *...We use it as a reference. It's a reference tool. We read it to go in and find out about the patient. What kind of meds he's on, how in the heck this happened to him, histories of things like bedsores, IV's and procedures that have been done.*

Other nurses commented:

Interviewer: *Do you also read – you're writing the admission notes – do you read others? Do you read the admission note from the prior shift or...*

Nurse: *Oh yeah...*

Interviewer: *So you end up reading the admission note for your patients even if you're not the one that's writing it. How efficient do you find the notes when you're reading them. The admission notes or other notes. How efficient or effective are they?*

Nurse: *I think it's very good because you get some information that you might not otherwise have time to get or you're not there to get it or the next day you're there, I mean, you want to know something about that patient that was admitted all you have to do is go back and read the note.*

Interviewer: *Do you have time to sit down and do that?*

Nurse 1: *You have to* ***make*** *time. (voices agreeing). Most days.*

Nurse 2: *Because, you're thinking of the patient.*

Nurse 1: *If I'd been off for two days and we had an admission on my day off, I'm not going to get a complete detailed report that I would get if they had just been admitted and I was just there and I was in report to hear it. So, if I want to know what's going on, I'm going to have to go back and read the progress notes.*

Nurse 2: *Because she's caring for the patient she's accountable for that information whether she's there or not.*

Using the Document System to Aid Communication

Another unexpected aspect of communication was nurses' adapting a capability in the documentation system to draw others' attention to a particular document. Designed to support multi-authored documents, the tool is now more frequently used as a communication device.

N: *What I find really helpful is that if something important happens over the weekend or on an off shift staff will add team members, people that are on the team as an additional signer. And so when you get into the system it comes up as a note that needs your attention.*

The nurses also speak of using the "addendum" feature, originally designed to allow correction of errors in notes, to coordinate team knowledge and planning.

Interviewer: *What about addendums? Is that like a little messaging back and forth? Is that something you use?*

Nurse 1: *Yes*

Nurse 2: *We use it a lot.*

Nurse 1: *Nursing staff use it. ...if an LPN has assessed a patient and has called my attention to the patient assessment: "see what you think about this." I will make an addendum to the LPN's note that says "met with patient concur with above note and assessment". To let the reader know that an RN is also involved in the care of this situation. And that the LPN's assessment is correct.*

Nurse 2: *Also to let the LPN know that you've been in and that your taking an action.*

DISCUSSION

Our original research goal was to increase understanding of the documentation process from the perspective of the practitioner, nursing and administrative stakeholders in order to identify "valued" characteristics of individual patient care documents in order to facilitate their retrieval for the benefit of users. A second goal was to use the insights gained from stakeholders to make recommendations for areas of design improvements in a future version of the CPRS system. Serendipitously, our initial investigation of user work experience with CPD reveals clues that warrant recommendations about how to think about the current CPD process, and suggests improvements that can be made using the configuration capabilities of the existing system in its present form. Perhaps not surprisingly, these recommendations have more to do with **how** and **why** the CPRS CPD system is used than changing the system greatly. In some ways, it would be easier to effect such changes under the cover of a major software change. Lacking that, we will doubtless confront the organizational currents that have fostered the present philosophy driving CPD usage. In the following discussion, we hope to demonstrate that nursing documentation is an especially apt area for incremental, but helpful, change in the VA CPRS system we have examined. Certain opportunities and dynamics in the nursing arena make this so. Not the least is that nursing manpower is a scarce and precious resource that must be optimally managed.

Our research is ongoing, and the work reported here is in the pilot stage, but some strong themes identified permit useful discussion now. We anticipate that as our study proceeds we will identify important areas where technology change can further enhance nursing performance and won't hesitate to make recommendations. We hope that keeping our focus on the **real work** of nurses will avoid the distractions of technological innovation. We assert, and hope to demonstrate with the results of our investigation so far, that a great portion of nurses' work is cognitive and social, and not well captured in the documentation that the VA nurses create.

Further, we expect that the principles we have identified are applicable across all settings, especially, to those deploying nursing informatics and nursing documentation systems using patient care information systems other than the CPRS. One consequence of examining a well-established, rather well-functioning integrated system is that the "noise" of a new system deployment has dissipated, and that some of the key issues that remain have more to do with management philosophy and policy than technology. These same issues, because they arise from nursing practice and human behavior, are likely to be evident in other patient care information systems, and may benefit from a similar review of the goals and costs of deployment decisions.

Issues Related to "Task-Technology Fit"

Our findings show that nurses have adopted a system not designed for them, but they have nudged its evolution toward greater functionality through creative workarounds, and no small measure of computer skill and sophistication. In so doing, they participate as peers in the information flux that surrounds an inpatient care episode and add value, by contributing their perspective to the treatment team in a variety of ways.

Their experience also demonstrates Varcoe's point (Varcoe, 1996) that the technology for documentation is still not a good fit with many aspects of the nursing process. This stems, at least in the VA case from the absence of documentation tools (such as the capability to document and track treatments) that are specifically needed for nursing. It would seem that they have done about as good a job as they could in adapting a system designed for office practice, with computers at the practitioner's desk and five minutes between patients to write an outpatient note. Our interviewees have commented poignantly on the difficulty of having to pull away from the patient's bedside to do their documentation.

A second consequence of using system designed for office work is that the VA CPD system forces nursing documents into the general document space (a "Notes" section of the CPRS). By default, this space (figure below) displays notes chronologically, with title and author information. Clicking allows only one note at a time to be opened. VA users in all work categories report that browsing to track the flow of care or find a needed piece of information is difficult. This creates difficulty when a user wants to focus on a particular theme.

One physician complaining about the difficulty of finding consultation reports remarked:

All these consults, they get buried in the notes section – the progress notes. Everyone writes a progress note – the nurses write 2-3 notes a day; the physicians write, if they're in the hospital, they write at least a note a day; PT, OT, everyone who has something to do with the patient writes a note!

Nurses experience difficulty with aggregation of documents as well, because it makes tracking the flow of nursing care challenging. Despite the barriers, nursing notes are valued by other caregivers. More than one nurse commented on positive feedback from physicians and others about the value of the nursing persepective in understanding the patient. In inpatient care, where nursing care is so important to the patient's safety and survival and nurses have the most contact with patients, the evolving flow of nursing observations should be especially supported. A separate section of the chart devoted to the flow of inpatient nursing care would avoid **diluting** the nursing documentation contribution, and make it easier for nurses to follow as well.

In a non-VA setting, Campion et al. (2007) analyzed usage of a tool built to produce a group of documents selected from the note space for the purpose of handing off the patient to another provider. The tool was designed for practitioner use, but unanticipated use by nurses and other staff was frequent. Among all the categories of staff who selected documents, the authorship of the selected documents was similar. Practitioners authored 90% of the documents they printed and Nurses authored only 8% of the documents they printed. Campion concluded, that for the purposes of sign-out, practitioners were "producers", and that nurses and others were "consumers" of sign-out content.

A broader view of using the "document space" was offered by a nurse we interviewed.

Interviewer: *"Do you use the documentation system for preparing for rounds? How do you prepare for rounds?"*

Nurse: *Basically, by the time the teams are making rounds you know your patients. When we first come in at the start of the shift we'll review almost all of the patients' records. We'll review the last note or so, we'll review our medication, we'll look at their orders and get to know it that* *way. Plus we do a face to face handoff when we do our reports. We sit there, we talk and we tell: "this is what's going on. This is the history" and that kind of thing. Because for a lot of the patients in the <inpatient care setting> they have a huge number of notes for their stay. That for us to sit there and read through everything in order to get the patient we'd never get the patient. So we do a really brief face to face handoff. We don't use CPRS for that. We use it when we admit a patient. We get a call saying somebody's coming in. We pull up usually the most recent history/physical notes by the surgical team - why this patient's coming in - that type of thing.*

We found this to be a recurring theme among inpatient nurses interviewed. The documents and other data in the PCIS provide a rich information resource which ward nurses absorb, verbally summarize and integrate into the care process. This constitutes the "juice" of nursing care information processing. It is efficient, fluent and current. We propose that "nursing documentation" serves more as a shorthand acknowledgement of care processes than a definitive journal or formulation of the care given.

Berg (2002, p. 34) anticipated this "undocumented" aspect of clinical documentation when commenting on furnishing full access of the electronic health record to patients:

Health care work requires continuous communication and coordination between professionals around and about patients; they order their thoughts in the record, and discuss potential hypotheses and next steps to take in the record. In this sense, records are working notes, written for a small group of peers or even only for oneself... Consequently, it can be easily predicted that any directive to really give patients complete access to the record will immediately result in a 'cleaning up' of these records, and in the emergence of a new layer of 'informal', 'grey' record keeping, for personal usage only.

Berg takes a physician's viewpoint here, but it appears that VA ward nursing practice has finessed the problem of lay people misunderstanding documentation by producing "cleaned-up" documents and communicating much of the essence vital care information verbally. In a previous paper, (Berg & Goorman, 1999, p. 51) he and Goorman remark on *the " (im)possibilities of the utilization of primary health care data for secondary purposes such as research and administration."* He makes the strong point that *"work is required to make data suitable for accumulation. We might phrase this as a 'law of medical information'... the more active the accumulation, the more work needs to be invested."* Our research observations of the documentation process show the impact of institutional demands on clinical documentation to support budgets, billing, quality reviews and compliance with government regulation.

Of all document authors, nurses may experience the greatest pull between meticulously journaling patient progress for a variety of institutional demands and attending to patients. In the VA setting we studied, it seems the pendulum has nudged slightly toward institutional recognition that nursing documentation is but a part of a broader, vital communication process. We see hints that the stored nursing "documents" are regarded by *most* caregivers, including nurses, as impoverished "footprints" of nursing care. Recognizing and adapting to this has taken most of a decade.

Was anything been lost when formalized nursing care planning was abandoned? Given the importance of care planning and nursing terminology to the academic side of the nursing profession, one might think so. Curiously, instead, we now see many examples of nursing concepts persisting in nursing documentation. Nurses, when they decide that it is important, still write care plans. Trained to use a contemporary conceptual framework, they document care plans when they are helpful, and seek on-line references for special situations. In the VA Nursing care planning continues as part of nursing care, but no longer consistently appears in nursing documentation. In the next section we will further discuss the forces that brought this situation about, and discuss directions our thoughts on how nursing could be more effectively integrated into nursing care processes.

Issues Related to the Nursing Process and CPD

Nurses also criticize nursing process-based documentation as burdensome. Varcoe (Varcoe, 1996) makes the point that the problem with theory-based nursing documentation may not be with the theory, but with its implementation. Lest nursing feel singled out, we should point to similar difficulties for physicians in strictly adhering to Weed's guidelines for a Problem-Oriented medical record, and similar efforts in mental health documentation based on the Diagnostic and Statistical Manual of the American Psychiatric Association. In all cases, it seems that a completely reasonable theoretical framework translates poorly to the information management tasks required for patient care.

Goosen, et al. (1997)summarized numerous reports of problems with introduction of computerized Nursing Process oriented documentation. Some of these included the possibility that information systems negatively affect nursing practice and nursing identity by creating tension between the aspiration to deliver "individualized" patient care and the goal of using "objective" language. Vivid terms used by Harris (1990) to describe this effect are "de-autonomisation", "de-individualization" and "de-professionalization" and "one size fits all". Harris's qualitative findings from 1990 anticipated many of the themes we heard in 2007. One of the nurses Harris interviewed stated:

The only nursing diagnosis that we can come up with for GI Bleed is ... Loss of Body Fluids. That's not quite it, but that's the idea. And that doesn't describe a GI Bleed. And yet, if you put that in there, "GI Bleed," that's a medical diagnosis [which is not acceptable] (Harris, 1990, p. 70)

Another observation Harris made was that nurses perceived the computer process to facilitate supervisory surveillance of work output and control of personal expressiveness.

Laduke (2001)noted problems with nurses using and understanding the language to describe nursing issues and the complexity of the concept space, stating, "While the created documentation system was well-grounded academically, we soon discovered it was too complex for bedside nurses... The large number of care plans made it difficult to become familiar with the contents and distinguish and the nursing diagnoses and interventions in one care plan from another." Other complaints noted were the time-burden of document entry and a lack of nurses' conviction that the documents they created were useful to others or clinically relevant. Allan and Englebright (2000) reported an effort to improve acceptance of computerized nursing documentation by simplifying tasks and lists. At baseline, "Nurses were frustrated that, although they were spending more time on documentation, chart audits continued to find discrepancies and omissions in the documentation. Physicians were complaining that nurses were spending more time with the computer than with patients. Managers and administrators were concerned about rising overtime costs and the lack of a reliable medical record" (Allan & Englebright, 2000, p. 91). LaDuke (2001) reported that nurses were as appreciative of efforts to simplify the system and there was a decrease in overtime.

Ammenwerth et al. (2003) reported a controlled longitudinal study of acceptance of nursing process documentation on four wards. Two were psychiatry wards, one was a pediatrics ward, and one a dermatology unit. Over the period of the study, acceptance of the theoretico-professional "nursing process" was unchanged by users. Acceptance of computers in the clinical setting was also essentially unchanged. Acceptance of the computerized document system was stable and "good" on three wards, but in the pediatric ward was lower, and worsened with time. The author noted that the pediatric ward required nurses to spend much more time at ill infants' bedsides, and that the required detail of computerized document was incompatible with the work pattern. The author also noted that computerized documentation required nurses to remove themselves to an office to complete their work. On the pediatric ward, nurses complained of doing double documentation, once on paper notes they kept with them in their rounds, and once again transferring this information to the computer. The burden of "double entry" was mentioned in numerous reported studies.

The most complete review to date of the impact of nursing process-based care documentation on nursing practice and outcome concludes that these documentation systems completely fail to demonstrate evidence of health outcome benefits. Currell and Urquhart (2003) conclude:

It would seem that the relationship between information, information systems and practice is poorly understood by practitioners and researchers. The questions addressed by the excluded studies and those rejected on methodological grounds were predominantly concerned with administration rather than clinical practice. The studies demonstrate the tension for practitioners between meeting the needs of clinical practice and the needs of management and administration. The results of the review suggest that the design of record systems to actively support nursing practice is a complex task, requiring synthesis of the knowledge of nursing practice, nursing organisation and nursing informatics. ... Nurses in practice now need to be ready to share information systems as well as information, with their patients and with their medical and health care colleagues.

FUTURE TRENDS

Considering the bumpy progress of computerized nursing process documentation, we are cautious about making sweeping recommendations. The current picture suggests the following changes in current CPRS CPD use can be made *now*.

1. Allow as much free text as possible in nursing documents
2. Keep nursing process language available to nurses as an on line reference but be parsimonious about its use in documents frequently viewed by non-nursing treatment team members.
3. Consider separating nursing documentation from general documentation to improve viewing the flows of care from both of these important perspectives.

Changes to consider for the future include:

1. Improved placement of computer equipment in patient rooms dictated by workflow ergonomics. For example, nurses viewing monitors should also be able to face the patient and instrument displays for the patient.
2. Develop mobile "smart clipboards" to capture treatment actions at the point of care. This almost certainly awaits deployment of portable mobile devices and software so that tracking treatments does not "steal time" from vital nursing activity.
3. Develop team based, multi-patient displays ("whiteboards") to assist nursing handoff and planning activity (Xiao, Schenkel, Faraj, Mackenzie, & Moss, 2007).
4. Develop mobile voice input and playback capabilities to allow asynchronous verbal communication among members of the nursing team.

CONCLUSION

Nursing documentation is important but can be improved, as our research in a mature setting has shown. More effort is needed to understand and exploit the benefits of staff to staff safety-promoting documentation that CPD in a PCIS provides. Consideration of the social aspects of nursing team coordination is important. In the PCIS studied, documentation of nursing treatments is haphazard and probably awaits better data capture at the point of care. Given the nursing manpower shortage, it is likely that more resources will be devoted to improving the efficiency of nursing process documentation.

ACKNOWLEDGMENT

This work was supported in part by the United States Department of Veterans Affairs Health Services Research and Development Service, Investigator Initiated Research Grant IIR 05-019. The opinions and conclusions in this chapter are the authors' own, and do not reflect official U.S. Department of Veterans Affairs Policy. All research was conducted under the auspices of the University of Washington Institutional Review Board, Committee V. We also acknowledge support of the University of Washington Information School and the following individuals who made valuable individual contributions to this work: Kenneth M. Cam, Ashley N. Hedeen, Peter J. Embi, and Stephen M. Thielke.

REFERENCES

Allan, J., & Englebright, J. (2000). Patient-centered documentation: An effective and efficient use of clinical information systems. *J Nurs Adm, 30*(2), 90-95.

Ammenwerth, E., Mansmann, U., Iller, C., & Eichstadter, R. (2003). Factors affecting and affected by user acceptance of computer-based nursing documentation: Results of a two-year study. *J Am Med Inform Assoc, 10*(1), 69-84.

Berg, M. (2002). Patients and professionals in the information society: what might keep us awake in 2013. *Int J Med Inform, 66*(1-3), 31-37.

Berg, M., & Goorman, E. (1999). The contextual nature of medical information. *Int J Med Inform, 56*(1-3), 51-60.

Bhasale, A. L., Miller, G. C., Reid, S. E., & Britt, H. C. (1998). Analysing potential harm in Australian general practice: an incident-monitoring study. *Med J Aust, 169*(2), 73-76.

Cam, K. M., Efthimiadis, E. N., & Hammond, K. W. (2008, January 7-10, 2008). An Investigation on the Use of Computerized Patient Care Documentation: Preliminary Results. *Paper presented at the 41st Annual Hawaii International Conference on System Sciences,* Waikoloa, Big Island, Hawaii.

Campion, T. R., Weinberg, S. T., Lorenzi, N. M., & Waitman, L. R. (2007). Analysis of a computerized sign-out tool: Identification of Unanticipated Uses. *Paper presented at the 2007 National Library of Medicine Fellowship Conference.*

Chaudhry, B., Wang, J., Wu, S., Maglione, M., Mojica, W., Roth, E., et al. (2006). Systematic review: impact of health information technology on quality, efficiency, and costs of medical care. *Ann Intern Med, 144*(10), 742-752.

Coiera, E. (2000). When conversation is better than computation. *J Am Med Inform Assoc, 7*(3), 277-286.

Currell, R., & Urquhart, C. (2003). Nursing record systems: effects on nursing practice and health care outcomes. *Cochrane Database Syst Rev,* (3), CD002099.

Effken, J., Loeb, R., Johnson, K., Johnson, S., & Reyna, V. (2001). Using cognitive work analysis to design clinical displays. *Medinfo. MEDINFO, 10*(Pt), 127-131.

Effken, J. A. (2002). Different lenses, improved outcomes: a new approach to the analysis and design of healthcare information systems. *International journal of medical informatics, 65*(1), 59-74.

Goodhue, D. L., & Thompson, R. L. (1995). "Task-Technology Fit and Individual Performance". *MIS quarterly : management information systems., 19*(2), 213.

Goossen, W. T., Epping, P. J., Dassen, T. W., Hasman, A., & van den Heuvel, W. J. (1997). Can we solve current problems with nursing information systems? *Comput Methods Programs Biomed, 54*(1-2), 85-91.

Harris, B. L. (1990). Becoming deprofessionalized: one aspect of the staff nurse's perspective on computer-mediated nursing care plans. *ANS Adv Nurs Sci, 13*(2), 63-74.

Hinshaw, A. S. (2008). Navigating the perfect storm: balancing a culture of safety with workforce challenges. *Nurs Res, 57*(1 Suppl), S4-10.

Kolodner, R. M., & Douglas, J. V. (1997). *Computerizing large integrated health networks the VA success*. New York: Springer.

LaDuke, S. (2001). Online nursing documentation: finding a middle ground. *J Nurs Adm, 31*(6), 283-286.

Miller, A. (2004). A work domain analysis framework for modelling intensive care unit patients. *Cognition, Technology, and Work, 6*, 207-222.

Nemeth, C., Nunnally, M., Connor, M. O., Klock, P. A., & Cook, R. (2005). Getting to the point: developing IT for the sharp end of healthcare. *J. of Biomedical Informatics, 38*(1), 18-25.

Perlin, J. B., Kolodner, R. M., & Roswell, R. H. (2004). The Veterans Health Administration: quality, value, accountability, and information as transforming strategies for patient-centered care. *The American journal of managed care, 10*(11), 828-836.

Rasmussen, J., Pejtersen, A. M., & Goodstein, L. P (1994). *Cognitive Systems Engineering.* New York: Wiley.

Varcoe, C. (1996). Disparagement of the nursing process: the new dogma? *J Adv Nurs, 23*(1), 120-125.

Vicente, K. J. (2003). Less is (sometimes) more in cognitive engineering: the role of automation technology in improving patient safety. *Quality & safety in health care, 12*(4), 291-294.

Weir, C. R., Nebeker, J. J. R., Hicken, B. L., Campo, R., Drews, F., & Lebar, B. (2007). A Cognitive Task Analysis of Information Management Strategies in a Computerized Provider Order Entry Environment. *Journal of the American Medical Informatics Association: JAMIA., 14*(1), 65.

Wilson, R. M., Harrison, B. T., Gibberd, R. W., & Hamilton, J. D. (1999). An analysis of the causes of adverse events from the Quality in Australian Health Care Study. *Med J Aust, 170*(9), 411-415.

Xiao, Y., Schenkel, S., Faraj, S., Mackenzie, C. F., & Moss, J. (2007). What whiteboards in a trauma center operating suite can teach us about emergency department communication. *Ann Emerg Med, 50*(4), 387-395.

KEY TERMS

CPD: Computerized Patient Care Documentation

CPRS: The PCIS used in the VA. Computerized Patient Record System

LPN: Licensed Professional Nurse

NP: Nurse Practitioner

PCIS: Patient Care Information System

RN: Registered Nurse

VA: United States Department of Veterans Affairs

Chapter VII
Nurses and Telehealth:
Current Practice and Future Trends

Sisira Edirippulige
University of Queensland, Australia

Anthony C. Smith
University of Queensland, Australia

Mark Bensink
University of Queensland, Australia

Nigel R. Armfield
University of Queensland, Australia

Richard Wootton
University of Queensland, Australia

ABSTRACT

Nurses play a pivotal role in the provision of healthcare. Home telehealth, the use of information and communication technologies to deliver and support healthcare directly to the home, is emerging as an important application for nurses. This chapter provides an overview of home telehealth and how it may be applied to the practical challenges nurses face everyday. We provide a summary of the evidence available to support its use in specific areas and a guide for those thinking of implementing telehealth in their own practice. The future of home telehealth lies in carefully considered and designed research, ongoing education and training and a multidisciplinary approach. This chapter aims to stimulate the consideration of home telehealth as an application that may improve nursing care and ultimately patient outcomes.

INTRODUCTION

The increasing incidence of chronic diseases (such as cancer, coronary heart disease, diabetes and dementia) and the growing aged population have added to the pressure on health care systems worldwide. The World Health Organization (WHO) predicts that chronic disease will be the leading cause of disability by 2020 and will be the most expensive problem facing health care systems (Belfield & Colin-Thome, 2004). For example, type II diabetes mellitus is becoming the most common chronic disease in the United States, affecting 7% of the adult population. Congestive heart failure affects about 5 million Americans each year and accounts for around 20% of hospitalised patients over 65 years (ATA, 2007). Studies show that caring for people with chronic diseases consumes approximately 78% of all health care spending in the United States – more than $1 trillion annually (ITAA e-Health Committee, 2004). The Centres for Medicare and Medicare Services estimated that total national health expenditure for home care was $40 billion in 2003, an increase of almost ten percent over the previous year. An additional $111 billion was spent on nursing home care (National Health Expenditures). With the ageing of the population, this rate of growth will increase.

Undoubtedly, these tendencies have put additional pressure on the already overburdened nursing community around the world. Nurses form the largest professional health care group and their role as a care provider has changed significantly since the last century. The lack of nursing professionals is a global phenomenon (Kingma, 2006). Producing more nurses is one answer that requires long term investment and policy implementation. Finding other complementary mechanisms to address these urgent needs is also required.

THE ROLE OF NURSES IN HEALTH CARE

Nurses play an important role in almost every sphere of health care from primary to tertiary care. Nurses have rapidly evolving roles and responsibilities. Terms such as district nurse, health visitor, school nurse, GP practice nurse, nurse consultant, clinical nurse specialist and nurse practitioner reflect just some of the diversity of nursing practice.

Among other roles, nurses are also responsible for delivering care to patients at home, especially elderly patients. There is a continuing demand for such a role. However, statistics show that the lack of nursing professionals and the growing aged population is a prime concern for health systems around the world (Flesner, 2004). Despite these challenges nurses have shown remarkable flexibility and adaptability. The nursing profession has been an early group to embrace home telehealth which offers an alternative to providing face-to-face care.

WHAT IS HOME TELEHEALTH?

Home telehealth is the use of information and communication technologies to deliver and support health care in a non-institutional setting – that is, at home or in an assisted-living facility (Wootton, Kvedar & Dimmick, 2006). Home telehealth applications may include real time techniques, for example videoconferencing (Figure 1) as well as store and forward techniques, for example email or web-based applications (Figure 2).

In addition, various devices such as alarms, sensors and monitoring equipment are being used in home telehealth applications (Darkins, et al, 1996). Telehealth gives an opportunity to contact

Figure 1. Real-time home telehealth using web cams and the Internet. Mother and child at home discussing care with an oncology clinical nurse consultant

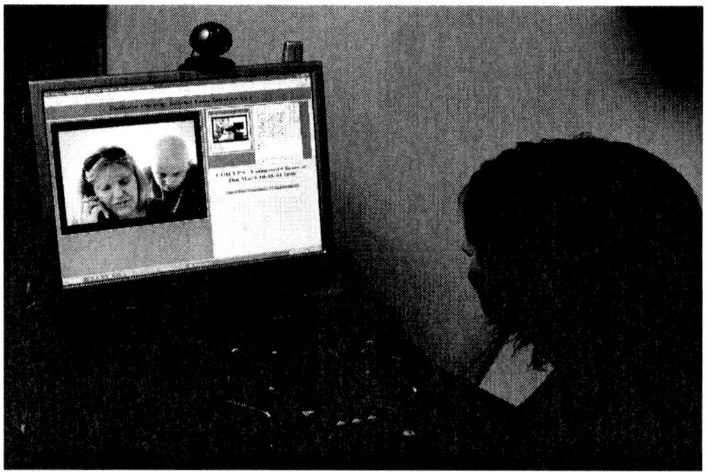

patients remotely augmenting and extending conventional care.

There are signs that interest in home telehealth is developing. Recent data shows that 20% of American based home health agencies employ some kind of telehealth in their day to day operations and another 20% plan to offer telehealth services in the next 12 months (Wootton, Kvedar & Dimmick, 2006). An increase has also occurred in the number of home health episodes. During 2001-2003 the number of Medicare home health users increased to 2.6 million and the number of episodes rose to 36 million. At the same time, the average number of visits per episode fell slightly to 17.3 (Wootton, Kvedar & Dimmick, 2006). The last few years have also seen an increase in the number of manufacturers of home telehealth equipment in the USA (mainly) and elsewhere.

Figure 2. Store and forward home telehealth. A nurse screening children with diabetes for eye problems sending clinical information and images to a specialist ophthalmologist via email

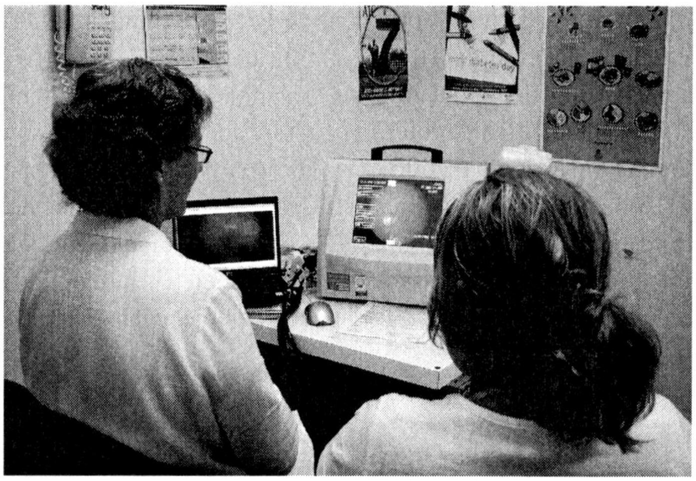

HOW CAN TELEHEALTH ASSIST NURSES?

The role of the nurse practitioner, a registered nurse educated to function in an advanced clinical role, (Darkins et al, 1996) has major implications for health services. Experienced nurses have more responsibility in managing patients, particularly where access to medical and health services is inadequate. Telehealth has been reported as a useful tool for nurse practitioners.

To Support Remote Nurses

For example in the United Kingdom (UK) nurse practitioner units have been established to provide care to patients with minor injuries. Telehealth is used in these units as a support for nurses (Darkins et al, 1996). They can use videoconferencing to contact emergency medicine specialists for advice and support. This has effectively reduced the need to refer patients to the tertiary emergency medicine department and to the local general practitioner, saving time and reducing costs. Home telehealth can assist nurses to expand their role, to access direct clinical support for this expansion, and to reach more patients and provide more services (Jenkins & White, 2001).

One nurse practitioner in the USA uses home telehealth to support other nurses in a remote medical facility by conducting patient consultations online (Reed, 2005). This allows the nurse practitioner, working with the remote nurse, to complete patient histories, assess patients using peripherals such as a stethoscope, a camera for viewing eardrums, nasal mucosa, mouths and throats as well as a dermascope used to view and magnify skin lesions. The nurse practitioner can remotely print prescriptions for the patient, order additional investigations or refer the patient to specialist care.

To Support the Patient in the Home

Another benefit of home telehealth is the ability to make more frequent visits to patients. Home telehealth provides a unique opportunity to maintain frequent interpersonal contact using information and communication technologies like videoconferencing. Nurses can 'visit' their patients more often, prioritising in-person visits and avoiding unnecessary travel (Ryan, Kobb & Hilsen, 2003; Kobb, Hilsen & Ryan, 2003).

One example of supporting patients in the home using telehealth is wound care. A pilot investigation used a combination of real-time consultation and the capture of digital wound images to provide specialist wound care (Moore, Britton & Chetney, 2003). Outcomes included earlier assessment of patients by a specialist wound care nurse, a reduction in healing time, fewer in-person home visits and an increase in productivity. Additional benefits included improved education of patients and improved education and professional development in the use of wound care protocols for generalist home care nurses. Home telehealth is an alternative means of delivering the knowledge and expertise of a wound care nurse to underserved patients.

Another development in patient in-home support is the smart-home concept. This idea focuses on autonomy and independence with the aim to give people (and those caring for them) added security, safety, quality of life and access to medical care without an in-patient admission (Rialle, et al, 2007). In some cases it may delay or avoid institutionalisation.

In the mid 1990's, smart-homes were equipped with sensors that turned on lights at night when movement was detected, turned off stoves if overheating or left on, unlocked doors and turned on lights if smoke was detected, alerted staff if residents were out of bed for prolonged periods and, for wandering people, alerted staff if external doors were opened (Bjorneby, 2000).

Newer developments in smart-home sensors include detectors worn by the resident to alert staff if a fall occurs (Gibson, 2003) or if a resident at risk of falling, sits-up in bed (Gelhaus, 2002) and to monitor the mobility and subsequent health status of residents (Prado, 2002).

To Promote and Support Self-Care

The role of home telehealth in helping patients to mange their own health is another growing area. Many elderly people live with at least one chronic disease or condition, such as diabetes or heart disease. On discharge from hospitals (particularly if the patient is newly diagnosed) patients need extensive support to manage their condition successfully. Traditionally this has been done with routine home nursing visits. However, home telehealth provides an opportunity to interact with and instruct patients at home. This may improve self-care, reduce subsequent readmissions and allow people to stay in their own familiar environment.

Telehealth units are available with the ability to add peripheral monitoring devices for tracking a patient's physiological status and providing this information to them as part of an ongoing education and self-management program. Peripherals can include a blood glucose meter, blood pressure cuff, pulse oximeter and other measuring/monitoring devices. Multimedia materials can also be integrated into home telehealth units. These materials may be used to remind patients to track their weight daily, to alter their fluid intake or increase their activity levels. Of course all of these activities require the support of an experienced and qualified health care provider. The use of this type of home telehealth requires frequent communication with patients to reiterate directions, educate and coach.

To Improve Medication Management and Compliance

There is also a growing body of literature on the value of home telehealth in medication management. Medication-related complications are a contributing factor in accidents and illnesses that lead to hospitalization (Joanna Briggs Institute, 2006). Research has shown that patients with greater than nine medications have at least a 22 percent incidence of medication errors which in turn contribute to adverse reactions and hospitalisation (Ahrens, Feldman & Frey, 2002). Home telehealth in medication management has proven effective. For example, a study by the Veteran's Administration in the USA demonstrated a 30 percent improvement in medication compliance after telehealth implementation (Kobb, Hilsen & Ryan, 2003). Medication reminders, interactive voice response (IVR) systems and telemonitoring solutions can improve medication management and enable nurses to improve the quality of care provided.

Given all of these benefits, what evidence is there to support the use of home telehealth?

The Evidence-Base for Home Telehealth

There is much hype surrounding home telehealth; a lot has been written about its potential and promise but little clinical research has been undertaken. A recent review of home telehealth (Bensink, Hailey & Wootton, 2006a) used a comprehensive search of electronic databases including Medline, PsychINFO, CINAHL, EBSCOhost and EMBASE to identify research in the area. These searches identified 769 references to home telehealth. Only 18% of these were controlled studies comparing a home telehealth alternative to a usual care control group. Despite the hype, there are still good to high quality studies in the area (Bensink, Hailey & Wootton, 2007a).

An Emerging Area of Research

The first reports of controlled investigations into the use of home telehealth began emerging in the early 1980s and there has been progressive interest in the area ever since. Not surprisingly, these early investigations used the ordinary home telephone to support patients. Topics of investigation included support after heart surgery; counselling hypertensive patients; and educating, counselling and monitoring patients after a heart attack. Since these early reports the number of published studies has steadily increased. Our review in 2006 identified 138 papers reporting on 130 home telehealth research projects.

The Technologies Used

Given its widespread operation in most areas of industrialised countries, the public switched telephone network (PSTN) continues to provide a readily available, affordable and reliable link to the home for home telehealth. The home telephone can itself be used or alternatively a variety of devices can interface with the telephone network. These devices can connect directly to computers or computer servers in a hospital or provide data over the Internet. Specifically designed devices are also available to provide transmission of vital signs data such as oxygen saturation, blood pressure and blood glucose level. Broadband Internet connectivity over home telephone lines is also emerging as a technology of interest to home telehealth providing higher bandwidth connections than the PSTN network. This is opening new areas of research allowing improved quality video-telephony amongst other applications.

Diseases/Conditions Studied

The majority of the published evidence (over two-thirds) has been from the United States with countries like the UK, Japan, Italy and France contributing a further 19%. The areas with the most supporting evidence are chronic conditions such as diabetes, heart failure, mental health problems and cardiac disorders although evidence exists in other areas such as high risk pregnancy monitoring.

Although the majority of studies have been completed in these areas, telephone counselling targeted at people trying to quit smoking, represents an interesting exception. In this area only six randomised controlled trials supporting the use of different technologies were identified. What set these studies apart was the sample size; over 10,000 people participated in these six trials. Results showed there is evidence that telephone counselling is an effective strategy for assisting self-quitters over and above self-quitting guides alone (Orleans et al, 1991).

Home Telehealth Evidence and Nurses

The primary care providers in over half of the studies identified in our review were nurses, most commonly providing a combination of remote patient monitoring, health counselling and education. One example of this is the use of a "dialogue box" for diabetes related patient monitoring in the home (Chumbler et al, 2005). This device attached to the home telephone line and allowed patients to answer basic questions on diabetes care and metabolic control using a simple key pad. Entered information was then relayed via the Internet and presented to a nurse who determined if any intervention was required for example, either health counselling over the telephone, a home visit or a clinic visit.

Neglected Areas

Some areas of health care are only emerging as topics of home telehealth research; these include paediatrics, neonatal care and obstetrics. Our own investigations in paediatric oncology are some of the first to appear in the literature (Bensink et al,

2004, 2005, 2006, 2007, 2007b) Here the use of videotelephony allows nurses to provide support to the patient and family at home, themselves or to coordinate support from other members of the specialist paediatric oncology team.

Economics

Another, more general area of neglect is the evaluation of the economic benefit of home telehealth. It is perhaps the economics of home telehealth that will encourage health care authorities to support projects as well as acting as a catalyst to the widespread adoption of home telehealth. In our review, only 17% of the 138 studies identified contained economic evaluations.

The care of patients with heart failure is one area where economic evidence does exist. Advanced practice nurses working with a cardiologist, were able to use data collected by the patient and relayed via the Internet, to provide treatment advice over the telephone (Benatar, Bondmass & Ghitelman, 2003). This study identified a reduction in readmissions to hospital and the overall cost of care for these patients. In another study, nurses provided telephone follow-up and received transmissions of one-lead ECG recordings from chronic heart failure patients at home (Scalvini et al, 2005). Again, a reduction in hospital admissions and a reduction in the corresponding cost of care were identified. There is an excellent overview of the main features of economic evaluation methodologies as applied to home telehealth in Scuffham et al, 2006.

Research Quality

Study design is an important point to consider in home telehealth, whether you are assessing the evidence available in a given area, or designing a study into a home telehealth intervention. As in any area of health research, large randomised controlled studies are the gold standard (Egger, Smith & Altman, 2001). Other non-randomised designs provide less reliable estimates of the relative effects of interventions (Clarke, 2004). Other study designs include case-controlled studies, matched cohort studies, time series studies and retrospective studies. Each provides a different level of evidence.

In the home telehealth studies we evaluated, 80% were randomised controlled trials. This, along with assessment of the quality of these studies, (Bensink et al, 2007) provides some reassurance on the level of evidence available for home telehealth in the areas identified. Some problems with the quality of published home telehealth research are still apparent. Patient selection, patient disposal and outcomes reported were areas where studies lacked sufficient information. The use of recognised guidelines, such as the CONSORT statement, (Moher, Schulz & Altman, 2001) can provide guidance not only when preparing trial results for publication, but also much earlier in the planning process when designing studies.

Research Challenges

One problem identified in some areas is the clear identification of exactly what the home telehealth alternative is and what usual care control group it is being compared against.

An example of where confusion can occur is the use of the Internet to provide support for a variety of mental health problems. A number of these studies compared two or more home telehealth interventions. For example, assessing home monitoring of lung transplant patients via the telephone versus an electronic diary (Mullan et al, 2003). Other studies compared a home telehealth alternative to a wait-list control rather than a usual care control group (Devineni & Blanchard, 2005; Andersson, Stromgren & Strom, 2002; Lange et al, 2003). These studies, although they provide interesting information, do not provide clear evidence to support the use of a home telehealth alternative over the care usually provided to patients as part of standard health care services (e.g. in-patient stays, out-patient visits or face-to-face home visits).

Even with a usual care control group, the comparisons are not always straight forward. An example of this is in the area of home uterine activity monitoring (HUAM). Despite the promise identified in early studies, one study found no difference in preterm birth rate, preterm labour incidence, average birth weight or the gestational age of infants with home monitoring (Iam, Johnson & O'Shaughnessy, 1988). The authors of this study concluded that the favourable outcomes credited to HUAM in earlier studies were related not to the home telehealth intervention, but instead to the increased contact with nurses, a focus on symptoms of preterm labour and perceived contractions. This sparked widespread debate in the field. A recent review identified that the use of control groups whose care was, in some studies, more similar to HUAM than the usual care available at the time, was an issue (Morrison & Chauhan, 2003). This set an artificially high standard to compare HUAM against.

What was the final conclusion? When HUAM is used correctly by patients at high risk for preterm birth, with suitable alarm rates and precise monitors, early diagnosis of preterm labour, prolongation of pregnancy, reduced incidence of preterm birth and reduced neonatal morbidity is always demonstrated when compared to a standard care control group. Specifically, for these studies, the authors noted that standard care was the care routinely available to obstetricians in the USA (Morrison & Chauhan, 2003).

Future Research

For health services to embrace home telehealth as a viable and sustainable method of health service delivery more evidence is required. A scientifically sound case requires more randomized controlled trials to be undertaken with appropriate methodological rigour and quality. In any particular area, for example care of patients with diabetes or depression, these trials will need to investigate the use of the same intervention in comparable populations. Ideally, studies will also provide information on the economic, as well as the clinical effectiveness of the intervention. Finally, subsequent meta-analysis of results will provide a clearer view of the evidence available for a particular intervention in a population with specific characteristics.

This process is beginning to occur. A recent review and meta-analysis of home telehealth for patients with chronic heart failure concluded that programmes which include remote monitoring have a positive effect on clinical outcomes (Clark, Inglis & McAlister, 2007).

IMPLEMENTATION

Given the above examples, home telehealth has some benefits. These may be interpreted from a range of perspectives including that of the patient, the health service provider – or society as a whole. It is also important to appreciate the underlying reason(s) for using telehealth in general, whether to the home or for other applications. According to Wootton (2006), there are two broad reasons which may influence the use of telehealth:

The first is that there may be no alternative. An obvious example is if the patient is on a ship at sea or on a space expedition. In these circumstances, it is not logistically possible to visit a medical facility in person, and therefore the patient will depend on information delivered from a distance. A more common example is if the patient lives in a very remote country location with no local health services within close proximity. If the patient is unable to travel it may be reasonable to consider the opportunities for delivering services using telehealth.

The second main reason to develop a telehealth service is that there may be evidence which shows that telehealth is 'better' in some way than the conventional services available. That is, telehealth may be more clinically effective, may provide patients with more regular contact with a specialist, may be cheaper and more sustainable than the alternative, and may be more useful for early intervention and preventative health care services.

In brief, there are a number of practical aspects to consider when starting a new telehealth service.

Getting Started

- Identify the need for telehealth. Why telehealth? What is the clinical problem to be solved?
- What is the best method – real-time; store-and-forward, or a hybrid? This will also depend on the type of information to be transmitted, i.e. live video, digital photographs, text only, audio etc.
- What equipment will be required for the telehealth service?
- Telecommunications – what will be required?
- Obtain funding? The amount of funding available will influence choice of application.
- What incentive is there for clinicians to do telehealth?
- What support will be provided to clinicians – technical, administrative, executive?
- Identify clinical coordinators at both ends. Who will be responsible?
- Give consideration to change management.
- Have an evaluation plan in place – i.e. evaluate the service – investigate feasibility, cost-effectiveness, satisfaction, clinical effectiveness etc.
- Start small – feasibility testing first and develop service incrementally.

Be Aware

- Identify previous successes and failures and learn from others experiences and mistakes.
- Don't duplicate known failures.

Logistical Factors

Telehealth should not automatically be viewed as a new service. Instead, telehealth may provide an alternative method of delivering services which already exist. It is very important when establishing a telehealth service, to understand the underlying requirements of the service. That is, what are the factors which support the need for telehealth (distance, limited access to specialist services); what telehealth methods are most suitable for the needs identified (real-time, store-and-forward); what is the service going to achieve (perhaps reduced travel for patients, improved recruitment of medical staff to rural areas or improved emergency responses from regional areas).

It is also important to consider how the telehealth service respects and integrates with established working practices (e.g. existing referral mechanisms, patient flows, and dischare support services).

Telehealth requirements in different areas should be judged on individual merit. What works well in one area, does not necessarily guarantee that it will work well in another. Review the literature first and learn from the experiences (positive and negative) reported by others.

The decision to use telehealth instead of conventional methods of service delivery may be directly related to the alternative services available. For instance, if the conventional referral process is easy to use, as is the case in many states in Australia (patients are reimbursed for travel costs), an even more convenient process (incentive) would have to be developed, before clinicians were likely to consider alternatives, such as telehealth. Even today, telehealth is often perceived as being more complex and time consuming for clinicians to set up than the conventional method of sending the patients to see the specialist in person. This may explain why very few clinical telehealth services have emerged as mainstream services in Australia and throughout the world.

Economics

Like any new service, if one is considering establishing a new telehealth service they ought to have a good understanding of the likely establishment and daily operating costs. In addition, one should investigate whether there are economic advantages in doing telehealth, instead of using conventional methods of service delivery, i.e. how do the costs of home telehealth compare to conventional methods of health service delivery such as nurse visits to the patient homes and appointments in specialist hospitals.

There are a various types of economic evaluation methods which may be selected subject to specific factors which need to be assessed. Common examples include cost-benefit; cost-effectiveness, cost-utility and cost-minimisation analysis (see Table 1) (Drummond, 1996).

Table 1. Types of economic evaluations (Drummond 1996)

Type of analysis	Definition
Cost-benefit	measures costs and benefits in monetary units and computes a cost-benefit ratio
Cost-effectiveness	compares interventions or programmes having a common measurement of health outcome in a situation where, for a given level of resources, the decision maker wishes to maximise the health benefits conferred to the population of concern
Cost-utility	measures benefits in utility-weighted life-years (QALYs) and which computes a cost per utility-measure ratio for comparison between programmes
Cost-minimisation	measures and compares the costs for each service whereby the health outcomes for both services are assumed to be equivalent

Perhaps the most common type of economic analysis reported in telehealth studies is the cost-minimisation analysis in which the total costs of two or more services (with comparable health outcomes) are compared to determine the most economical choice of service at a given workload. This type of analysis is also useful to determine what workload (i.e. number of consultations) must be achieved in order for one service to cost the same as another. This point is often referred to as the threshold.

In order to do a cost-minimisation analysis, you will need to identify all of the costs associated with operating your telehealth service and the costs of operating the alternative service. These costs are usually categorised as fixed and variable costs. Fixed costs include equipment, installation and rental of telecommunications, managing staff salaries and facility costs. Variable costs are related to the volume of activity and include telecommunication (call) costs, clinician salaries, travel and accommodation costs. Once these costs are determined, you are then able to calculate the total costs of each service based on a selected workload. It will be possible to calculate the average cost per consultation by dividing the total cost of operating the service by the number of consultations. More importantly, you will be able to determine the cost of providing one additional consultation, assuming all establishment costs are in place. This is referred to as the marginal cost.

Case Example

Although not a home telehealth application, instead providing links between a tertiary paediatric referral centre and regional hospitals, the experiences of the telepaediatric service in Queensland, provides a valuable insight into telehealth implementation.

As an incentive to use telehealth, clinicians at selected regional sites throughout Queensland were given exclusive access to a centralised referral centre - contactable by a single toll-free telephone number. By calling this number, clinicians had a direct link to a telehealth coordinator based in Brisbane. Once a referral was made to the telepaediatric service, the telehealth coordinator took full responsibility for the case, liaised with the appropriate specialists and guaranteed a response within 24 hours. The single point of contact model has been a critical factor leading to the uptake and integration of telehealth services into the routine component of outreach service delivery.

A cost-minimisation analysis was conducted to compare the cost of providing telepaediatric services to two hospitals during a five year period. These costs were compared to the potential cost of transporting patients to the nearest hospital to see their specialist in person. During this period a total of 1499 consultations were conducted. In this analysis, we assumed that all patients would have had to travel to see the specialist in person, had the telepaediatric service not been available.

All costs are reported in Table 2.

In the above example (at the reported workload actually experienced) telepaediatrics was a much cheaper method of delivering the specialist service, mainly due to the high costs associated with potential travel. Had the workload (number

Table 2. Telepaediatric service costs and potential costs had all patients travelled to Brisbane

Expenditure	Telepaediatrics ($)	Outpatients ($)
FIXED COSTS		
Equipment (5-year total annuatized cost)	128,191	0
ISDN Installation	2655	0
ISDN Line rental	32,400	0
Coordinators salaries	475,000	0
Sub total (fixed costs)	***638,246***	***0***
VARIABLE COSTS		
Telecommunications *ISDN Line charges*	65,400	0
Staff salaries:		
RCH Consultants ($200 per h)	109,000	109,000
RCH Nursing / Allied Health ($50 per h)	27,250	27,250
RCH Admin Support ($30 per h)	0	16,350
Regional presenter ($150 per h)	81,750	0
Regional admin support ($30 per h)	16,350	0
Patient travel subsidy scheme: *Travel* *Accommodation*	 0 0	 1,391,670 8,994
Project costs	18,000	0
Sub total (variable costs)	***317,750***	***1,553,264***
TOTAL COST	**955,996**	**1,553,264**
Average cost per consultation (Divide total cost by the number of consultations)	637.76	1036.20
Marginal cost (Divide the total variable cost by the number of consultations)	211.97	1036.20

of consultations) been significantly lower, the overall economics of doing telehealth would have been less attractive. Similarly, had the workload been higher, the economics would have been even more favourable.

BARRIERS

Given that home telehealth has the potential to assist health service provision in a number of ways, that evidence exists to support its use in a number of areas and the success demonstrated by a number of telehealth projects, what other factors may be impeding the uptake of home telehealth?

Education and Training

In line with other developments in health care, education and training is a key factor in uptake. Like advances in medical imaging, ongoing education and training are critical for patient safety and for staff to use these systems efficiently and effectively. Advances in telehealth should be no different.

Very little attention has been paid to education and training in telehealth. Research has shown that despite the fact that health practitioners are familiar with computers and other electronic devices the practice of telehealth requires systematic education and training (Edirippulige, Smith & Young, 2006). The lack of knowledge of telehealth, its basic concepts and application is a result of the absence of systematic education (Edirippulige, Smith, Beattie, Davies & Wootton, 2007). Unless students are given education in basic concepts, principles and the variety of applications possible, then it is unlikely that telehealth will become a part of their practice. The potential benefits of telehealth can only be realised if students are provided with formal education as part of their curriculum.

In addition, integrating telehealth into ongoing professional development and support is also important. Health and medical professionals must be supported to acquire (until telehealth is integrated into curricula) and maintain their knowledge and practical skills in telehealth via continuing professional development (CPD) programmes. For this to occur, these courses will need to be recognised by relevant professional bodies through formal accreditation and support provided by employers for staff to attend.

A Multidisciplinary Approach

Another barrier to ongoing development in telehealth is the lack of interdisciplinary collaboration. Successful home telehealth implementation depends fundamentally on the ability to form, and lead, a multidisciplinary team through a lifecycle from initial analysis to the eventual day-to-day routine delivery of the service. It is important to remember that, whilst home telehealth uses technology as the vehicle for delivery of clinical services, there are other important non-technical aspects that must be given equal attention to ensure uptake and successful operation. This of course includes clinical aspects as mentioned previously, but also includes administrative aspects associated with coordination and ongoing operation.

Although the composition of a telehealth team will change over time, the underlying membership of the team must consist of skilled individuals in three key areas:

1. Clinical (e.g. nurses, doctors, social workers)
2. Technical (e.g. application developers, networkers)
3. Administrative (e.g. telehealth service coordinators, medical records staff).

Because these areas are closely interlinked, all members of the team need to be involved from initial inception of the project. The team, and its leader, must posses an uncommonly wide range of skills and experience in both project management and operational service management.

In common with general technology projects, a successful telehealth implementation will result from a delicate balancing act of both project-oriented and operational tasks carried out by a skilled team. In contrast with most general technology projects, the telehealth project requires a multidisciplinary approach and the necessity for each of the disciplines to be represented at all stages of the project. In addition, the project manager must have a broad understanding of all of the issues across clinical, technical and administrative boundaries and be able to manage various demands of the team to successful implementation.

CONCLUSION

Home telehealth is the use of information and communication technologies to deliver and support health care directly to the home. For nurses, home telehealth provides an opportunity, amongst other applications, to support other nurses at a distance, to support patients in the home through direct communication or via passive monitoring techniques, to promote and support self-care and to help patients with medication management and compliance.

Despite the hype, home telehealth is still an emerging application. As in all areas of health service, evidence is required to establish the worth of investing in home telealth examining both the clinical and cost-effectiveness of interventions.

Nurses have an opportunity to place themselves at the forefront of these developments. To achieve this, nurses will need to identify, in their own practice and area of expertise, how telehealth may play a role and why it might be of benefit, which methods are most appropriate and what outcomes might be achieved.

Nurses are also well placed (clinically, practically and historically) to play a key role in multidisciplinary telehealth teams. This collaborative approach is required to bridge the gap between patients and the clinical, administrative and technical aspects inherent in care delivery via telehealth techniques.

Finally, as a catalyst for this type of development, nurses need to know more about telehealth through systematic education as an integral part of undergraduate and graduate nursing curricula.

REFERENCES

Ahrens, J., Feldman, P. H., & Frey, D. (2002). Preventing medication errors in home care. *Centre for Home Care policy & Research Policy Brief, 12*, 1-6.

Andersson, G., Stromgren, T., Strom, L., & Lyttkens, L. (2002). Randomized controlled trial of internet-based cognitive behavior therapy for distress associated with tinnitus. *Psychosom Med.,* 64(5), 810-816.

ATA's Federal Policy Recommendations for Home Telehealth and Remote Monitoring. (n/d). Retrieved October 20, 2007, from http://www.americantelemed.org/news/policy_issues/FINA_%20DRAFTHome_Telehealth_Policy_ver3.5.pdf

Belfield, G., & Colin-Thome, D. (2004). *Improving chronic disease management.* Department of Health, UK National Health Service. Retrieved October 20, 2007, from http://www.dh.gov.uk/en/Publicationsandstatistics/Publications/PublicationsPolicyAndGuidance/DH_4075214.

Benatar, D., Bondmass, M., Ghitelman, J., & Avitall, B. (2003). Outcomes of chronic heart failure. *Arch Intern Med., 163*(3), 347-52.

Bensink, M., Hailey, D., & Wootton, R. (2006a). A systematic review of successes and failures in home telehealth: preliminary results. *Journal of Telemedicine and Telecare, 12*(Suppl. 3), 8-16.

Bensink, M., Hailey, D., & Wootton, R. (2007a). A systematic review of successes and failures in home telehealth. Part 2: final quality rating results.

Journal of Telemedicine and Telecare 2006 13 (suppl 2) 10-14.

Bensink, M., Shergold, J., Lockwood, L., Little, M., Irving, H., Russell, T., et al. (2006b). Videophone support for an 8-year-old boy undergoing paediatric bone marrow transplantation. *Journal of Telemedicine and Telecare, 12*(5), 266-268.

Bensink, M. E., Armfield, N., Russell, T. G., Irving, H., & Wootton, R. (2004). Paediatric palliative home care with Internet-based videophones: lessons learnt. *Journal of Telemedicine and Telecare, 10*(Suppl. 1), 10-13.

Bensink, M., Wootton, R., Irving, H., Hallahan, A., Theodoros, D., Russell, T., et al. (2007b). Investigating the cost-effectiveness of video-telephone based support for newly diagnosed paediatric oncology patients and their families: design of a randomised controlled trial. *BMC Health Services Research, 7*(38):doi:10.1186/1472-6963-7-38.

Bjorneby, S. (2000). Smart houses: can they really benefit older people? *Signpost.* 5, 36-38.

Clark, R. A., Inglis, S., C., McAlister, F. A., Cleland, J. G. F., & Stewart, S. (2007). Telemonitoring or structured telephone support programmes for patients with chronic heart failure: systematic review and meta-analysis. *BMJ* (Clinical research ed.) *334*(7600), 910-911.

Clarke, M. (2004). Systematic reviews and the Cochrane Collaboration. Retrieved November 12, 2007, from http://www.cochrane.org/docs/whycc.htm.

Chumbler, N. R., Vogel, W. B., Garel, M., Qin, H., Kobb, R., & Ryan, P. (2005). Health Services Utilization of a Care Coordination/Home-Telehealth Program for Veterans With Diabetes: A Matched-cohort Study. *J Ambul Care Manage, 28*(3), 230-240.

Darkins, A., Dearde, C. H., Rocke, L. G., Martin, J. B., Sibson, L., & Wootton, R. (1996). An evaluation of telemedical support for a minor treatment centre. *Journal of Telemedicine and Telecare, 2*(2), 92-99.

Devineni, T., & Blanchard, E. B. (2005). A randomized controlled trial of an internet-based treatment for chronic headache. *Behav Res Ther, 43*(3), 277-92.

Drummond M. F., & Jefferson T. O. (1996). Guidelines for authors and peer reviewers of economic submissions to the BMJ. *British Medical Journal,* 313, 275–83.

Edirippulige, S., Smith, A. C., Young, J., & Wootton, R. (2006). Knowledge, perceptions and expectations of nurses in e-health: results of a survey in a children's hospital, *Journal of Telemedicine and Telecare, 12*(Suppl. 3), S3, 35-38.

Edirippulige, S., Smith, A., Beattie, H., Davies, E., & Wootton, R. (2007). Preregistration nurses: an investigation of knowledge, experience and comprehension of e-health. *Australian Journal of Advanced Nursing,* 25(2), 78-83.

Egger, M., Smith, G., & Altman, D. G. (2001). *Systematic Reviews in Health Care: Meta-analysis in Context.* 2 ed. London: BMJ Publishing Group.

Flesner, M. K. (2004). Care of the elderly as a global nursing issue, *Nursing Administration Quarterly*, 28(1), 67-72.

Gelhaus, I. (2002). High-tech homes mean a brighter future for seniors. *Provider*, 28, 40-42.

Gibson, F. (2003). Seven Oakes: friendly design and sensitive technology. *Journal of Dementia Care, 11*, 27-30.

Iams, J., Johnson, F., & O'Shaughnessy, R. (1988). A prospective random trial of home uterine activ ity monitoring in pregnancies at increased risk of preterm labor Part II. *Am J Obstet Gynecol., 159*, 595-603.

Information Technology Association of America E-Health Committee (2004). *Chronic care improvement: How Medicare transformation can save lives, save money and stimulate an emerging technology industry*, ITAA May 2004. Retrieved October 20, 2007 from http://www.itaa.org/isec/docs/choniccare.pdf

Jenkins, R. L., & White, P. (2001). Telehealth advancing nursing practice. *Nursing Outlook, 49*(2), 100-105.

Joanna Briggs Institute. (2006). strategies to reduce medication errors with reference to older adults. *Aust Nurs J, 14*(4), 26-9.

Kingma, M. (2004). *Nurses on the move, Migration and the global health care economy*, Cornell University Press, Ithaca.

Kobb, R., Hilsen, P., & Ryan, P. (2003). Assessing technology needs for the elderly: finding the perfect match for home. *Home Healthc Nurs, 1*, 666-73.

Kobb, R., Hilsen, P., & Ryan, P. (2003). Assessing technology needs for the elderly: finding the perfect match for home. *Home Healthc Nurse, 1*, 666-73.

Lange, A., Rietdijk, D., Hudcovicova, M., van de Ven J-P., Schrieken, B., & Emmelkamp, P. M. G. (2003). Interapy: A controlled randomized trial of the standardized treatment of posttraumatic stress through the internet. *Journal of Consulting and Clinical Psychology, 71*(5), 901-999.

Moher, D., Schulz, K., & Altman, D. (2001). Revised recommendations for improving the quality of reports of parallel group randmoized trials. *Annals of Internal Medicine, 134*(8), 657-662.

Moore, R. S., Britton, B. & Chetney, R. (2005). Wound care using interactive telehealth. *Home Health Care Manage Pract, 17*(3), 203-12.

Morrison, J. C., & Chauhan, S. P. (2003). Current status of home uterine activity monitoring. Clinics in Perinatology, *30*, 751-80.

Mullan, B., Snyder, M., Lindgren, B., Finkelstein, S. M., & Hertz, M. I. (2003). Home monitoring for lung transplant candidates. *Prog Transplant, 13*(3), 176-82.

National Health Expenditures Aggregate Amounts and Average Annual Percent. Retrieved October 15, 2007 from http://www.cms.hhs.gov/NationalHealthExpendData/downloads/tables.pdf

Orleans, C., Schoenbach, V., Wagner, E., Quade, D., Salmon, M., Pearson, D., et al. (1991). Self-help quit smoking interventions: effects of self-help materials, social support instructions, and telephone counselling. *J Consult Clin Psychol, 59*(3), 439-448.

Prado, M., J. Reina-Tosina, and L. Roa (2002). Distributed intelligent architecture for falling detection and physical activity analysis in the elderly. In: *Proceeding of the Second Joint EMBS/BMES Conference, 3*, 1910–1911.

Reed, K. (2005). Telemedicine: Benefits to advanced practice nursing and the communities they serve. *Clinical Practice*. 17(5), 176-180.

Rialle, V. Rumeau, P, Ollivet, C. & Hervé, C. (2006). Smart homes. In Wootton R, Kvedar J & Dimmick SL. *Home Telehealth: Connecting care within community*, 65-75. RSM, London,

Ryan, P., Kobb, R., & Hilsen, P. (2003). Making the right connection: matching patients to technology. *Telemed J E Health, 9*, 81-8.

Scalvini, S., Capomolla, S., Zanelli, E., Benigno, M., Domenighini, D., Paletta, L., et al. (2005). Effect of home-based telecardiology on chronic heart failure: costs and outcomes. *J Telemed Telecare, 11*(Suppl 1), 16-8.

Scuffham, P. (2006). Economic evaluation. In: Wootton R, Dimmick S, Kvedar J, editors. *Home telehealth: connecting care within the community*. London: Royal Society of Medicine Press Ltd, 21-35.

Smith, A. C., Scuffham ,P. & Wootton, R. The costs and potential savings of a novel telepaediatric service in Queensland. *BMC Health Services Research* 2007, 7:35, available online at http://www.biomedcentral.com/1472-6963/7/35

Wootton, R., Kvedar, J., & Dimmick. S. L. (2006). *Home Telehealth: Connecting care within community.* RSM, London.

Wootton, R. & Patterson, V. (Eds.). (2006). *Introduction to Telemedicine* (2 ed.). London: Royal Society of Medicine Press.

KEY TERMS

Telehealth: The delivery of health-related services and information over distance via telecommunications technologies.

Home Telehealth: The use of telehealth techniques in a non-institutinal setting such as the home or residential care facility.

Evidence: The collection of data through observation and experimentation used to determine or demonstrate the truth of an assertion.

Telepaediatrics: Telehealth applications relevant to the health and wellbeing of children, young people and families.

Real-Time Mode: The use of telecommunications allowing instantaneous two-way interaction between participants e.g. videoconferencing.

Store-and-Forward Mode: The delayed exchange of data requiring first capture using for example a digital camera, voice recorder, X-ray machine or video camera, sub sequent storage and latter transmission.

Health Economics: A specialist field of economics related to the demand and supply of health and health care.

Multidisciplinary: The collaboration of individuals and groups with specialised education and expertise in distinct and different areas.

Telehealth Education and Training: The formal and systematic imparting of the knowledge and skill required to apply best practice principles to the application of telehealth in practice.

Chapter VIII
Successful Online Teaching and Learning Strategies

Mary D. Oriol
Loyola University New Orleans, USA

Gail Tumulty
Loyola University New Orleans, USA

ABSTRACT

This chapter presents a theoretical framework and research base for the successful transition of an established Master of Science in Nursing program from that of traditional classroom delivery to one that is Web-based with no geographic limitations to students. The application of ***socio-technical systems*** *theory to facilitate creation of a positive learning environment for future nurse leaders is described. Use of social processes and application of technology to optimize learning is explained and the latest research on content presentation and student engagement in an e-learning environment are presented. The authors hope that through examination of successful online teaching/learning strategies, readers will have a clear understanding of the competencies necessary for students and faculty to be successful in* ***online education****.*

INTRODUCTION

In the United States, there were approximately 116,000 registered nurse vacancies as of December, 2006 (American Hospital Association, 2007). A recent survey confirmed that over half of all health care organizations have difficulty in recruiting nurse managers, and shortages are most severe in community hospitals. Further, there is a critical need to prepare nurses with graduate degrees in nursing to serve as nursing faculty (Fang & Wisniewski, 2007). Thus, the impact of nursing education is becoming clearer, placing increased responsibility upon educators to address this important issue. Through the availability and accessibility of online courses, more nurses are encouraged to enter graduate programs, providing sorely needed masters prepared nurses for both leadership and faculty positions. Ultimately, the health and safety of patients will benefit from a strong online curriculum designed to prepare nurses for leadership positions in a managed care environment and for faculty positions in nursing education that will increase the number of adequately prepared nurses at the bedside.

The **Health Care Systems Management (HCSM) program** at **Loyola University New Orleans,** the first of its kind in Louisiana, was designed to prepare nurses for advanced education and practice in leadership roles in managed health care. Graduates of the **HCSM program** earn a Master of Science degree in nursing and are prepared to take the American Nurses Association Certification Exam in Nursing Administration, Advanced, the American Nurses Association Certification Exam in Case Management, and the Commission for Case Management (CCM) Exam. The curriculum follows the Graduate Core Curriculum Content as outlined in the *Essentials of Master's Education* (1996) from the American Association of Colleges of Nursing and the supplement to The Essentials of Master's Education, *The Joint Position Statement on Nursing Administration Education (*1997), issued by the American Association of Colleges of Nursing and the American Organization of Nurse Executives as well as Standards of Practice for Case Management developed by the Case Management Society of America. The **HCSM** curriculum contains significant content on health system management, leadership, finance, quality improvement, health promotion, disease management, integrated delivery systems, and managed care strategies to prepare nurse leaders to better meet the needs of the population. The **HCSM program** began in 2001 as a traditional on-campus educational program with a non-web-based distance learning option. After several years of planning and implementation, the distance learning option was transitioned to a fully online program attracting students throughout the United States.

This chapter will present a theoretical framework and research base for the successful transition of an established Master of Science in Nursing program from that of traditional classroom delivery to one of web-based delivery with no geographic limitations to students. The objectives of this chapter are to:

1. Apply **socio-technical systems theory** to facilitate creation of a positive learning environment for future nurse leaders.
2. Explain the use of social processes and application of technology to optimize learning.
3. Present the latest research on content presentation and student engagement in an online learning environment.

TRANSITION FROM CLASSROOM TO ONLINE

Health care professionals seeking to further their education desire a convenient and flexible environment that enables them to manage multiple employment and personal responsibilities while providing opportunities for participation and exchange of ideas with other professionals. Lee and Nguyen (2007) refer to online learning as an "AEM", Automated Educational Machine, because educational services are conveniently delivered with few time and physical boundaries.

However, an online curriculum must be more than just an alternative educational delivery system developed to provide accessible, student-friendly learning experiences. It must be a strong curriculum grounded in distance learning pedagogy that will provide student-centered learning experiences and improve learner productivity (Britt, 2006). And like traditional courses within a curriculum that are linked by a conceptual framework, the online courses within the curriculum must demonstrate the same conceptual linkages (Ryan, Carlton, & Ali, 2004). Conversely, **online education** differs in that a shift in emphasis is required from traditional classroom memorization and understanding to analysis, synthesis, and application of information to situations that resemble the demands of contemporary practice (Billings, 2007).

THEORETICAL FRAMEWORK

Socio-technical systems theory is a systems perspective focused on the internal organizational processes of interdependencies and relationships. As such it is the ideal theoretical framework to support curriculum development for a technologically-rich learning environment. Any system requires both a work-relationship and a technology structure that relates humans to technology and to each other. Especially in hospitals, but in almost all health care settings, nurses are organized into groups whose individual and collective action and technical performance produce patient care. It is through the nursing staff interaction with professionals from other disciplines, and with the use of modern technology that care is delivered (Green & Kenyon, 1991; Griffin, 1980; Tumulty, 1980).

A series of reports from the **Institute of Medicine (IOM)** tell us that the nation's healthcare delivery system requires fundamental change (Institute of Medicine, 2001). The first phase of the **IOM**'s quality initiative documented the serious and pervasive nature of errors due to health care system issues (Institute of Medicine, 1999). Phase II laid out a vision for radical reform. Health Professions Education: A Bridge to Quality (2003) represents the third phase of the **IOM** initiative and makes the case that reform of health professions education is critical to enhancing the quality of health care in the United States. Just as the health system must be transformed in order to advance quality, so must the education of health professionals. The overall vision for health professions education in the 21st century is that "All health professionals should be educated to deliver patient-centered care as members of an interdisciplinary team, emphasizing evidence-based practice, quality improvement approaches, and informatics" (Institute of Medicine, 2003, p. 3).

Health care is overwhelmingly a people business. Its product, delivered by people, is the most personal one imaginable. This personal relationship of nurse and patient will remain at the heart of quality patient care regardless of the explosion of new technologies into the healthcare workplace (Numerof, 2004). Thus, the modern health care manager must be able to manage both the social and the technical: the people and the technology. Human factor approaches alone are no longer optimum due to the basic limitations of human information processing and information overload. Accordingly, the ability to manage and manipulate information must be increasingly machine assisted. Information technology can be both a vital tool and critical link in the modern health system (Magruder, Burke, Hann, & Ludovic, 2005). Even before the emergence of the Health Insurance Portability and Accountability Act (HIPAA), health practitioners and leaders were aware that information technology (IT) was changing the health landscape. In Healthy People 2020 (http://www.healthypeople.gov/), there is a focus on information systems, data collection, and data management, along with system communication and integration. Information technology has now taken center stage in many health discussions because of its ability to provide ways to monitor health, track disease, increase efficiency and promote quality.

HEALTH PROFESSIONS EDUCATION

As the health care system is in need of fundamental overhaul, health professions education must reinvent itself to better prepare the professionals to function in a different environment. Five core competencies recommended by IOM (2003) for implementation by all organizations involved in the education of healthcare professionals are: (a) Patient-centered care; (b) work in interdisciplinary teams; (c) employ evidence-based practice; (d) apply quality improvement; and (e) utilize informatics to reduce errors, manage information, make decisions and facilitate communication. In 2005, in collaboration with the American Association of Colleges of Nursing, the American Organization of Nurse Executives (AONE), working with the Council on Graduate Education for Administration in Nursing (CGEAN), a revised and more in-depth set of competencies integral to the practice of nurse executives was published (Harris, Huber, Jones, Manojlovich, & Reineck 2006). The competencies include the broad categories of communication and relationship building; knowledge of healthcare environment; leadership; professionalism; and business skills, including information management and technology (American Organization of Nurse Executives, 2005). These competencies should be utilized along with the IOM recommendations as a guide in the development of curricula for the education of the next generation of nurse leaders.

INFRASTRUCTURE AND DELIVERY SYSTEM REQUIREMENTS FOR ONLINE EDUCATION

When the decision is made to develop an online course or program, it is essential to complete a comprehensive evaluation of administrative support, available technical resources, student support services, and faculty development needs (Baldwin & Burns, 2004). The following outlines some of the issues within these areas that must be addressed before a firm commitment to online program development is made.

Administrative Support

The highest levels of university administration must firmly support online program development before significant financial and human resources are invested by the program. Currently, development of online learning opportunities is very attractive to university administrators because it offers solutions to some of the most pressing problems they face. First, the portability and flexibility of **online education** provides increased access for students, thus potentially increasing enrollment numbers. In a survey done by Allen and Seaman (2007), the growth rate for online enrollment in higher education is 9.7%, far exceeding the 1.5% overall higher education growth rate. The Generation Xers who thrive on quick results and independent activities, those employed full-time and those bound by geographic limitations all provide an expanded pool of potential students from which to draw. Next, online education provides an option for addressing faculty shortages. High profile leaders in content areas can be hired as adjunct faculty or on a per diem basis with their salaries being structured to their teaching load. Finally, the issue of limited classroom space experienced on most campuses is eliminated for online courses (Kenner, Androwich, & Edwards, 2003).

Even after 25 years and despite the acknowledged advantages of **online education**, university administrators have been unable to completely resolve issues concerning workload credit, faculty role, class size, course ownership and the blend of on-campus and online classes (Billings, 2007; Ryan, Carlton, & Ali, 2004). All of these pose both financial and workload equity issues that affect faculty university-wide. For instance, online courses can take up to twice as long as traditional classes to prepare and implement (Britt, 2006). Thus, administration must decide if it is appropriate to provide additional compensation or work release time for faculty to prepare and teach online courses. In addition, it is recommended that online class size not exceed 20 students. This brings into question workload equity concerns (Cuellar, 2002; Ryan, Carlton, & Ali, 2004; Ryan, Hodson-Carlton, & Ali, 2005)) where one might ask if an on-campus faculty teaching a three-credit class with 50 to 100 students is credited with the same workload as a faculty teaching the same three-credit course online with 20 students. Clear administrative policies that address class size and workload for both on-campus and online courses will clarify expectations and provide guidance for planning and budgeting anticipated course offerings.

Technical Resources

Course Delivery System

A very important decision that has to be made early in the planning process is the selection or re-appraisal of the online **course delivery system** to be utilized. Often, universities already have one in use, but with the implementation of an **online education** program, system capabilities and requirements must be reassessed.

Some of the most frequently used online **course delivery systems** are Blackboard (WebCt has now merged with Blackboard) (http://www.blackboard.com), Moodle (http://moodle.org/), Intellum (http//www.intellum.com/), Scholar360 (http://scholar360.com), Angel Learning Management Suite (http:/www.angellearning.com) and Desire2Learn (http://www.desire2learn.com). All of the systems offer such basic features as the ability create student and faculty accounts, deliver online courses, send email, track student performance, automate testing, store documents, and network with others in the class both synchronously and asynchronously. Each system purports to be user-friendly and flexible.

Every online **course delivery system** has hardware and server software requirements that depend on the number of expected enrolled users, number of expected concurrent users, number of courses, anticipated growth rates, and desired speed. In addition, plans for hardware replacement as well as performance and redundancy expectations must be considered. For instance, Blackboard Academic Suite (2004) makes institutional recommendations for the amount of RAM, internal and external storage, and number of servers based on the university's chosen server software for web and database processors. The recommendations are tiered for small (1,000-5,000 users), moderate (10,000-25,000 users), and large institutions (50,000-100,000 users). Most of the course management systems base their price on a range of the number of users while others price their product per unique user.

Technical Support

Prior to beginning online course development, a partnership should be formed with an internal or external entity that can lend technological expertise and on-going support. Faculty who develop courses are generally content and curriculum experts rather than technology specialists. Therefore, it is imperative that technical support be available from the outset to assure that appropriate software and hardware are in place for the selected course management system and for individual faculty who will be teaching online (Beitz & Snarponis, 2006; Ryan, Hodson-Carlton, & Ali, 2005). Further, on-going technical support must be readily available for technology changes, software updates, and troubleshooting when technical problems are incurred by users. Finally, system security must be initiated and maintained to protect all users.

Technology requirements must be determined and communicated to students before they begin their coursework (Jairath & Stair, 2004). For students to be successful and satisfied with their **online educational** experience, minimum computer hardware requirements, minimum acceptable internet speed, internet browser requirements, and necessary software must be explicitly stated. There must also be a plan for responding to technological problems. Guidelines should be in place for contacting technical support when computer access in unavailable or for alternative means for computer access (Keockeritz, Malkiewicz, & Henderson, 2002). The guidelines should include a toll-free contact number and the time of day/night that technical support is available. Typically, a minimum of 12 to16 hours per day of technical support availability is considered acceptable. At **Loyola University New Orleans**, the **HCSM** online program began with 16 hours per day of technical support. As the program grew, technical support was expanded to 24 hours per day. Without appropriate computer resources and a plan for addressing technical problems, students will be frustrated with the performance and speed of the equipment and software they are using, discouraged when technical problems occur, and ultimately dissatisfied with their online learning experience.

Student Support Services

Accrediting bodies for higher education require that on-campus and distance learning students have access to the same support services as all other students enrolled in the university. Some of the basic support services that must be provided to online students include admissions, registration, links to university offices, faculty directories, bookstore, writing assistance, and library resources such as electronic databases, online and electronic journals, and email delivery of interlibrary loan materials (Cuellar, 2002; Baldwin & Burns, 2004; Jairath & Stair, 2004; Ryan, Hodson-Carlton, & Ali, 2004). The mechanism through which support services are provided will vary from one university to another. The consistent requirement is that the services are comprehensive, readily available and easily accessible. When a problem with services arises, students want prompt access to a live person prepared to give them individualized attention.

Faculty Development

The success of an online learning program is largely dependent on faculty development initiatives that meet the needs and priorities of online faculty. Many faculty are transitioning from lifelong classroom instruction with a defined physical space and scheduled teaching time to the **online educational** environment that is 24/7, portable, and virtually without geographic or environmental limitations (Ryan, Carlton, & Ali, 2004). It cannot be assumed that faculty who are considered expert classroom teachers have the knowledge necessary regarding technical requirements (**course delivery systems**, video conferencing, **video streaming**, chat rooms, etc.), online pedagogy (collaborative learning), and principles of online course design (Billings, 2007).

While there are many resources available to faculty that address online teaching strategies, few speak to the "art of teaching" online (Cuellar, 2002). Providing resources and support for faculty to make a smooth transition from classroom teacher to the role of online facilitator is necessary for the development of clear and comprehensive online courses, thereby reducing the stress of both faculty and students.

Faculty development initiatives must include instruction in online pedagogy, particularly strategies for student engagement and design of learning experiences that will draw on individual creativity and use of personal and professional knowledge and expertise. Faculty must also be educated on the use and appropriateness of online tools and technology, online etiquette and communication skills, time management, and avenues for faculty support (Ali, et al., 2005).

The transition of the **HCSM program** at **Loyola University New Orleans** to online was built on the existing expertise and continuing efforts of faculty to provide a flexible and effective curriculum for future nurse leaders in a first-class distance-learning environment. Initially, a series of seminars, technical workshops and hands-on training sessions were held for faculty to increase their awareness of and involvement in Internet technology. A great deal of enthusiasm for Internet technology was generated by these activities and the goal of transitioning the **HCSM program** to total online accessibility was on its way to becoming realized.

Several developments supported progress toward this goal. The university purchased Blackboard as its online course management system to provide educators with comprehensive and flexible e-learning software platform designed to enhance teaching and learning environments through the use of the Internet. Faculty originally used its set of web-based tools to facilitate course preparation and enrich students' learning experiences in on-campus courses. However, moving from periodic use of the Internet to enhance regular live classes to offering courses and ultimately an entire program online was a significant undertaking for faculty.

Faculty soon realized that while they were the content experts, they needed help to assist with conversion of the curriculum to an online format. To effectively plan and implement the curriculum online, **HCSM** faculty utilized the **Competency Assessment in Distributed Education (CADE)** model for the design of the MSN online courses (Jesuit Distance Education Network, n.d.). The **CADE** model approaches course design by beginning with expected competencies and moving to evidence of achievement to instructional task accomplishment. Thus, the assessment of student competency within instructional tasks is an explicit requirement of course development. The **Jesuit Distance Education Network (JesuitNET)** was created in 1999 as a collaborative effort of 25 U.S. Jesuit colleges and universities to develop, share, and deliver a broad range of online academic programs and services for a national and eventually international audience. **JesuitNET** seeks to meet the diverse, growing needs of both traditional and non-traditional learners by providing a flexible and convenient way to learn, and by complementing classroom learning on Jesuit campuses. **JesuitNET** is part of the Association of Jesuit Colleges and Universities (AJCU). The AJCU President, JesuitNET Advisory Board and the JesuitNET Staff collectively set policies and ensures representation from a broad range of AJCU constituencies to guide JesuitNET activities. In 2001, the U.S. Department of Education selected **JesuitNET** as a Distance Education Demonstration Program participant to test the quality and viability of the innovative **CADE** competency-based approach. Thus, Loyola faculty embraced the **CADE** model for development of online courses.

Phase 1 of course development began with Loyola nursing faculty working intensively with **JesuitNET**'s Director of Curriculum Development for two days on-campus. Faculty were led through the **CADE** design portfolio process by preparing the portfolio's initial worksheets and narratives for the courses. Faculty used backward design to develop strategic knowledge competencies, evidence and cognitive apprenticeship strategies for each of the courses.

During Phase 2 in the subsequent six week period, **JesuitNET** staff and nursing faculty responsible for creating and teaching the courses continued the **CADE** workshop in a well-developed online environment. Faculty worked with the Director of Curriculum Development in an iterative process of course development. Working together in an asynchronous discussion space, faculty completed the remaining portfolio worksheets and narratives for their courses. Following completion of course competencies, outlines, learning activities and other content items, a second two-day, on-campus **JesuitNET**-led **CADE** course design session was held to finalize the content development phase.

At the end of Phases 1 & 2, faculty began to work on Phase 3 which focused on the activities required for the production of multimedia elements in the online courses. In this session, faculty created a plan for completing the development of the course through the following production activities:

Interface Design

- Implement the web design parameters, style guides and visual standards.
- Working with a Loyola videographer to assist in planning and producing original graphics for course materials, key frame art for animations, print-based and video-based instructional materials.

Multimedia Production

- Create interactive web-based multimedia learning objects to enhance instructional activities using Flash, Director, and other relevant applications.
- Provide basic non-linear video editing support for web-based courses.

ONLINE TEACHING/LEARNING STRATEGIES

Presentation of Course Materials

Online course content is mastered by guiding students in the discovery and comprehension of concepts. Material is presented so that, ideally, students will approach content as active participants in the learning process, individually adapting the educational experience to meet their individual needs (Baldwin & Burns, 2004).

Online presentation format should be visually attractive, consistent, simple and clear across all courses within the curriculum. Using the same organizational format, colors, and fonts assist students to focus on and process the information rather than the design elements (Parker & Howland, 2006). Adult learners are seeking quick answers to their questions. So, content and method of presentation that is relevant to their professional challenges is highly valued and engaging.

Multimedia is considered an effective method of presentation for those with many competing demands for their attention (Smith-Stoner & Willer, 2003). **Power Point presentations** are one popular mechanism for communicating content. When developing **Power Point presentations**, it is important to ensure that there is contrast between background and text. Clip art and animation should be used only if it supports content. Otherwise, it becomes distracting to the online learner. A simple slide design is often more stimulating and focuses the learner on the material (Smith-Stoner, & Willer, 2003). If slides are narrated, it is important for the instructor to speak slowly and clearly. Asking questions that require reflection followed by a pause provides students time to think about their answer before the presentation continues.

Video streaming (incorporating digitalized videos into a presentation) has become a very popular mechanism for presenting content online. **Power Point presentations** are often considered the "backbone" of **video streaming** where the instructor presents **Power Point** slides in a video or where the slide presentation is accompanied by only the instructor's narration (Smith-Stoner & Willer, 2003). On the other hand, Skiba (2007) discourages use of **Power Point presentations** as their use produces limited student **engagement**. She advocates more interactive methods of online learning.

It is important to note, however, that digitalized video files are generally very large and are time-consuming to download. So, it is advisable to create video streams that are limited to 10 to 15 minutes in length. Video streams that can be watched by several students simultaneously generally need to reside on a server. In addition, for the student to be able to view the video, it is necessary that they download a media player from providers such as Microsoft, Apple, or Real Networks.

Smith-Stoner and Willer (2003) recommend the following guidelines for instructors filming a video presentation:

- Look directly into the camera
- Smile genuinely and often
- Wear extra make-up (even males) to avoid looking pale
- Wear solid colors—prints can be very distracting
- When filming more than one presentation at a time, bring along different outfits
- Practice, practice, practice before actually videoing.

On the other hand, faculty at **Loyola University New Orleans** have found that extensive practice has not been of great benefit. Rather, a written script and teleprompter are used to reduce presenter anxiety, thus making presentations more conversational.

Since health professionals need to become familiar with popular software programs used to enhance decision-making, **video streaming** is an effective mechanism for demonstrating different applications. Smith-Stoner & Will (2003) recommend the following techniques to facilitate student learning of unfamiliar software applications:

- As each function of the software program is presented, go through the steps slowly and deliberately. Even though there are shortcuts that can save students time in the long run, it is important that each step in the function be demonstrated and explained so that the underlying rationale for the function is explicit. It is helpful if written instructions for each step are posted prior to the presentation so that students can prepare beforehand and follow along as the demonstration proceeds.
- Move the mouse very slowly from function to function. Remember, students are watching this on video where it is more difficult to follow and there is no opportunity to request that the instructor repeat the step.
- Use default setting for the computer. Background themes distract from the presentation.
- Include pauses in the demonstration so that the student can practice the activity before going to the next function.
- Limit tutorials to 10 minutes. If it takes longer to present a function, break it up into multiple presentations, each covering a segment of the function.

Many of these techniques are used to teach software applications in the **HCSM program**. For example, in the Outcomes Assessment and Data Management course, students are taught SPSS, a statistical and data management software package (http://www.spss.com/spss/index.htm). While only the very basic functions of the program are utilized to make decisions based on data analysis, students are often challenged and intimidated by a new and sophisticated software application. To put students at ease in performing analyses using SPSS, several supportive techniques are used to facilitate the learning process.

- For each statistical function presented, there are clear and concise step-by-step written instructions. In addition, students are provided with additional resources such as web-based tutorials and readings that support learning each function.
- Students are provided with sample raw data files and asked to complete assigned exercises associated with each statistical function. These exercises require that students use the appropriate SPSS function to analyze the data and then present their analysis and interpretation of the findings for extensive faculty feedback.
- Rather than requiring students to work in isolation on the exercises, they are encouraged to collaborate and support one another in the online learning activities.
- Faculty are available for support and consultation via Blackboard, email, or by telephone when students have difficulty completing the exercises. As learning new software

applications can be stressful for students, active faculty engagement is a must.

Discussions

Group **discussions** can be used for both academic and social purposes (Koeckeritz, Malkiewicz, & Henderson (2002). For academic purposes, **discussions** can be used to share resources, expertise, observations, and clarification of course materials. Getting to know classmates, developing support systems, and sharing common problems provide social support for students. The richness and inclusiveness of online **discussions** facilitate collaborative relationships among faculty and students, enhance critical thinking skills, provide opportunities for creative problem sources, and have demonstrated a more efficient use of resources than **discussions** utilized in classroom teaching (Kenner, Androwich, & Edwards, 2003). An added advantage is that experts can be invited as guests to discuss a specific topic with students (Britt, 2006).

Discussions online can be synchronous, as in chat rooms, or asynchronous, as in threaded **discussions**. Chat rooms provide an opportunity for real-time interaction on a topic or issue. However, since online learners generally engage in course work at times that do not interfere with personal and professional responsibilities, it is difficult to hold a chat session where every student is available to participate. Asynchronous discussions allow students to post their responses at a time convenient for them. Varying levels of participation can be expected where some students participate actively throughout the discussion and others only post infrequently.

Regardless of whether faculty choose synchronous or asynchronous **discussion** as the preferred mechanism, guidelines for acceptable levels of participation must be made explicit. Further, clearly stated expectations that students will remain respectful of the postings of fellow students and that the **discussion** will be limited to the topic at hand are imperative (Jairath & Stair, 2004). Students who may be reluctant to participate in classroom **discussions** are usually not as inhibited to share their individual views online. The open forum is an avenue for exchange of ideas (Kenny, 2002). And while continued **engagement** of students in online activities requires faculty to maintain an online presence, Parker and Howland (2006) recommend that faculty limit their participation in **discussions** so as to encourage independent learning and avoid inhibiting student interaction. They advise that faculty respond to the initial **discussion** posting but avoid commenting on subsequent threads unless the **discussion** needs to be clarified or redirected.

While the majority of **discussion** should enhance content presentations through provocative dialogue among students, there should also be the a designated forum for students to ask faculty questions about assignments, course requirements, and clarification of any other issues of concern (Moore & Hart, 2004). Additionally, some faculty provide a forum designated only for student social **discussion** which allows them to dialogue about personal issues, common problems, and to provide support and helpful suggestions. Finally, students must be made aware that discussions are open to all enrolled and, thus, are not confidential (Fulton & Kellinger, 2004).

Written Assignments

Written assignments are part of every education program. In **online education**, faculty and students must rely on written dialogue as their major form of communication. Without face-to-face interaction, the level of respect communicated in written responses will determine the quality of the connection made between faculty and students in an open online learning environment (Diekelmann & Mendias, 2005).

Many of the challenges faced in on-campus classes are also found in online classes. For instance, Internet sites that sell pre-written papers are becoming more common but so are the resources, such as Turnitin.com, to monitor the submission of "canned" papers. Plagiarism should be addressed from all angles including an analysis of whether assignments are overwhelming to students or whether they might just need help with organizational skills (Moore & Hart, 2004). Students should also be given support in their writing assignments through access to online writing laboratories available through most universities and access to a 24-hour library help line. The requirement for use of only one word processing program for submission of written assignments helps faculty and students to exchange information without needing multiple programs to open files.

Whatever **course delivery system** has been selected by the online program, it must include mechanism for secure submission of files by both faculty and students. Unlike discussions which are open to all users, students must feel secure that when an assignment for grading is sent via the course delivery system, it will be seen only by those for whom it was intended. When faculty return graded assignment files with their comments and suggestions to students, they too must be confident that the exchange is secure.

ENGAGEMENT OF ONLINE PARTICIPANTS

Health professionals enter **online educational** programs with a wealth of personal and professional experiences that can enhance their learning experience. Most are self-directed and internally motivated to learn (Cuellar, 2002). Even so, many who enter online programs expect that the courses are easier that traditional classes only to find that online courses are harder and the independent learning experience is more time consuming (Britt, 2006).

Orientation

Before students begin their first online course, a concise and visually attractive orientation is essential to provide necessary information and dispel myths (Beitz, & Snarponis, 2006; Tips, 2002). Moreover, the orientation should remain accessible online for students as a readily available reference to which they can return throughout their time in the program. It should include resources such as the student handbook as well as comprehensive information about the library, support services, and technical assistance, including hours of availability and contact numbers.

An important part of the orientation to online learning is an introduction to ethical guidelines and tenets of online etiquette (Fulton, & Kellinger, 2004; Koeckeritz, Malkiewicz, & Henderson, 2002; Ryan, Carlton, & Ali, 2004; Tips, 2002). There must be a clear expectation that the views of others will be respected and responses to students and faculty will remain professional. Since control over postings on the Internet lie with the user, an explicit code of ethics can provide the framework for student decision-making without the necessity for continual oversight.

Students need the most support before a course begins and during the first two weeks of the course (Parker & Howland, 2006). They are often overwhelmed with the amount of information available to them over the Internet. A good orientation to managing the amount of time necessary to complete course work helps students to plan their time (Koeckeritz, Malkiewics, & Henderson, 2002). They must also be made aware from the outset that information on the Internet is not confidential and instruction must be provided on how to verify and evaluate the legitimacy of sources (Fulton and Kellinger, 2004). Faculty have the opportunity to act as role models in legitimizing all information posted by thoroughly documenting their sources.

Faculty Role

A climate where active learning is involved leads to more student **engagement** in online courses (Billings, 2007; Cuellar, 2002; Keockeritz, Malkiewicz, & Henderson, 2002). This environment where faculty act as facilitators but students are in control of the learning process requires vigorous participation and stimulating activities to foster continued involvement in course activities.

Clear and open communication through **engagement** and reassurance are key to helping students adapt to online learning, thus, increasing the probability of success in the course (Tips, 2002). Like all students, online students need feedback about their progress in a course. Beginning a course with a welcome email or announcement that includes directions for getting started and outlining general expectations for the course allays anxiety and initiates a connection with students. When a course first goes online, faculty must expect that additional time will be needed to assist students in logging on, navigating the **course delivery system**, or addressing technical problems with their own personal computers. Student response to the online experience can often be attributed to the preparation and attitude with which faculty respond to these initial student problems (Cuellar, 2002).

It is important to correspond frequently with students, always anticipating information students might need to proceed through their course activities. Faculty should publish their anticipated timeframe for responding to student emails and returning graded assignments. Student satisfaction with a course often wanes when prompt and appropriate individual feedback is not provided (Parker & Howland, 2006). Even though the course is online, phone calls to students to further clarify an issue or to encourage participation is an effective method for engaging students having difficulties (Britt, 2006). Faculty replies should have a caring tone and comments to students should be consistent with intended meaning (Koeckeritz, Malkiewicz, & Henderson, 2002; Moore & Hart, 2004). Faculty should always re-read their comments before sending them to students. When a pattern of student questions or problems is identified, clear and concise announcements directed at the whole class are effective in clarifying issues and allaying anxiety.

CONCLUSION

The transition of the Health Care Systems Management Program at Loyola University New Orleans to an online delivery method has been exciting and challenging. Faculty have learned from experts in the field and have developed successful strategies on their own. As the use of technology becomes increasingly important in our health care system, online education provides an avenue not only for readily accessible advanced preparation in nursing education, but for the use of technology as a primary learning tool.

REFERENCES

Ali, N. S., Hodson-Carlton, K., Ryan, M., Flowers, J., Rose, M. A., & Wayda, V. (2005). Online education: Needs assessment for faculty development. *The Journal of Continuing Education in Nursing, 36*(1), 32-38.

Allen, I. E., & Seaman, J. (2007). Online *nation: Five years of growth in online learning.* Needham, MA: Sloan Consortium.

American Association of Colleges of Nursing (1996). *Essentials of master's education.*

Retrieved December 11, 2007 from http://www.aacn.nche.edu/education/mastessn.htm.

American Association of Colleges of Nursing (1997). *Joint position statement on nursing administration education.* Retrieved December 11,

2007 from http://www.aacn.nche.edu/Publications/positions/nae.htm.

American Hospital Association (2007). The *2007 state of America's Hospitals: Taking the pulse.* Retrieved November 24, 2007 from http://www.aha.org/aha/research-and-trends/index.html

American Organization of Nurse Executives, (2005). AONE nurse executive competencies. *Nurse Leader.* February 2005, 15-21.

Baldwin, K. M., & Burns, P. G. (2004). Development and implementation of an online CNS program. *Clinical Nurse Specialist, 18*(5), 248-254.

Beitz, J. M., & Snarponis, J. A. (2006). Strategies for online teaching and learning: Lessons learned. *Nurse Educator, 31*(6), 20-25.

Billings, D. M., (2007). Optimizing distance education in nursing. *Journal of Nursing Education, 46*(6), 247-248.

Blackboard Academic Suite hardware sizing guide (2004). Retrieved November 7, 2007 from http://library.blackboard.com/docs/r6/6_1/admin/bbls_rel61_hardware_sizing_guide.pdf

Britt, R. (2006). Online education: A survey of faculty and students. *Radiologic Technology, 77*(3), 183-190.

Cuellar, N. (2002). The transition from classroom to online teaching. *Nursing Forum,37*(3), 5-13.

Diekelmann, N., & Mendias, E. P. (2005). Being a supportive presence in online courses: Knowing and connecting with students through writing. *Journal of Nursing Education, 44*(8), 344-346

Fang, D., & Wisniewski, S. W. (2007). American Association of Colleges of Nursing: Special survey of AACN membership on vacant faculty positions for academic year 2007-2008. Retrieved November 25, 2007 from http://www.aacn.nche.edu/IDS/pdf/vacancy07.pdf.

Fulton, J., & Kellinger, K. (2004). An ethics framework for nursing education on the Internet. *Nursing Education Perspectives, 25*(2), 62-66.

Green, D., & Kenyon, B. (1991). Rigidity and fragility of large socio-technical systems: Advanced information technology, the dominant coalition, and paradigm shift at the end of the 20th century. *Behavioral Science, 36*(1), 64-79.

Griffin, R. (1980). Relationships among individual, task design, and leader behavior variables. *Academy of Management Journal, 23*, 665-683.

Harris, k., Huber, D., Jones, R., Manojlovich, M., Reineck, C. (2006). Future nursing administration graduate curricula, part 1: Call to action. *Journal of Nursing Administration, 36*(10), 435-440.

Institute of Medicine (2001). *Crossing the Quality Chasm: A New Health System for the 21st century.* Washington, D C: National Academies Press.

Institute of Medicine (2003). *Health Professions Education: A Bridge to Quality,* Washington, D C: National Academies Press.

Institute of Medicine (1999). *To err is human: Building a Safer Health System.*Washington, DC: National Academies Press.

Jairath, N., & Stair, N. (2004). A development and implementation framework for Web-based nursing courses. *Nursing Education Perspectives, 25*(2), 67-72.

Jesuit Distance Education Network. (n.d.). *Competency Assessment in Distributed Education.* Retrieved November 10, 2007 from http://www.ajcunet.edu/index.aspx?sid=21.

Kenner, C., Androwich, I. M, & Edwards, P. A. (2003). Innovative educational strategies to prepare nurse executives for new leadership roles. *Nursing Administration Quarterly, 27*(2), 172-179.

Kenny, A. (2002). Online learning: Enhancing nursing education? *Journal of Advanced Nursing, 38*(2), 127-135.

Koeckeritz, J., Malkiewicz, J., & Henderson, A. (2002). The seven principles of good practice: Applications for online education in nursing. *Nurse Educator, 27*(6), 283-287.

Lee, Y., & Nguyen, H. (2007). Get your degree from an educational ATM: An empirical study in online education. *International Journal on E-Learning, 6*(1), 31-40.

Magruder,C., Burke, C., Hann, N., and Ludovic, J., (2005) Using information technology to improve the public health system. *Journal of Public Health Management Practice, 11*(2), 123-130.

Moore, P., & Hart, L. (2004). Strategies for teaching nursing research online. *International Nursing Review, 51,* 123-128.

Numerof, R., Abrams, M., & Ott, B., (2004). Building a nursing leadership infrastructure. *Nurse Leader, 2*(1), 33-37.

Parker, E. B., & Howland, L. C. (2006). Strategies to manage the time demands of online teaching. *Nurse Educator, 31*(6), 270-274.

Ryan, M., Carlton, K. H., & Ali, N. S. (2004). Reflections on the role of faculty in distance learning and changing pedagogies. *Nursing Education Perspectives, 25*(2), 73-80.

Ryan, M., Hodson-Carlton, K., & Ali, A. S. (2005). A model for faculty teaching online: Confirmation of a dimensional matrix. *Journal of Nursing Education, 44*(8), 357-365.

Skiba, D. (2007, November). Engaging students through on-line learning. Paper presented at the meeting of the American Association of Colleges of Nursing, Leadership Networks, New Orleans, LA.

Smith-Stoner, M., & Willer, M. (2003). Video streaming in nursing education: Bringing life to online education. *Nurse Educator, 28*(2), 66-70.

Tips to increase success for teaching online: Communication! (2002). *CIN Plus, 5*(1), 1, 3-4, 6.

Tumulty, G. (1980). The relationship of heal nurse role characteristics, job satisfaction and unit outcomes, Unpublished doctoral dissertation, University of Texas, Austin.

KEY TERMS

Competencies: Expressed desired results of an educational program.

E-Learning: The process of learning online.

Engagement: Active participation in learning activities.

Nursing Education: Formal educational programs to prepare individuals to enter the nursing profession or to advance their professional nursing careers.

Online Curriculum: The aggregate of courses in a web-based program of study.

Online Education: The act or process of imparting or acquiring specific knowledge through a web-based delivery system.

Online Pedagogy: The whole context of instruction, learning, and educational operations utilizing a web-based delivery system.

Socio-Technical Systems Theory: A systems perspective focused on the internal organizational processes of interdependencies and relationships, requiring both a work-relationship and a technology structure that relates humans to technology and to each other.

Teaching Strategies: Plans or methods for providing instruction.

Chapter IX
Shaping Funding Policy for Nursing Services

Virginia Plummer
Monash University, Australia

ABSTRACT

This chapter is about the major policy issue of nursing resource allocation for hospitals. Health service executives have different views about whether systems based on ratios or those based on patient dependency are more accurate. This chapter reports on a statistical analysis of almost 2 million hours of nursing data provided by 22 acute care public and private hospitals in Australia, New Zealand, and Thailand. The TrendCare informatics system was selected because it has the capacity to simultaneously measure nurse patient ratios and nursing workloads by a dependency method of nursing hours per patient day. The results showed that TrendCare predicts actual direct nursing care requirements with greater accuracy than ratios for all hospital and patient types, facilitating better allocation of nursing resources and demonstrating that the cost of nursing care would be less for hospitals using that system than for ratios. This is an important outcome for nursing informatics.

INTRODUCTION

The principal reason for admitting patients to hospital is because they require nursing care (Diers, 2004; Sovie, 1988). Nursing care is one of the most costly care items in a hospital operating budget (Hovenga, 1994; Diers, 2003) and in a policy context, accounting for nursing care should be high on the agenda for hospital managers and funding agencies. Nurses represent the largest professional group in the health care workforce in most Western economies (Diers, 2000; Cockerill,

O'Brien-Pallas, Bolley and Pink; 1993; Bennett, 1990; Sovie, 1988; Barr, 1984). Careful management of the wages and conditions of this important section of the healthcare workforce could be expected to protect an organization's clinical and financial future, especially since the outcomes of nursing work impact upon so many stakeholders. Despite the need for enhanced accountability in hospital service provision, most nurses and their managers continue to experience difficulties in accounting for & allocating nursing work.

Many health care commentators and leading health industry officials would suggest that the nurses' contribution to patient care simply cannot be measured; let alone predicted. A dearth of credible evidence for a measure or quantification of nursing care raises the question of how hospital managers are accounting for nursing in hospitals in the current economic climate of accountability and resource rationalization. The complexity of nursing resource allocation is exemplified in the following quotes which show the diametrically different views of two expert Australian nurses. *'Equitable resource allocation for the provision of hospital nursing services is dependent upon the use of valid and reliably used nursing workload monitoring systems'* (Hovenga, 1994:6), & *'Dependency systems cannot provide certainty of nurse staffing numbers, unlike nurse patient ratios which are linked to Government funding and are enforceable'* (Morieson, 2003:4). These two experts have advanced two contrasting practices for measuring and managing nursing workloads. The two practices are patient dependency systems and nurse patient ratios.

INSIGHTS INTO AN INFORMATION DEFICIT

The objective of this chapter is to illustrate the influence nurses can have on policy development and refinement in a climate of contrasting views and practices, using data and trends analysis from an Australian patient level workload informatics system. A study was designed to inform the debate about future policy directions in workforce planning. It is expected to be of interest to all stakeholders and notably to funding agencies that have established nursing policy using either of these two systems to measure and allocate nursing workloads. Examples of these policies include the introduction of mandated nurse patient ratios in Victoria (Australia's second most populated state) by the Department of Human Services (DHS), the Safe Staffing Law governing hospitals and nurse patient ratios in California, USA and a staffing by TrendCare agreement incorporated in the Enterprise Bargaining Agreements of some regional Victorian public hospitals (Plummer, 2005)..

This study was set in the policy arena of the Victorian public hospital experience where a staffing ratio law had been passed that trumped acuity based staffing. It was conducted from the perspective of an observer, attempting to understand the political and clinical landscape of mandated nurse patient ratios and was designed to shed light on a situation where policy has been established in the absence of data and the alternative was never tested. The study was grounded in nursing resource allocation and costs frameworks and is in effect a simulation of two different policy approaches. This was a correlational study of a retrospective cohort of nursing workload reports for the same patients and staff, during the same cross-sectional period of time. It was a study that will inform policy decisions on workloads.

The primary aim of the study was to examine the variation between predicted and actualized nursing care for two contemporary nursing workload allocation practices. The analysis was undertaken to determine if a correlation exists between predicted and actualized hours per patient day for mandated ratios (as in Victorian public hospitals) and/or the dependency system known as TrendCare. The analysis also examined whether each practice reliably predicts the nursing resources appropriate to the variations in patient requirements in 22 acute care hospitals in Australia, New Zealand and Thailand.

The chapter reports on a 3 year study to measure nursing services required for in-patients in acute care hospitals, for the purpose of calculating consumption and costs of nursing and the application of the study outcomes to generate a reliable costing model for Australian and international public and private hospitals. Conceptual, methodological and measurement information literacy are important aspects of the research design and interpretation of the findings (Hebda, Czar and Mascara, 2005).

NURSING AS A RESOURCE

Nursing was once considered 'invisible because it was difficult to measure' (Doncliff, 2001). Optimum nursing resource management is now known to be the essence of sound clinical and financial outcomes (Wood, 2001). Two contemporary management practices which purport to address an issue which has historically been difficult for nurse managers are examined, i.e. predicting the nursing resources appropriate to the variations in day-to-day patient requirements in acute care hospitals. These nursing resource requirements usually occur in a random pattern. The practices examined are a computerized dependency system that calculates nursing hours per patient day by various patient types and nurse patient ratios. The practices underpin key nursing resource management policies.

This policy study includes an analysis of actual acute hospital data and seeks to inform the development of knowledge for nursing resource management and the evolution of sound nursing policy. The TrendCare system was selected to facilitate this analysis because it is a computerized system which has the capacity to simultaneously measure nursing workloads through both of these practices i.e. a dependency method of nursing hours per patient day (HPPD) by various patient types and nurse patient ratios. These practices have recently been incorporated in policy and Enterprise Bargaining Agreements (EBA) in Australia and other international settings. The study is significant because it is the first empirical analysis of patient dependency and nurse patient ratio data on the same patient and staff cohort. It was designed to inform the debate about future policy directions by providing data for the first time about nursing hours in a simulation of the Victorian public hospital nurses' experience.

MEASURING AND ALLOCATING NURSING WORK

Some attempts to measure nursing work have focused on patient requirements. Others have focused on nurses' work or on the costing of nursing services or a combination of these. Over the past fifty years, a wide variety of methods, systems and technologies have been developed at local and international levels. Nursing workload measurement systems are known as nurse dependency, patient dependency, patient classification, nursing acuity systems or patient dependency systems. The meanings and definitions of these terms vary to some extent, however each measurement system attempts to measure nursing work. In this chapter, 'patient dependency system' is used when such systems are referred to, including TrendCare.

Patient dependency systems measure the nursing resources required for the care of a given classification of patient types. Different patient types occur in various ways, such as by medical or nursing diagnoses, length of stay or severity of illness. For introductory purposes, the concepts of high and low patient dependency can be explained by variations in patient requirements for nursing care. Patients with high dependency have complex or extensive care needs and may require care for long periods of time and often by nurses with high skill levels. In contrast, patients with low dependency have less extensive or less complex care needs, and may require less nursing time and/or nurses with less specialised skills.

Patient dependency systems were commonly used for predicting nursing care requirements and contemporary systems now enable nurses to update or 'actualize' the record to include the care actually provided. This ability to actualize provides nurses with the opportunity to analyse and address the variance between predicted and actualized care. In the past, prediction-only systems were often paper-based. Hospital managers generally ignored them and preferred to operate with the indicator of 'wages paid' in an equivalent historical period. In other words, managers compared the payrolls of a ward or unit rather than the care requirements of patient types or the workload of nurses (Plummer, 12005)..

As an indicator of nursing activity this method is often flawed. The wages paid could have been considerably higher than required. They could be higher in a ward with a majority of patients with a low dependency or where there is an unplanned reduction in occupancy i.e., a number of discharges and no admissions after the commencement of a shift. Equally, the wages paid could be considerably lower than required, as in a ward with a majority of high dependency patients or in wards that experience severe shortages where not enough nurses are available to meet predicted needs. Nursing shortages are of world wide concern, especially in rural areas. Prolonged shortages of nurses would establish a pattern of lower payrolls (Diers, 2003).. The payrolls would reflect the reality of sub-optimal nursing levels, yet hospital managers continue to use them as the cornerstone for fiscal planning for future financial periods. These future periods would forseeably include increased patient dependency associated with an ageing population and a growth in demand for acute services with subsequent limitations on the availability of convalescent care in acute hospitals. In short, retrospective data that is based on inadequate staffing levels is still commonly used to determine the prospective nursing care requirements of patients (Diers, 2003).

Hospital managers, who used the patient dependency system data, would often over-ride the results of the measurements by nurses. In response to this practice, nurses sometimes 'fudged' the data, especially when data input time was limited or there was a perceived unfairness in workload. Data fudging, or up scaling, is used to classify patients at a higher dependency level than would be expected, in order to increase nursing resources and ease a poorly defined workload. The practice may occur either deliberately or incidentally. An example of incidental up-scaling may be where higher than expected dependency levels are perceived for patients cared for by overloaded, inefficient or junior nurses. The nurses know they are busy yet the measurement system fails to demonstrate that satisfactorily. Up-scaling is most common in settings where budget cuts are customary and where associated policy has been implemented without consultation (Diers, 2003). Such policy, for example, could be the reduction of nursing hours by 10% across the hospital or on public holidays or towards the end of the financial year. Up-scaling is also common where the patient dependency system has little or no credibility with hospital managers, accountants or nurses and serves no major function.

Many nurse managers consult their nursing team but continue to allocate nursing resources using what Finnigan, Abel, Dobler, Hudon and Terry (1993) describe as the 'gut override' or an intuitive approach. Essentially, these managers continued to rely on experience as a way of harnessing nursing resources with varying degrees of success. Sometimes this method can be accurate, though it is lacking in a scientific approach and struggles to achieve credibility with hospital finance managers. Clearly, nurses need empirical data for decision-support for their expert opinion, which will legitimately continue to be the predominant workload management tool.

Emerging technologies are now available to record patient dependency and nursing workloads in a way which is increasingly valid, reliable, retrievable and comparable for nurses and their managers. Important enhancements include incorporating the capacity to actualize care requirements, in addition to those predicted, together with the ability to predict and actualize the nursing skill mix. The nursing skill mix is the number, qualifications, experience, competencies and efficiencies of rostered nurses. If information on the trends and variances in patient dependency can be linked appropriately to nursing services, then managers may be able to more accurately predict nursing resource requirements both in nursing time and skill mix. Enhanced accuracy of prediction of nursing resource requirements, according to variations in patient type, has some significant advantages when compared to the inflexibility of allocation in accordance with historically similar periods such as monthly nursing payrolls or bed occupancy levels. These advantages are;

- Patients receive their fair share of nursing according to clinical need;
- Nurses are allocated a fair share of the work; and
- Funders or payers receive what they paid for.

An optimum match of nursing resources to patient requirements facilitates sound management of one of the most costly care items in the hospital operating budget. The ability to predict this match with a high degree of reliability is essential under prospective payment systems (PPS) of contemporary casemix funding environments.

PER DIEM TRADITIONS, DATA MINING AND CASEMIX

For many years nursing resource requirements have been predicted by hospital managers who have calculated an estimate on a per diem basis, using retrospective information such as ‘wages paid’ and ‘occupied bed days’ from previous years. Nursing resource requirements per patient were calculated by dividing the wages of the total staff resources of the nursing unit over each year, by the total number of occupied bed days. This calculation was referred to as the daily or ‘per diem’ cost for nursing. However, wages paid in the calculation is an entirely different concept to that of nursing resources measurement since it is a reflection of payment for the nurses who actually ‘turned up for work’ rather than the nurses who were required. As already discussed, in some cases the wages will be higher and in others it will be lower than required. In any case the wages are likely to have been an unreliable estimation of nurse staffing and do not reflect actual nursing care requirements.

The per diem estimate calculates each nurse’s working day as though patients had similar requirements and required similar resources. Per diem thus implies the same costs were incurred. Whilst this may be a reasonable assumption for accounting purposes, nurses know that patient dependency varies significantly and that resources must vary according to the level of care to be provided and skill mix of staff available. Most hospitals continue to use the ‘per diem’ method for estimating nursing resource requirements which is usually based on the patient census at midnight. The census is the denominator in per diem calculations, purporting to reflect the number of patients in the ward. It is often the number of inpatients at midnight but this fails to reflect the true number of patients cared for in the previous 24 hours period and the dependency of those patients. The true number of patients would additionally include same day admissions and separations.

The absence of a reliable and universally accepted method of allocating nursing resources means that the resources continue to be approximated by local and international funding agencies with little input from nurses delivering the care. Nurses and hospital managers know that the per diem method is flawed because all patient days do not have similar nursing resource requirements.

Patient dependency and nursing care requirements, can vary significantly vary from shift to shift, ward to ward, hospital to hospital and year to year (Gillet, 2001). As a result of such variance, nursing resource allocation is often inadequately linked to an organizational financial framework (Finnigan et al, 1993) Further; nursing resource allocation is poorly integrated with other hospital information systems (Goossen, 2000; Diers, 1999).

The implementation of prospective payment systems (PPS) in the USA during the early 1980s brought attempts to measure nursing resource requirements prospectively, although to date the payment rate remains prospectively based on retrospective casemix data. Prospective payment systems were introduced into Australia and New Zealand during the 1990s. Data mining conducted by the Victorian Department of Human Services (DHS) on estimating nursing resource weights for diagnosis related group (DRG) casemix classifications established that nursing resources significantly varied between hospitals, for the same DRG (Gillett, 2001). Private health insurers conducted similar comparative studies. Data showing variations in patient dependency within or between DRGs or between hospitals had not been available until that time. Researchers at the DHS suspected that DRGs may be generally resource homogenous in terms of length of stay (LOS) but nursing heterogeneous (Gillett, 2001). Picone, Phillips, Hathaway and Parkes (1993) observe that the outcome of research on nursing resource weights by DRG is that they are limited in many respects, since DRGs do not:

- Fully describe actual work done by nurses;
- Recognise the complexity of care for patient co-morbidities for example obesity and dementia;
- Recognise different or changing environments for example pre-admission clinics;
- Acknowledge the patients' contribution to their own care, or lack of contribution for example compliance with physiotherapy exercises or conversely continuing to smoke during respiratory illness.

Diers (1992:139) sums this up by observing that '*DRGs provided a way to pay for care that was defined by what patients need, rather than what was done for them.*'

Nursing dependency systems of the past were paper-based and often without permanency within the patient record. While it seems extraordinary now, it was then common practice to record in pencil to facilitate erasure for the next shift. The nursing dependency records formed no part of the medical record, or the financial reports, and were eventually stored away in an office for many years before disposal, neither informing any one or in any retrievable state should access to the data be requested. Some research has been published on the Australian experience to provide dependency-based costing information for nursing services (Hovenga, 1983; Picone et al, 1993). However, we now have the technology to mine financial and clinical data to provide integrated information by DRG or other methods which best measure patient dependency and the management of nursing resources in casemix and other environments.

AN AUSTRALIAN SYSTEM

An example of this technology is the Australian TrendCare system. It is the most widely used method of providing nursing resource information in public and private hospitals in Australia, New Zealand, Thailand and Singapore. The system captures both clinical and non-clinical data and records nursing information in two ways, by nurse patient ratio and by hours per patient day. Nurses at over 100 sites routinely collect data on each patient on each shift and reports can be generated for use at the ward or operational level and for research. The system includes comprehensive variance tracking and reporting and all reports have print-preview ability. These report features have been essential elements of the data collection methodology.

The system measures the nursing time required to care for specific patient types and for specific dependency categories. There are approximately 60 different patient types including for example surgical, paediatric oncology, forensic mental health, medical high dependency, maternity and cardiac patients and this number is constantly under review in response to user feedback. There are up to 6 categories of dependency, depending on the patient type or category and which are calculated by the system for day, evening and night shifts. The category level timings for patients include every aspect of nursing care for that patient for each shift. These aspects of care are known as 'indicators' See left hand yellow highlighted column in Figure 1 to follow

The base line hours for each patient type are the Category 1 hours. These hours give an average time allowance for a patient who is generally independent in activities of daily living (ADLs). Category 1 average time allowance also includes nursing time for documentation, patient inquiries, doctor's rounds, simple medications, simple treatments, routine teaching and counselling for patients and relatives (under 30 minutes), general care and attention. See Figure 2 on the next page.

The system will allocate a higher category when more complex care requirements with higher timings are recorded following prediction or actualization, according to prescribed indicators. The timings allocated for the prescribed indicators in TrendCare, vary between patient types. For example, the indicator 'mobility' will have less time allocated for care of day surgery patient types than mobility for rehabilitation patient types. Expert TrendCare hospital sites validate these timings at least every two to three years.

The system has the capacity to provide comprehensive empirical data on nursing workflow processes to develop accurate nursing cost weights for specific Diagnosis Related Groups (DRGs). TrendCare data can be linked to ICD-10 and DRG data, collected in hospitals, through its Patient Master Index (PMI) and is HL7 compliant. The development of HL7 interfaces, within TrendCare, to other hospital systems enables a seamless transfer of patient information from hospital information systems, such as theatre bookings or payroll, into the TrendCare System. Patient

Figure 1: Example of indicators for analysis of requirements using TrendCare

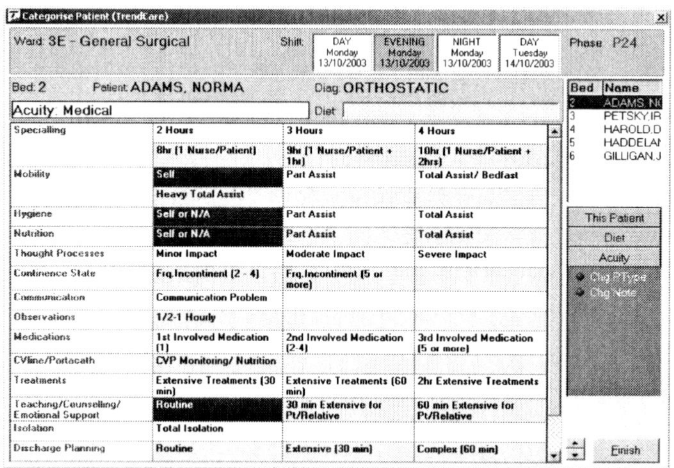

Figure 2. Patient category and care timings in TrendCare (simulation)

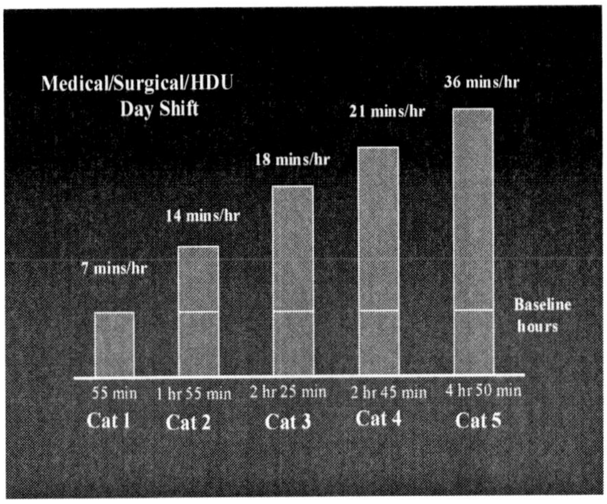

details are automatically updated from PMI via HL7 messaging on admission and after a change in compulsory fields.. The system provides a variety of data export capabilities for clinical costing and DRG analysis (TrendCare, 2008).

Both predicted and actual nursing care requirements for acute in-patient care are recorded in TrendCare and work allocation by the Nurse Unit Manager is based on decisions about the variables of nursing time and nursing skill mix. The system provides managers with present time patient dependency data for decision support. It measures patient dependency and predicts the nursing hours required. TrendCare also records care actually provided to individual patients on each shift. It provides data which can be used by hospitals preparing to develop dependency based budgets, re-engineer rosters, measure nursing resources for specific episodes of care, track variances and patient outcomes, and distribute equitable nursing workloads (TrendCare Systems Pty Ltd,. Training Manual 2007).

RATIOS

Where data are ignored by hospital managers on the basis of poor quality or quantity, patients and nurses perceive themselves to be at risk of unfair workloads. When nurses perceive that their workloads are unfair, patient care may be compromised, potentially affecting patient outcomes. Nurses also become dissatisfied with their working conditions and in Victoria they have been proactive in lobbying governments for workloads that are manageable and fair. In response to this lobbying and industrial action on pay and conditions by nurses, Commissioner Blair recommended a review of nursing workload conditions in the August 2001 Public Sector Agreement (Blair,2001; Watson, 2001). Under the terms of the Agreement and in an effort to increase the retention of nurses in the Victorian public hospital sector, the Victorian State Government in 2001 introduced mandated nurse patient ratios and also conducted a pilot of a dependency system in 20 Victorian hospitals in 2003.

The dependency system agreed upon was the TrendCare system since it was already implemented in 14 of the 74 Victorian public hospitals (the highest number with a common system) and was highly regarded within the industry. The decision to pilot TrendCare was part of a three-year agreement between the Victorian State Government, the Australian Nursing Federation (ANF) Victorian Branch and the Victorian Hospitals Industrial Association (VHIA).

The ratios were minimum levels and additional nurses were to be rostered for patients of higher dependency. Data on patient dependency would seem to be essential, even in this negotiated and 'controlled' ratio environment, however the ANF remains opposed to the use of dependency systems. A history of nurses inadequately accounting for nursing work and management overriding the results of dependency reports, would account for this opposition. The introduction of nurse patient ratios in Victorian public hospitals was a world first. Mandated ratios are employed in relatively few locations elsewhere in the world.

RESEARCH DESIGN AND RESULTS

The research involved empirical testing of the two practices, using correlation, to test the hypothesis that both ratios and TrendCare can predict a fair allocation of nursing resources to patients, since they were both designed to do this, but that TrendCare predicts with greater accuracy as it has more detailed data inputs. A detailed analysis of 103, 269 valid shifts of care that represented 1,998,902 nursing hours showed that TrendCare predicts a fair allocation of nursing resources to patients. The study conducted by Plummer (2005) is proof of concept for the application study as it established the accuracy of TrendCare for measuring nursing work and the reliability and validity of the TrendCar*e* database for sophisticated cost analysis.

In summary, the study limitations which mattered were limitations to ratio practices which would be expected to decrease the accuracy of prediction of care requirements and increase the cost of care using ratios, further than that reported in the results, if the hospitals were located in Victoria. These variations could be quantified with further analysis of the same data in future studies

The key findings in this study were:

- Both ratios and TrendCare showed a high correlation between the hours of care predicted by each practice and the care actually provided;
- There is a higher correlation between TrendCare predicted hours and actualized hours than for ratios for each hospital level, for both public and private hospitals, for all patient type categories, for day, evening and night shifts. There is no category of variable where ratios have a higher correlation than TrendCare; an example is shown for a patient category group in Figure 3 below where there is a close correlation for TrendCare illustrated by a slim 'cigar-shaped' pattern at 45 degrees on the right.
- TrendCare predicts more of the variability than ratios for each hospital level, public and private hospitals, for Australian and New Zealand hospitals, metropolitan and rural hospitals, all patient type categories and morning, evening and night shift, with 95% confidence intervals. There is no category of variable where ratios predict more of the variability than TrendCare;
- Actual HPPD decreases as occupancy increases. This means that TrendCare users become more efficient as occupancy

Figure 3. Correlation between predicted and actualized hours, by shift, for adult, non-critical care, non-med/surg patient types, by Victorian mandated nurse patient ratios (left) and by TrendCare (right)

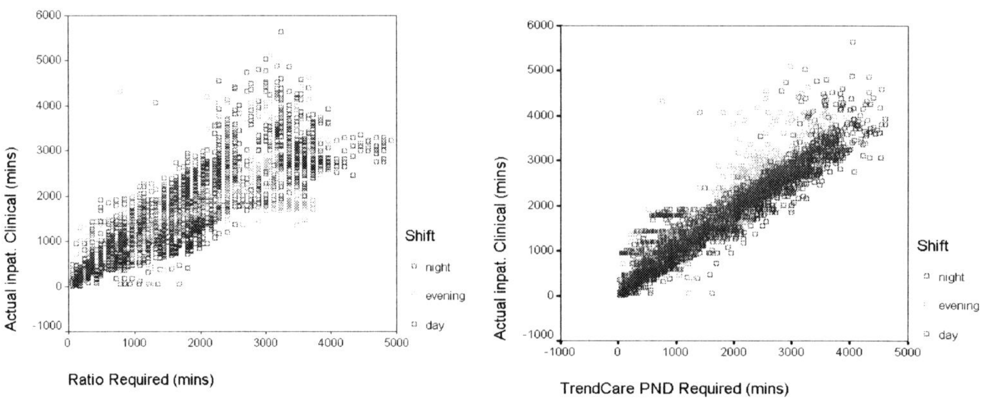

increases. In Victorian public hospitals and in Thai private hospitals, more nurses are rostered as occupancy increases. Ratio practices are likely to be less efficient in use of resources as occupancy increases;

- Mean actual hours are higher for metropolitan hospitals than rural. This means that metropolitan and rural hospitals of the same level may be allocated the same ratios under Victorian mandated ratio rules, but have significantly different patient requirements in wards and shifts of the same type;
- Mean actual hours is higher for level 2 hospitals than for level 1 hospitals (larger hospitals). This result may be due in part to lower occupancy in level 2 hospitals but that could not be analyzed on the data available. This means that level 2 hospitals may be disadvantaged under Victorian mandated ratio rules where level 1 hospitals attract lower nurse patient ratios.
- Ratios predict less of the variability in the majority of the shift types for which they were they were designed, than for other shift types i.e. shifts in Australian, public metropolitan, level 1 hospitals, in medical/surgical wards for morning shifts. This means that, as well as for the ward and shift type variables, TrendCare predicts more of the variability in Australian public hospitals. Therefore TrendCare is also likely to predict more of the variability in Victorian public hospitals. This means that ratios perform least well, not only in the settings for which they were designed, but also in the settings in which they are most popular. This suggest that the popularity with ratios may not be the accuracy, but other factors such as the legal enforceability of the practice ensuring that staffing cannot be manipulated by hospital managers without agreed process. Another factor may be the relatively higher cost of ratios compared to the actual cost of care. This suggests that at least some nurses are being paid for more work than they do. The popularity would arise from the satisfaction of the majority of nurses. Most nurses would be employed in level 1 hospitals which have lower ratios than level 2 hospitals despite having a lower mean HPPD.
- TrendCare under predicts the costs of the actual hours of care by about as much as ratios over predicts those costs. This demonstrates that the cost of nursing care would be less for hospitals using TrendCare than for ratios. The over prediction by ratios is likely to be higher in Victorian public hospitals due to the reasons described earlier about limitations to the interpretation of the costing analysis results. This means that the actual cost of nursing care by ratios is likely to be higher in Victoria than anywhere else in Australia. Multiple costing scenarios were analyzed, see an example in Table 1.

The most important interpretation of the cost analysis is as follows; the provision of nursing care at lower cost using a dependency system rather than ratios, can be organized to meet patient requirements by using less nursing hours and better management of the allocation of hours and skill mix. This is an important outcome for the costs of care and for distribution of the limited nursing resources experienced by most countries in a worldwide shortage of working nurses.

Other findings are:

- Mean actual hours of care are highest for Thailand and lowest for Australia.
- The patient type category with both the lowest mean actual hours and standard deviation is ante/post natal;
- The patient type category with both the highest mean actual hours and standard deviation is non-adult critical care.

The results also revealed that some anticipated associated results were not supported in

Table 1. Cost analysis - all hospitals, all shifts by patient type category

Patient Type Category		N	Sum	Mean	Std. Deviation	Total Cost
Medical/Surgical	Actual inpatient hours	63363	1279878.05	20.1991	18.45949	$51,195,122
	TrendCare predicted hours	63363	1283228.98	20.2520	19.90268	$51,329,159
	Ratio predicted hours	63363	1360295.40	21.4683	20.37116	$54,411,816
Paediatric	Actual inpatient hours	7209	118770.15	16.4753	13.69405	$4,750,806
	TrendCare predicted hours	7209	112598.27	15.6191	14.80118	$4,503,931
	Ratio predicted hours	7209	95865.87	13.2981	12.39210	$3,834,635
Ante/Post Natal	Actual inpatient hours	15197	234189.23	15.4102	13.37345	$9,367,569
	TrendCare predicted hours	15197	207556.28	13.6577	14.27377	$8,302,251
	Ratio predicted hours	15197	176592.10	11.6202	12.34282	$7,063,684
Adult Critical Care	Actual inpatient hours	9319	223229.87	23.9543	17.88241	$8,929,195
	TrendCare predicted hours	9319	225356.83	24.1825	19.64746	$9,014,273
	Ratio predicted hours	9319	263585.88	28.2848	24.19768	$10,543,435
Non-Adult Critical Care	Actual inpatient hours	1431	47746.48	33.3658	28.50000	$1,909,859
	TrendCare predicted hours	1431	47417.85	33.1362	28.21746	$1,896,714
	Ratio predicted hours	1431	30112.08	21.0427	26.08304	$1,204,483
Other	Actual inpatient hours	6750	147235.45	21.8127	16.47870	$5,889,418
	TrendCare predicted hours	6750	143042.08	21.1914	17.74230	$5,721,683
	Ratio predicted hours	6750	161633.70	23.9457	18.62731	$6,465,348

the data, although of a lower order than those which fulfilled the research aim. The data did not show more variability in actualized hours for hospitals where there are dynamic departments which influence the peaks and troughs of activity levels throughout those hospitals; for example, departments such as delivery suites or accident and emergency departments. The data also did not demonstrate more variability for smaller hospitals where the peaks of actualized care are less able to be provided for by the recruitment of indirect care staff mid shift as would be available to larger hospitals: for example, the mid-shift recruitment of the night nurse supervisor, clinical teachers or nurse quality managers. Indirect care staff is more readily available in larger hospitals. They may also be more readily available in the not for profit sector, but this was outside the scope of the study. Finally the data did not show more variability in public hospitals rather than private hospitals despite the trend of latter hospital type to be procedural, i.e. surgical. Public hospitals tend to be medical, 69.7% of separations are for medical DRGs in 2001 compared to 36.3% in the private sector (Dept of Health and Ageing, 2003:10, 11). It was anticipated that a predominance of surgical wards would account for less variability for an individual hospital but this was not demonstrated.

What the data didn't show also supports the argument that the greatest influences on the acuity and variability of patient requirements are not hospital type or size. Hospital size, or level, and occupancy are key features of the ratio formula and both have been found to be unrelated to acuity and variability of patient requirements. The theoretical framework underpinning the development, use and implementation of ratios is the concept of fair and equitable workloads for nurses achieved by the allocation of an *equivalent number of patients per nurse*. The theoretical framework underpinning the development, use and implementation of patient dependency systems is to assign the *right nursing resources to the right patient.*

A NEW UNDERSTANDING

The results have offered a new understanding of patient dependency and workload allocation. They have revealed a greater than expected difference between the frequencies of ward type and patient type categories. This demonstrated that the label associated with ward type does not accurately capture the range of nursing care requirements of the range of patient types admitted to those wards. The frequency by ward type reveals that 83% of the sample was shifts for medical/surgical wards. This leaves only 17% of ward types which have an alternative ratio formula. By contrast medical/surgical patient types account for just 63% of the shifts. That means that 20% of patients in medical/surgical wards, by ratio rules, have another patient type classification in TrendCare. This significant proportion of patients is likely to have different requirements to medical/surgical patients and may be allocated different ratios if they were accommodated in another ward type.

Ratio allocation by ward types also does not adequately capture the range of requirements for several other patient types. For example low acuity medical patients are allocated the same ratios as high dependency surgical patients, antenatal patients who are essentially self care are allocated the same ratios as postnatal mothers and babies and there are no psychiatric or paediatric ratios. In the current environment of bed shortages and limited bed access, there are likely to be many wards and departments experiencing a mix of patient types, as beds are allocated on a priority basis, regardless of whether their accepting unit attends that ward. See Figure 4. Think about how a system based on ratios by ward type would be flawed if it was applied in this example.

In general ratios are reliable and useful where there is no alternative and have been one factor in the recruitment of additional nursing staff in Victoria and California. It would also be reasonable to assume that as length of stay decreases, there may be more homogeneity in nursing care but at higher levels of patient acuity. This means that ratios may have a place, at least for same day cases. While it is true that same day cases have risen from 30.6% in 1991 to 50.6% in 2001 (Dept of Health and Ageing, 2003:10, 11), the acuity of those same day patients may continue to remain highly variable despite their short stay. Ratio practices would require the support of dependency to determine that homogeneity, or lack of it.

Nurses need to understand their work and they need to record it in a retrievable format to participate fully at the policy table. Nurses need the information and knowledge to advocate for patients so that they receive their fair share of nursing and to negotiate their wages and conditions including fair and equitable workloads. Payers also need to receive what they paid for. It is reasonable to assume that many payers (outside Victoria at least) are getting more than they pay for. At the opening of the Asia Pacific nursing Congress in Sydney in November 2004, Australian Federal Health Tony Abbott praised Australia's nurses

Figure 4. Ward acuity by HPPD

Ward Acuity HPPD per Patient Type

Printed: 30/03/2004 11:12:29 AM

Ward: **Ward 3 East**
Month: **May, 2003**

Patient Type		Average Patient Days	Required Clinical Hours	Part Specialled Hours	Required Clinical HPPD
HDS	High Dependency - Surgical	26.33	252.04	4.00	9.57
	- Specialled	0.67	16.00		24.00
MED	Medical	250.00	988.12	5.00	3.95
	- Specialled	0.33	8.00		24.00
PCU	Palliative Care	11.00	67.67		6.15
SHM	Short Stay - Medical	5.33	16.08		3.02
SHS	Short Stay - Surgical	54.33	185.42		3.41
SUR	Surgical	477.33	2033.03	7.00	4.26
	TOTALS:	825.33	3566.36	16.00	4.32

(and doctors) after his one and only first hand experience of nursing, after admission to hospital during the 2004 Federal election campaign. He said that *'sometimes we in government tax and try that on-going commitment and idealism'* (Arlington, 2004). He observed that nurses are central to the heath system but the wages and conditions have resulted in approximately 23,000 qualified nurses not working nationally and 20% of nursing students leave the profession one year after graduating. While it is heartening that the health minister now has a new understanding of patient dependency and workload allocation for nursing, it was prompted by a kidney stone and not strategic inquiry within a policy framework. Nurses must continue to actively research and develop tangible and timely information for policy makers.

In Australia we have a vast amount of expertise in data management and data analysis in the health system. We have a national minimum data set, national coding standards, and standard chart of accounts, national diagnosis, and procedure and DRG classification system and on-going monitoring and analysis by commonwealth and state health departments, the Australian Institute of Health and Welfare, the Australian Bureau of Statistics, the Commonwealth Department of Veteran's Affairs, various compensation and insurance organizations, the Health Insurance Commission and the Private Health Insurance Administrative Council. There is little to support nursing, the reason people are admitted to hospital and central to the operations of hospitals. So those accountable for managing the budgets of the nation's hospitals have few details other than wages paid, to quantify nursing care in acute hospitals.

Prior to this study, data showing variations in patient acuity and dependency was not routinely available for comparison, because nursing care is not coded and often not directly comparable for workload or cost analysis. The system quantifies uncertainty and makes nursing visible and accountable for nurses and other consumers. It provides an opportunity to re-develop trust between management and nurses, supported by data rather than inflexible legislation. The mandated aspect of ratios has been an overriding factor of their success, rather than the ratios themselves. Yet, staffing by dependency system also works well for some EBAs i.e. Djerriwah, Colac and Hamilton public hospitals in Victoria. Buchan summarized the situation very well when he said 'R*atios are a blunt instrument for achieving employer compliance, where reliance on alter-*

native, voluntary (and often more sophisticated) methods of determining nurse staffing have not been effective' (2004:3).

TECHNOLOGY, AN ESSENTIAL POLICY PARTNER

As a result of this research, there is now a whole new way of looking at things; a new understanding of our ability to predict actual hours of care and better provide for patients nurses and payers. We can provide the data that removes the need for ratios. Where it was difficult to account for and allocate nursing work in the past, it's now easy, accurate and better understood using the visibility provided by TrendCare and probably similar systems in the future. The information means that we can also better manage where there are not enough nurses or where there is a skills shortage. This information will also enhance our ability to develop establishing trends in conversion of clinical documentation into dependency classifications and shape associated policy.

We now know, as a result of the research, that there is a need to determine the acuity of the patients, not simply the numbers of patients to determine dependency. We also know that the acuity of patients is not affected by the location, type or size of the hospital. For example, the acuity of a patient requiring post-operative care post prostatectomy, with no other complications, co-morbidities or age factors, is the same in a level 3 rural hospital in New Zealand as for a level 2 metropolitan hospital in Australia. The variables are captured in the indicators in TrendCare. Ratios which are dependent on patient numbers and hospital size or level make no sense.

Patient dependency systems provide decision support and provide the option for overruling the predictions by clinical judgment. Fixed ratios dampen the notion of decision support. Where some ratio flexibility has been introduced, documentation or justification of the rounding to ensure patient care is not compromised, is still not required. The clinical judgment used in partnership with patient dependency systems can flow on to contribute to up-dated indicator timings. Timings in TrendCare are up-dated on this basis in addition to formal timing studies every 2-3 years.

When patient dependency is understood, the patient requirements can be matched with the skills and competencies and preferences of the nursing team. For example, Nurse Managers may choose to allocate 7.5 hours to each graduate nurse and 8 hours to each experienced nurse on the same shift. Nurse Managers can ensure that graduate nurses do not run on negative variances but may decide that experienced nurses can. Unpredicted and unproductive care allowances can be adjusted to suit the mix of patients and staff. Matching the dual requirements of the patients and the nurses takes patient dependency and workload allocation to the next step. It is not just about nurses' workloads and unreliable mathematical equations which are the focus of mandated nurse patient ratio systems. It is about matching the right patient to the right nurse, who will be paid the right amount of money for that care and about nurses feeling valued, not like numbers in an equation. Some strong conclusions have been drawn from the research and may be applied to other settings, including Victoria. The results are on a limited sample but it is appropriate to extrapolate to all in the same population in the future. The results show that we are now able to predict reasonably well using either practice. What really matters is what should be allocated and what should be paid. If we can filter out where both practices are equally successful in predicting care requirements, we can concentrate on identifying the characteristics of those extreme cases. This will enable better management of the shifts for which ratios are not hitting the mark, resulting perhaps in dependency driven ratios in the future.

Beat observed that the old system of determining departmental staffing levels purely on the number of beds occupied had no place in modern management technique. She asked, '*How can a matron convince a group of lay people that a certain number of nurses are required for her hospital? How can she convince the medical staff that her nurses can no longer cope with further admissions? How could all this information be recorded and be put forward in a graph form so that anyone looking at it, either professional or lay could understand what he saw*' (1970:1)? And 38 years later we now have the graphs, so that a lay person, or even a health minister, can understand that nurses can now predict their work with high levels of accuracy, regardless of the variables, and they have the data to rightfully take their place at the policy table.

The 2004-2007 EBA for nurses in Victorian public hospitals included provision for ratio variation according to the clinical assessment of patient needs, environmental demands such as ward layout, occupational health and safety, workloads and occupancy. The current EBA includes provision for the use of dependency systems, weighted in-lier equivalent separations (WIES), skill mix, DRGs, separations or LOS to determine these variations. Short shift provision has been re-introduced, which is an indicator of acknowledgement of peaks and troughs in workload by the ANF. The DHS has conducted a series of meetings with managers of Victorian public hospitals since the agreement was finalised and advised that ratios such as 1:4 can be averaged over 4 week roster period, e.g. 1:6 on Sunday or Public Holiday and 1:3.5 on 'post–op' mornings. It would be reasonable to suggest that TrendCare was used by DHS and hospitals to negotiate this. This means that the ratios are no longer rigidly fixed, but how do nurses in Victorian public hospitals determine the variable ratios, or record and track them? Will the last of the 4 weeks be unfairly 'ratioed' if that is the balance after 3 busy weeks or poor allocation practices? Will nurses make arbitrary decisions or use another system to achieve new ratio mixes within the 4 week averaging rule? Mandated ratio practices in Victoria have now adopted some of the features of dependency systems and will probably need a dependency system to support decisions made within it. Perhaps it is now easier to 'game' a ratio system than TrendCare.

The increasing frequency of high dependency type patients has many implications for acute care nursing. Higher numbers of high dependency patients is associated with advances in complex medicine and surgery, the increasing age of patients, higher levels of co-morbidities and risk of complications, shorter LOS and the trend is likely to be sustained. Higher dependency nursing such as that provided in high dependency units (HDU), special care nurseries (SCN) and dialysis, are highly resource intensive. This means that more nurses with specialized skills will be required to care for the same number of patients in the future. The limited beds available in these units means that many patients who cannot be accommodated will increasingly be accommodated on general wards. Accordingly, there will also be higher demand for more nurses with specialized skills for the general wards. The care of older Australians and other influences such as defensive medicine, advances in technology and communications, delayed discharge for non-acute medical reasons, and the declining health of indigenous populations are further examples of impending nursing demand. The future demand for nursing is expected to be compounded by a decreased capacity to provide the nurses required. This combination of circumstances demands strong and informed nursing leadership, to manage the working conditions and the distribution of current and future nursing resources.

What it means for nursing is that we must go beyond ratios and analyzing data and link workload allocation practices to clinical pathways, skill mix, variance analysis, clinical indicators, patient outcomes and population based care in the future. We must illuminate the key concepts of acuity, dependency and workload allocation, so that we can move onto bigger agendas such as realistic nursing budgets and the achievement of sound financial and clinical outcomes within the context of existing government policy. Nurse dependency systems can provide the rudder for future policy direction.

ON-GOING RESEARH DIRECTIONS

The future is funding policy for quality. This is a welcome rebound from the financial focus of the formative casemix years in Australia, which purported to address many of the past efficiencies. I argue that efficiencies in nursing were gained by stealth since there was little reliable information to do otherwise. Nurses now have access to that information and can realistically focus on quality outcomes and associated funding issues. Quality outcomes require integrated, co-coordinated and reliable data. Success in the industrial relations setting does not equate to quality nursing care. Nursing cannot stand alone and claim that there is no need to record data for acuity, dependency or workload purposes because mandated nurse patient ratios have been successfully re-negotiated. Nurses know they need to record data about their work and interface with the care systems of the rest of the multi-disciplinary team. They also know they need to provide documented publicly accountable quality care. Securing fair workloads by arbitration was a logical first step and moved hospital managements 'off the case', so that nurses could re-establish control of their working conditions. With that control secured, it is now time to return to the quality agenda and research is an integral part of the process.

It is clear that nursing requirements can now be predicted with a high level of accuracy and that this can be provided more equitably and at lower cost using a dependency system rather than ratios. Nursing in acute hospitals is influenced significantly by funding policy. The challenge for nurses is to steer that policy. The researcher proposes a shift from maintaining and supporting a centralized policy based on prescribed ratios, towards a decentralized policy of staffing to demand, which is now possible using systems as described in this chapter. The consequences are considerable, including change to the amount of government and ANF control and a threat to workload equity for nurses between wards and between hospitals. These are significant hurdles.

The cost analysis was the first reasonable estimate of a comparison between the two practices using routinely collected data. On-going analysis of this type of data, rather than ad hoc trials, will establish a database for routine and more sophisticated cost and clinical analyses. The use of live data also enhances the ability to predict accurately. Reliable nursing cost data needs to be linked by DRG to the financial systems for costing and budgeting.

Unfortunately, Victorian public hospitals are still funded for nursing costs which are reported inclusive of ward nursing, ward consumables, ward catering, patient transport as well as direct care (Clinical Costing Standards of Australia CCS 2 version:10.9). All Victorian public hospitals report nursing and are funded in this way under the standard chart of accounts which was effective from 1 July 2004. Reliable nursing cost data cannot be buried in ancillary costs and retain it's newly identified high levels of predictability.

Australian and New Zealand governments' model acute care costs by DRG unit level but they are not a nursing classification by definition. There is no reason why we can't measure according to smaller or more nursing appropriate units, for example, shifts of care as undertaken in this study. On-going research in interfacing nursing costs by dependency of shift of care to the DRG financial systems is highly recommended

The Commonwealth Government acknowledges that there is no hard evidence about acuity of care and is planning future research in this area. The government is considering the inclusion of predominantly nursing procedures in the ICD-10 classification. (Dept of Health and Ageing,

2003:93). This will begin building the pathway to coding, costing and accounting for nursing more precisely at the federal level. It is recommended that future research is planned for interfacing clinical pathways and dependency reports to identify trends, frequencies and the capacity to code nursing procedures and practices.

CONCLUSION

Ratios had their place in rescuing failing health systems in Victoria and California; they were simple, inexpensive and required no training or technology.

This was the first international empirical study, of the world first introduction to mandated nurse patient ratios in Victorian public hospitals and experience has been established for future studies in this area. The Victorian model is fair for ratios but there are differences in some areas and TrendCare is better able to predict those differences. The findings also concluded that TrendCare can provide fairer and more equitable workloads, and at lower cost, than the Victorian mandated nurse patient ratios. Although expressed differently, ratios and HPPD essentially mean the same thing. They are both about averages by categories. We need to review the way we use them and focus on developing policy based on co-operative relationship between the two practices. For example, in Victoria, the future may include negotiated ratios based on the data provided by dependency HPPD.

One of the most important innovations from this research will be the releasing of hospital costing from the current crippling definition of nursing costs using wages paid and replacing it with accurate data on the demand for nursing from a computerized nursing workload informatics system. The data will arise from the real time nursing care provided to actual patients using TrendCare or similar systems which interfaces with all other hospitals systems at administrative and clinical levels. The increased ability to predict patient requirements accurately, in an environment with a corresponding decrease in ability to actually provide for those requirements, complicates the landscape for nursing resource management. However, long term management solutions for the shortage of nurses remain in the policy area (Diers, 2004).

ACKNOWLEDGMENT

TrendCare: Permission to use the trademark within the manuscript has been provided by Ms Cherrie Lowe, Director of TrendCare Systems Pty Ltd – Nursing Support http://www.trendcare.com.au/contact.html

REFERENCES

Arlington, K. (2004). Health Minister gets stony awakening to nursing care. *Nursing Review*. Canberra: 3.

Barr, A. (1984, January). Hospital nursing establishments and costs. *Hospital and Health Services Review*, 31-37.

Beat, J. W. S. (1970). Ward analysis. *Nursing Times* 66(29), Supp 101-104.

Bennett, M. (1990). Nursing research in Australia: development of patient dependency scales. *Nursing Research for Nursing Practice*. Melbourne, Australia, Chapman and Hall: 145-161.

Blair, W. (2000). Australian Industrial Relations Commission – Record of Proceedings. Cited on ANF Victoria website Retrieved April 6 2004 from www.anfvic.asn.au/news_briefs/news_ratios.htm

Buchan, J. (2004). A certain ratio? Royal College of Nursing: 3. United Kingdom.

CCSAA (2001). *Clinical Costing Standards Version 5.* Frankston, Vic, Australia, Clinical Costing Standards Association of Australia.

Cockerill, R., O'Brien-Pallas, L., Bolley, H., & Pink, G. (1993). Measuring nursing workload for case costing. *Nursing Economic$* 11(6), 342-349.

Commonwealth, Department of Health and Aging (2003). Trends in hospital activity Australia, 1991-2 to 2000-2001. *Occasional papers.* Canberra.

Conrick, M. (2006) Health informatics, transforming healthcare with technology, Thomson, South Melbourne, Victoria..

Diers, D. (1992). Diagnosis-Related Groups and the measurement of nursing. charting nursing's future, Agenda for the 1990's. L. Aiken and C. Fagin. Philadelphia, J. B. Lippincott: 139-156.

Diers, D. (2003). Personal communications.

Diers, D. (2004). Speaking of Nursing. Sudbury, MA: Jones and Bartlett.

Doncliff, B. (2001). Making nursing visable and valueable. *KAI TIAKI nursing New Zealand* December/January.

Finnigan, S., Abel, M., Dobler, T., Hudson, L., & Terry, B. (1993). Automated patient acuity. linking nursing systems and quality measurement with patient outcomes. *Journal of Nursing Administration, 23*(5), 62-71.

Gillett, S. (2001). *Nursing intensity in Victorian public hospitals.* Unpublished.

Goossen, W. T. F. (2000). *Towards strategic use of nursing information in The Netherlands.* The Haag, Gegevens Koninklijke.

Hebda, T., Szar, P., & Mascara, C. (2005). Handbook of informatics for nurse and health care professionals 3rd Ed, Pearson Prentice Hall, New Jersey.

Hovenga, E. J. S. (1983). *Patient dependency and nurse staffing for Victorian hospitals.* Victoria, Health Department.

Hovenga, E. J. S. (1994). *Casemix, hospital nursing resource usage and costs: The basis for a nurse staffing and costing system.* Sydney, The University of New South Wales: 269.

Morieson, B. (2003). *Secretary of the Victorian Branch of the Australian Nursing Federation.* Personal Interview. South Melbourne.

Picone, D., Phillips, K., Hathaway, V., & Parkes, R. (1993). *National nursing service weight study.* Canberra, Commonwealth Department of Human Services and Health, Casemix Development Program.

Plummer, V. (2005). *An analysis of patient dependency data utilizing the TrendCare system.* Monash university, Melbourne, Australia

Sovie, M. D. (1988). Variable costs of nursing care in hospitals. *Annual Review of Nursing Research, 6*, 131-150.

TrendCare Systems Pty Ltd (2007). *Training Manual Queensland.*

TrendCare (2008). www.trendcare.com.au/trendcare/documents/TrendCare_2008.pdf

Watson, J. (2000). *Australian Industrial Relations Commission – Record of Proceedings*, Melbourne AG2001/771423

Wood, S. (2001). *National nursing workload measurement.* Wellington, Ministry of Health, New Zealand.

KEY TERMS

Actualize: A function of the TrendCare system: the direct care nurse reviews and updates the indicators. The 'hours predicted for nursing care' are then automatically adjusted to reflect actual nursing hours currently being worked. An update in the categorizing of patients also automatically follows. Actualization facilitates a variance measurement. This variance in the actual hours worked by the nurse that are above or below the hours predicted for nursing care and is recorded as 'Total Variance by hh: mm' in TrendCare reporting.

Acuity: A term used in slightly different ways throughout the literature and used in this thesis to describe the relative requirements for nursing care for patients with a given medical condition or conditions.

The term acuity has a patient centred focus. There are several variables in addition to nursing time. Additional variables may be the requirement for nurses with certain qualifications or experience for example, there may be environmental variables such as a need for a monitored bed, private room, darkened room, specialized equipment or medication.

Acuity is affected by the reason for admission, complications, co-morbidities, variances, standards of care, length of stay and the practices of the senior clinician (See Figure 3.1 Data Flow in TrendCare). The contribution, or otherwise, of a patient to their own care also affects acuity.

Acuity is not affected by occupancy, staff shortages, staffing inexperience, missing stock or location of care. See also dependency.

Casemix: The mix of different patient types in a specific ward/unit or hospital.

Dependency: Nurse dependency, patient dependency, nursing acuity and patient acuity are terms which have been used to refer to the same or similar phenomenon within the literature. In contrast to the patient centred term 'acuity', the term dependency is commonly viewed as nurse centred. The acuity of the patient needs to be measured or determined before describing the dependency. This thesis analyzed patient dependency data, because of the intention to compare two nurse centred practices related to nursing workload.

In the past dependency systems implied that nursing resources were fixed and only patient variables were recognized. In contemporary dependency systems such as TrendCare, a patient's acuity is determined and then the nurse dependency. The nursing resources are no longer seen to be fixed and dependency is measured in hours and minutes (hh:mm) and skill mix. The skill mix may comprise qualifications, experience, competencies, team models, mentoring and leadership qualities, even languages spoken. For example; a nurse may be proficient in AUSLAN sign language for the hearing impaired. See also acuity.

Direct Care: Direct care is a component of nursing care which includes all aspects of the patient's specific care requirements. The direct care requirements may vary from shift to shift with changes in patient acuity. Care given to a patient through direct contact with that patient e.g. hygiene care, administration of medications and treatments. (TrendCare 2003) *Generally care in the presence of the patients. (PSCU, 1997:11)* This thesis focuses on direct nursing care because it is variable and the most difficult to measure and predict.

Nursing Resources: Nursing resources are the available hours and skill mix of nurses. See skill mix.

Ratios: Nurse patient ratios are a nursing resource allocation methodology. There are various methods of application including formal and informal ratios and mandated nurse patient ratios as applied for example, under the Victorian Public Sector Heads of Agreement. The principal is to ensure that the number of nurses available is commensurate with the number of patients requiring care and that nurses in similar settings care for the same number of patients. Also known as occupancy based nurse patient allocation.

Skill Mix: Skill mix refers to the mix of nursing team skill. These skills include knowledge, competencies (formal and informal), and experience and time management practices. The skill mix affects patient care, staff development, staff satisfaction and costs. An effective team leader and a skill mix of senior and junior staff working together, provides leadership, mentorship, teaching and learning experiences and role models, to ensure quality patient care.

The skill mix can be manipulated by the Unit Manager. For example, an unavoidably poor skill mix may be supplemented by additional nursing hours, or supplemented according to identified deficiency, for example, additional clinical hours, clinical nurse specialist, educator, lactation consultant, stomal therapist or by changing the model of care. It is also possible to enhance the staff skill mix over time. For example, the provision of targeted education for the development of staff competencies and time-based experience.

Chapter X
Simulations to Assess Medication Administration Systems

Elizabeth M. Borycki
University of Victoria, Canada

Andre W. Kushniruk
University of Victoria, Canada

Shigeki Kuwata
Tottori University Hospital, Japan

Hiromi Watanabe
Tottori University Hospital, Japan

ABSTRACT

A range of new technologies/information systems are increasingly being used by nurses in healthcare organizations. These technologies/information systems are being implemented in clinical settings in order to reduce errors associated with the medication administration process. At present, few published articles report empirical findings on the effects of using electronic medication administration systems where nurses' work is concerned. This chapter reports that there are both intended and unintended consequences, associated with implementing such systems in the clinical setting. Simulation methods can be used to assess the impact of integrating new technology/information systems into the nurses' work environment prior to full-scale implementation of a health technology/information system. Simulations as an evaluative tool emerged from a direct need to assess unintended and intended consequences of health information systems upon nurses' work before systems are fully implemented. Simulations, as an evaluative methodology, emerged from the cognitive-socio-technical literature. Methods for analyzing workflow and conducting simulations of user behavior can be used to assess and improve the cognitive-

socio-technical fit of technologies/information systems. They can be used to identify work and workflow problems (i.e. unintended consequences) involving health technologies/information systems as they are designed, developed, procured, purchased and implemented. Nurse informatician use of simulations to assess and test health technologies/information systems will allow nurses to determine the impact of a new software and/or hardware upon aspects of nurses' work before its implementation to allow for appropriate system modifications.

INTRODUCTION

A recent focus on reducing medication error during the medication administration process has led to the introduction of many new technologies aimed at streamlining and supporting nurses' work in order to reduce errors made in the clinical setting. This streamlining has led to the use of new technologies such as the medication administration system (MAS), bar code reader, radio frequency identification device (RFID) and wireless medication administration cart. Although there have been many publications that have espoused the benefits of using each new technology, few studies have examined the implications of integrating these technologies into the work environment (e.g. Borycki, Kushniruk, Kuwata, & Kannry, 2006; Kushniruk, Borycki, Kuwata & Kannry, 2006). For example, a recent search conducted by the authors involving the search engine Medline using the key terms "electronic", "medication administration system" and "nurse" (i.e. May 2008), revealed few published articles (i.e. less than 10) reporting empirical findings about the effects of using electronic MAS upon nurse's work. In contrast, a plethora of opinion pieces and anecdotal accounts have been published. Furthermore, only a few studies have attempted to identify empirically based methods that could be used to predict the effects of MAS upon nurses' work before implementation.

Simulation methods are a promising methodology that can be used to assess the impact of integrating a new technology/information system into the work environment prior to its implementation (e.g. Kushniruk et. al., 2006). Simulation as an evaluative tool emerged from a direct need to assess unintended and intended consequences of health information systems upon health professional work. Historically, simulations have been used in a number of industrial settings including aviation. Simulations can be used to evaluate device functionality, a software's ability to integrate into the work environment, and the interactions between software, hardware and its human operators in real world situations (Gaba, 2000; Issenberg, McGaghie, Petrusa, Gordon & Scalese, 2005). Industries that have effectively employed simulation in the development and testing of hardware and software for the real world include aviation (e.g. use of flight simulators to train pilots on the use of new aircraft), nuclear power (e.g. simulations of nuclear accidents to maintain software and hardware user competency and skills in responding to a unique or unusual crisis) and the education of health professionals (e.g. using programmable mannequins to train nurses on clinical skills and develop competencies prior to entering real world settings) (Issenberg et al., 2005). The use of simulations in the study of health technologies/information systems upon nurses' work prior to their being implemented in clinical settings is a relatively new application. Even so, simulations show considerable promise as a tool for studying the effects of technology/information systems upon nurse cognition and social interactions before their implementation.

In recent years, simulations of clinical activity have been developed to assess how users interact with systems in realistic clinical environments. As such work has emerged from the cognitive-socio-technical literature; there is a need to understand this literature before one can understand the use of simulations as an evaluative methodology. Therefore, before we discuss how simulations can be used to assess nurses' work and workflow involving the use of MAS, we will briefly review relevant cognitive-socio-technical research from the general, health and nursing informatics literatures. Specifically, the purpose of this chapter will be to describe:

a. The emergence of a cognitive-socio-technical framework in the nursing and health informatics literature,
b. The use of simulations to improve cognitive-socio-technical fit in medication administration systems.

A BRIEF OVERVIEW OF THE EMERGENCE OF COGNITIVE-SOCIO-TECHNICAL FIT: FROM THE GENERAL TO THE NURSING INFORMATICS LITERATURE

Over the past several years, a number of studies have outlined the unintended and intended consequences of poorly designed and implemented health information systems (e.g. Koppel et al., 2005). As a result, nurse informaticians have recognized that there is a need to assess and evaluate the impact of emerging technology upon aspects of nurses' work (i.e. social and technical). In the general literature, the notion that there are socio-technical aspects of work is not a new one. Socio-technical aspects of work or those parts of work that emphasize an "understanding of the social and the technical system" have their origins in research conducted by academics from the Tavistock Institute of Human Relations (Preece, Sharpe, Benyon, Holland & Carey, 1994). In the early 1950's Tavistock Institute researchers conducted a number of studies. This research concluded that there is a relationship between the organization, the work environment, and the social system of human relations among and between workers. Tavistock researchers found that the design of technical systems by organizations, whether they are changed by the implementation of a new technology, the organizational context or the style of management, influence the quality of work performed by human workers or actors in their work environment (Preece et al., 1994).

Early work in this area, involved the study of the mechanization of coal mining. Here, Trist and Bamforth (1951) examined the implications of mechanizing human work processes and outcomes. In this seminal work, the researchers found that mechanization altered coal mining practices and human interactions in intended and unintended ways. The researchers reported that prior to mechanization miners were able to work in small independent units. These units were composed of one or two miners. Prior to mechanization, miners were able to decide: (1) with whom they worked, (2) their own goals and objectives, and (3) the pace with which work was completed. With mechanization, the researchers found that each of the above mentioned aspects of work were disrupted.

With the introduction of mechanization, small independent units of miners were replaced with larger units. Workers were organized into larger groups (i.e. more than two people). Each larger group had less autonomy in deciding: (1) how to perform and (2) how to organize work. Mining tasks became fractionized. Workers were less able to maintain relationships between themselves and other miners. This impacted on worker ability to coordinate work (Trist & Bamforth, 1951). Management researchers consider coordination an important antecedent to effective and efficient team performance and positive team and organizational outcomes (Lemieux-Charles & McGuire, 2006). This work led researchers to conclude that there is a need to match social (i.e. working relationships between workers) with technical systems (i.e. the mechanized components of work) in the work environment and that such matching would improve the effectiveness and efficiency of workers (i.e. socio-technical fit).

Since this early work, a number of studies have been conducted in several industries (e.g. paper production, banking, nuclear power) involving the use of differing technologies (e.g. computers, robots) with similar results (Preece et. al., 1994; Zuboff, 1988). Following this work, researchers agreed that attention needs to be paid to aligning the social and technical aspects of work to ensure positive outcomes in all incremental and radical redesign of work using technology (McLaughlin & Kaluzny, 2006; Preece et. al., 1994). This research has been mirrored in the fields of health and nursing informatics.

In the health and nursing informatics literature, it was recognized that health information systems and their associated technologies (e.g. workstations, wireless devices) needed to be designed and implemented in such a way as to ensure good socio-technical fit (Berg, 1998a; Berg, 1998b). Health informatics researchers began to explore and identify the ideal means or "best practice" approaches towards effecting seamless or highly integrated socio-technical fit between health care worker social systems and the technologies/information systems used to support worker's task completion as new technologies were designed and implemented in the health care work environment (Lauesen, 2007; McLaughlin & Kaluzny, 2006).

In the early 1980's with the introduction of computers to many industries, a new dimension was added to the design and implementation of technology. Researchers found that it was also important to address cognitive fit in order to assess the impact of information systems upon workers cognition (i.e. workers' decision-making, reasoning processes and understanding of work) (Preece et. al., 1994). Workers' decision-making and reasoning had to be supported by the technology. Workers also needed to understand how technology could be employed in their work. Workers' ability to comprehend how a technology could perform work became an essential aspect of ensuring the quality, efficiency and effectiveness of workers when using new technologies/information systems. For example, Zuboff (1988) identified that workers who were able to comprehend how work tasks were performed in a newly mechanized pulp and paper mill (i.e. workers understood how people, machinery and computers could interact to produce paper) were better able to diagnose production problems and improve the productivity of the technology than those workers who did not. Workers who were able to comprehend the technology, its potential uses and its interaction with the work environment were also better able to improve the quality and efficiency of the technology in producing paper. These workers, when given some autonomy by the organization's management to make decisions about production processes, harnessed the power of the technology because of their understanding and awareness of the integration of technology and work. In summary, workers were able to understand how technology and others in the work environment could work together (i.e. the social system) and use this knowledge to optimize work and workflows. Workers were then able to optimize the technical system (i.e. the machines on the pulp and paper mill floor using the computers in the control room) through discussion and coordination of activities among individuals in the control room (i.e. the social aspects of work) (Zuboff, 1988). Similar examples are present in the management literature and across other industries such as banking, nuclear power and telecommunications (Preece et al., 1994; Zuboff, 1988). Unlike banking and other industries, few cognitive studies were conducted in health care in the 1980's.

Since the 1980's a number of evaluative methodologies have attempted to examine the social and technical aspects of design. For example, the Multiview methodology proposed by Avison and Wood-Harper (1990) characterizes the steps in developing socio-technical systems involving analysis of both social and technical aspects in a series of stages. Other similar methodologies include the Open Systems Task Analysis (OSTA) method (Eason, 1988; Eason & Harker, 1989), Soft Systems Methodology (Checkland & Scholes, 1990) and earlier work by Checkland (1981) and Wilson (1984) which attempt to give formal definitions of what systems should include from both a technical and social perspective. However, prior to the 1990's there continued to be little consideration given to the cognitive aspects of health information systems design and their possible influence upon social aspects of work.

THE EMERGENCE OF A COGNITIVE-SOCIO-TECHNICAL FIT FRAMEWORK IN NURSING AND HEALTH INFORMATICS

In the mid 1990's a number of researchers began to explore the effects of technology/information systems upon health professional cognition (e.g. Kushniruk et al., 1997). Researchers identified that technology (e.g. computer patient record systems) could affect cognitive processes (i.e. understanding, comprehension, decision-making and reasoning). Over the years, these researchers have extended this research and have found that health information system attributes (as designed by technology designers) could affect health professional diagnosis of disease (Kushniruk et al., 1997), organization of health professional knowledge (Patel et al., 2001), commission of medical errors (Koppel et al., 2005; Kushniruk et al., 2004), health professional learning (Patel et. al., 2001) and the nature and ability of health professionals to obtain and utilize information in their work with patients (Borycki & Lemieux-Charles, 2008). In summary, these researchers identified a relationship between differing aspects of health information systems and cognition.

Researchers did not identify socio-technical fit as an issue in health and nursing informatics until the late 1990's (e.g. Berg, 1999a; Berg, 1998b; Berg Langenberg, Berg & Kwakkernaat, 1998). In the 1990's health information systems were disseminated on a widespread basis in health care facilities. Although many of these information systems were successfully implemented, others failed to be implemented or they did not achieve their expected outcomes (e.g. Massaro, 1993; Koppel et al., 2005; Kushniruk et al., 2004). For example, researchers found that in many cases there was resistance among health professionals to the introduction of such systems. In other cases, where there was acceptance of these systems, health professionals (i.e. nurses and physicians) were bypassing system functions or health professionals chose to use only a limited set of system functions because of the difficulties associated with integrating the technology with their work and workflows (e.g. Lapointe & Rivard, 2006; Massaro, 1993). Berg (1999a; 1999b) proposed that these health information system failures were a direct result of poor socio-technical fit. Berg (1999a; 1999b) argued that there was a need to match health information systems to the clinical setting where health professionals practiced. This observation was similar to those made by researchers in other industries (e.g. Orlinkowski, 1992; Trist & Bamforth, 1951; Zuboff, 1988). Unlike research in other industries, health care placed less emphasis upon the potential impact of the roles of organizational context and management upon work. As well, little attention was given to integrating the cognitive aspects of work (as outlined above) into socio-technical fit.

In nursing and health informatics two streams of research emerged: (a) research involving health technologies/information systems and cognition, and (b) research involving socio-technical fit of health technologies/information systems. More recently, health care researchers have chosen to focus upon the intended and unintended consequences associated with implementing such technologies/information systems in the health care setting. Their findings have revealed poor cognitive-technical or socio-technical fit can lead to unintended consequences (e.g. Ash et al., 2007; Berg, 1999a; Berg, 1999b; Berg et al., 1998; Koppel et al., 2005; Patterson, Rogers, Chapman, & Render, 2004).

Other researchers have advocated an integrated approach towards the evaluation of technologies/health information systems in the work context. The approach would address the cognitive in addition to the socio-technical aspects of work (i.e. cognitive aspects of fit involving nurses' cognition, technology and social interactions in the clinical setting or cognitive-socio-technical fit). For example, Borycki and Kushniruk (2006), Kushniruk et al. (2006) and Kuwata et al., (2006) found that a nurses' cognitive processes, the organization's social system and the technology/health information system could lead to intended as well as unintended consequences when new technologies/information systems are introduced to the work environment. In this work they demonstrated how specific features of user interface design could lead to errors in medication administration (Kushniruk et. al., 2004). These researchers have argued for the need to consider cognitive aspects of work in addition to social context when designing and implementing health technologies/information systems. They have also suggested we have only begun to integrate the cognitive aspects of health care work (i.e. understanding the impact of systems on learning, information seeking, the organization of knowledge, reasoning and decision-making) with socio-technical aspects arising from the implementation of new technologies/health information systems (e.g. RFID and bar code scanners) in health care organizations. Consequently, there is a need for researchers to identify and solve cognitive-socio-technical issues and develop "best practice" approaches towards implementing technologies/health information systems in the clinical settings to better support nurses.

Lastly, much of the research in health and nursing informatics has focused upon the socio-technical implications of health technologies/information systems after they have been implemented in clinical environments (Anderson et al., 2005; Friedman & Wyatt, 2007). The emphasis of nursing and health informatics research has been upon the evaluation of systems post implementation (e.g. Anderson & Aydin, 2006; Friedman & Wyatt, 2007; Shortliffe & Cimino, 2006), when less can be done to change the technology/health information system to meet the cognitive-socio-technical demands of work (Borycki & Kushniruk, 2006; Kushniruk et al., 2006). This has led some to conclude that in some cases health technologies/information systems may need to be redesigned or even re-implemented after their initial implementation (Ash et al., 2007).

According to the software development literature, it is more costly to make changes to an information system later in the software development lifecycle (SDLC) (Kaner, Falk & Nguyen, 1999; Patton, 2001). As well, according to information system redesign and re-implementation research changes after implementation can be a costly endeavour for organizations (Kaner et al., 1999; Patton, 2001). This is especially the case for health care organizations that must also consider the implications of such expenditures upon patient care during periods where governments are attempting to curb health care spending or limit hospital budgets. A few researchers have suggested assessing and/or testing health technologies/information systems for cognitive-socio-technical fit using simulations prior to their implementation is a less costly alternative to evaluating the intended and unintended consequences of health technology/information systems after their implementation (e.g. Borycki & Kushniruk, 2008; Kuwata et. al., 2006; Patton, 2001).

Such assessment and testing could take place during the SDLC, during procurement or prior to organizational implementation of the technology/information system using simulations (Anderson et. al., 2005; Kushniruk, 2002). In recent years there has been a steady increase in the number of publications where simulations have been effectively used to assess new technologies/information systems prior to their implementation in the clinical setting. Assessment and testing prior to implementation using simulations may allow for radical redesign as well as iterative optimization of technology/health information systems in terms of cognitive-socio-technical fit between health care workers and the clinical environment prior to implementation.

In summary, the contribution of cognitive and social research is recognized in the nursing and heath informatics literature as a foundation on which nursing and health informatics may be built. This work involving the evaluation of health technologies/information systems may form the basis for understanding the implications of a new model for cognitive-socio-technical fit that employs simulations prior to implementation to assess the impact of technology/information systems upon workers'cognition as well as the social interactions that take place between the worker, other workers in their organization environment.

Research has found that nurses observe and cognitively integrate aspects of their environment such as social interactions between themselves, other workers, their patients, and technology. In order to support such work there is a need to ensure cognitive-socio-technical fit between nurses' cognitive representation of work, work tasks, workflow, social interactions and the technology (i.e. software, hardware and associated technological devices used when undertaking direct patient care) (Berg, 1998a; Berg, 1998b; Goodhue & Thompson, 1995). This is illustrated in Figure 1. Figure 1 shows that there is a need to integrate the social and technical aspects of work. This involves comprehending the aspects of work that are undertaken by the technology, the technology's limitations and the workflows arising from the technology that affect social interactions with others (i.e. health professionals and patients) in the health care setting. It is argued that a good socio-cognitive-technical fit will lead to nurse effectiveness and efficiency (i.e. intended consequences) in completing work.

Figure 1. Socio-cognitive-technical aspects of nurses or health professional work

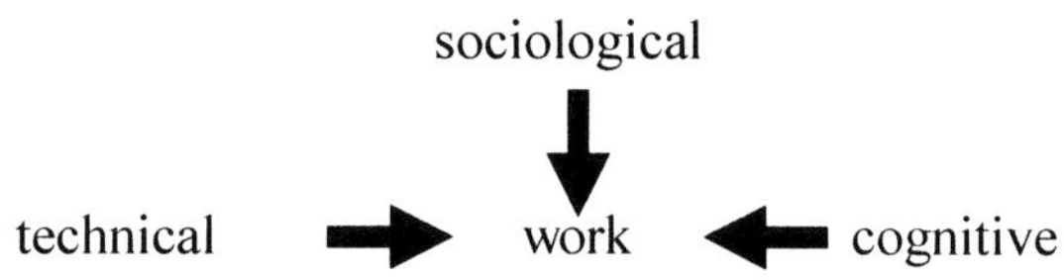

USING SIMULATIONS TO IMPROVE COGNITIVE-SOCIO-TECHNICAL FIT

Before a simulation can be effectively used to understand the impact of introducing a new technology/information system into the work environment, there is a need to understand the nurses' current work. One needs to outline how work is performed (i.e. cognitive-socio-technical) using existing paper and/or technological processes. This involves documenting the following:

- Routine and non-routine nurse tasks
- The frequency of nursing tasks
- How tasks are performed
- The order in which those tasks are performed
- The methods of synchronizing tasks with other tasks
- The information flows and activities used to support nurse tasks.

Figure 2. Typical workflow for a nurse using an electronic medication administration system

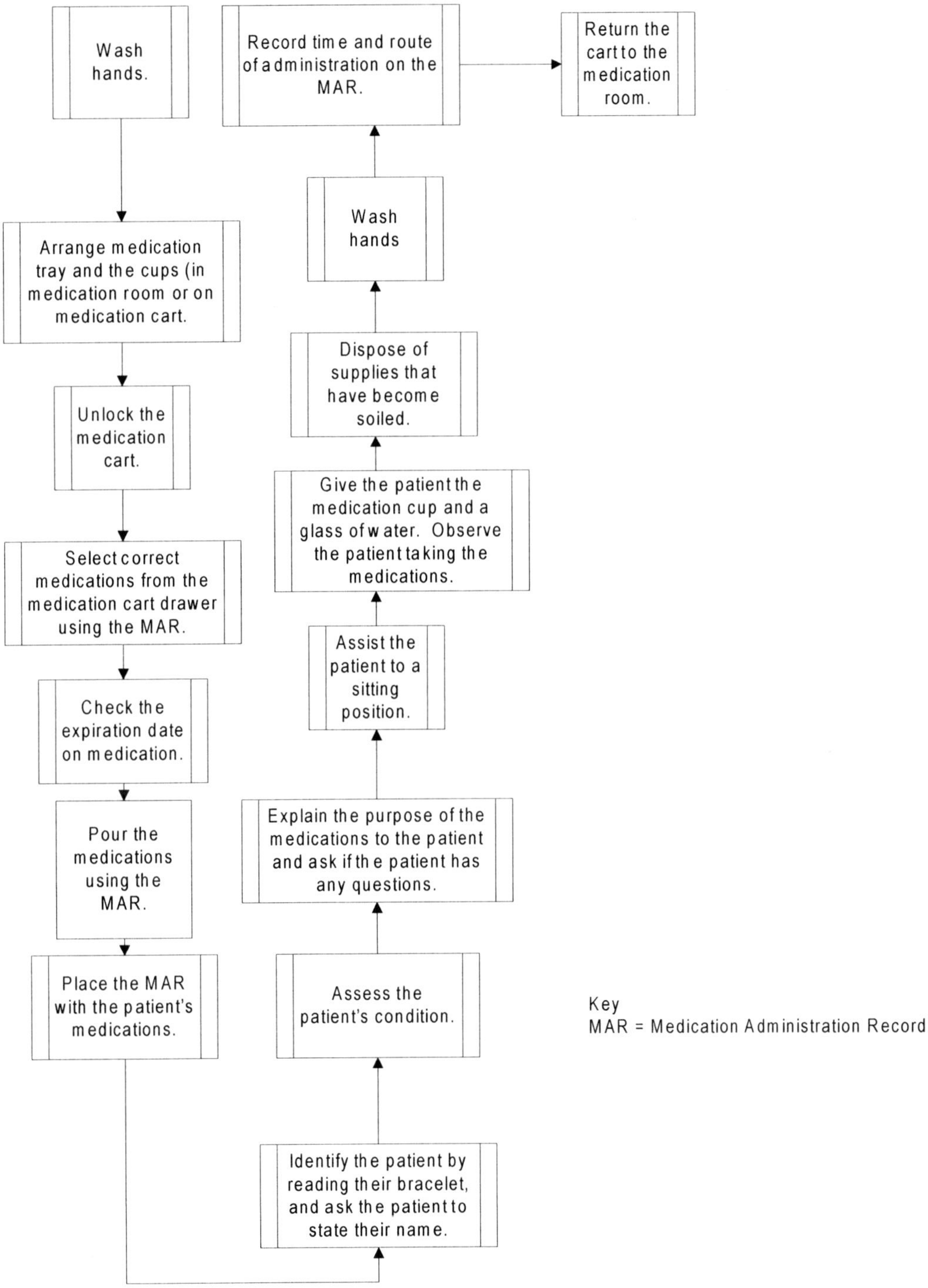

In addition to this, there is a need to document how nurses understand tasks within the context of the nurses' social system at work (Borycki & Kushniruk, 2006; McLaughlin & Kaluzny, 2006; Kushniruk et al., 2006; Kuwata et al., 2006). This can be done by describing work processes or activities (i.e. cognitive-socio-technical aspects of work) using flow diagrams. Flow diagrams are frequently used to document processes in the quality improvement and systems analysis and design literature (McLaughlin & Kaluzny, 2006; Satzinger & Orvik, 2001). For example, Figure 2 represents a typical workflow for a nurse using a medication administration cart and a paper based documentation system. Here, we see the individual steps that a nurse typically works through from washing her hands, to pouring and administering patient medications (Altman, 2004). The process is easy to understand and represents the activity associated with the process that integrates the cognitive, social and technical elements of nurses' work (Altman, 2004; Borycki & Kushniruk, 2006; Kuwata et al., 2006). Once the nurse has completed each step in the task as outlined in Figure 2 she undertakes the next step in performing the task.

Such a work process has good cognitive-socio-technical fit because of its simplistic workflows and the balance between both sequential and parallel processes. Simplistic workflows allow the nurse to integrate the cognitive and social aspects of work. Cognitively, the nurse is aware of each stage in the work process and his/her progress through the task and the potential outcomes. The nurse is able to coordinate and integrate his/her social interactions with the patient with her own cognitive processes within the social context of the clinical setting. The ability of the nurse to perform activities such as pouring several medications at the same time allows the nurse to integrate parallel (i.e. pouring all medications at the same time) and sequential processes (i.e. administering medication processes). This in turn reduces cognitive load or demands placed on the nurse's memory (i.e. estimated to hold five plus or minus two items) (Preece et al., 1994).

In addition to documenting existing cognitive and social workflows (as outlined in Figure 2) nurse informaticians need to outline the nurse processes and workflows once a technology/information system is introduced. This is especially the case in environments where a health information system and/or a technology have already been integrated and radical rethinking of nurse work processes and workflows involves additional changes arising from the introduction of a new health technology/information system (Borycki et al., 2006; Hammer & Champy, 1993). This helps the nurse informatician to obtain an understanding and representation of the integration of nurses'cognitive-socio-technical work involving existing and newly introduced health technologies/information systems (Borycki et al., 2006; Kushniruk et al., 2006; Kuwata et al., 2006). This also helps nurse informaticians to understand the implications of introducing a new technology/health information system that replaces, supports or changes nurses' work. It also affords nurse informaticians the opportunity to identify potential unintended consequences prior to the full scale implementation of a new technology/information system when an existing constellation of paper and technological tools is already being used in the clinical setting to support work.

A cognitive and social representation of work as well its integration with existing health technologies/information systems devices (represented through the use of flow diagrams that emerge from observation of current nurses' work during simulations involving the use of a new information technology) are key to understanding the possible intended and unintended consequences that may arise. Diagramming or mapping workflows through the use of flow diagrams observed during simulations both prior to and after introducing changes involving technology/information systems may: (a) illuminate the possible implications of significantly changing work, and (b) identify the presence of unintended consequences. Therefore, the mapping of workflows and work processes pre and post technological/information design change help to highlight those aspects of the new work or workflow that may be cumbersome, complex or may lead to errors that need to be improved (poor socio-cognitive-technical fit). In summary the mapping of workflow and work processes using flow diagrams can help nurse informaticians to understand the implications of redesigning how work is done from a cognitive-socio-technical perspective and helps to identify potential unintended consequences. Such advanced knowledge may help nurse informaticians to optimize cognitive-socio-technical fit during the design process and prior to implementation (Borycki et al., 2006).

Impact of systems on nurses' work can be assessed using low cost simulations. In our work we have developed a range of simulations that have involved recording nurses interacting with new information technologies (including recording all physical activities, verbalizations and computer screens). In our simulations we record and analyze video data of individuals interacting with their environment to map out (i.e. using flow diagrams) and understand the impact of technologies/information systems (e.g. Kushniruk et al., 2006). In conducting our simulations we typically video record all interactions (e.g. nurses giving patients medications) as well as the computer screens of associated technology (e.g. medication administration systems). We typically carry out such simulations in the real clinical setting in which the system will be introduced. By analyzing the resultant video recordings using principled methods of video coding (as described in Kushniruk & Patel, 2004; Borycki & Kushniruk, 2006) we can timestamp and analyze activities of interest, problems and changes to cognition and workflow as well as assess the impact of systems upon the number and quality of interactions with other health professionals and patients. We have had a number of successes in predicting workflow issues arising from the introduction of new technologies/information systems in the redesign of processes using health information systems and preventing unintended consequences from arising.

The resultant data obtained has been used as the basis to create flow diagrams in order to assess and predict cognitive-socio-technical fit (see Kushniruk et al., 2006 for details). For example, Figure 3 shows a typical workflow documented after the introduction of new and primarily electronic approach towards nurse medication administration (as assessed during simulation testing that involved asking nurses to give to a mannequin patient their medications). In this workflow a medication administration cart and bar code scanning device are linked to a portable laptop that provides access to an electronic medication administration system. The patient also now wears a bar coded bracelet that must be scanned. In addition to this the medication administration cart acts as a storage facility for medications and a workstation for preparing medications for their administration. In the workflow we see that superficially the medication administration process continues to be sequential (much as was outlined earlier). Each step in the process from pouring a medication to scanning the patient's bar code bracelet using the bar code scanner, to administering a medication follows an ordered sequence. In a situation where a patient receives a single oral medication, such a workflow appears simple and parsimonious - easily comprehendible from a cognitive perspective (by the individual undertaking the work process) and physically not difficult to move through.

Alternatively, deeper examination may be required and more complex tasks may need to be given to subjects during simulations. For example, in North America patients receive, an average, 8-10 medications in hospital. In addition to this, if the patient is acutely ill, he or she may also receive intravenous (IV) medications and/or intra muscular (IM) and/ or subcutaneous injections (S/C) in conjunction with their oral medications

Figure 3. Typical workflow from an electronic medication administration system

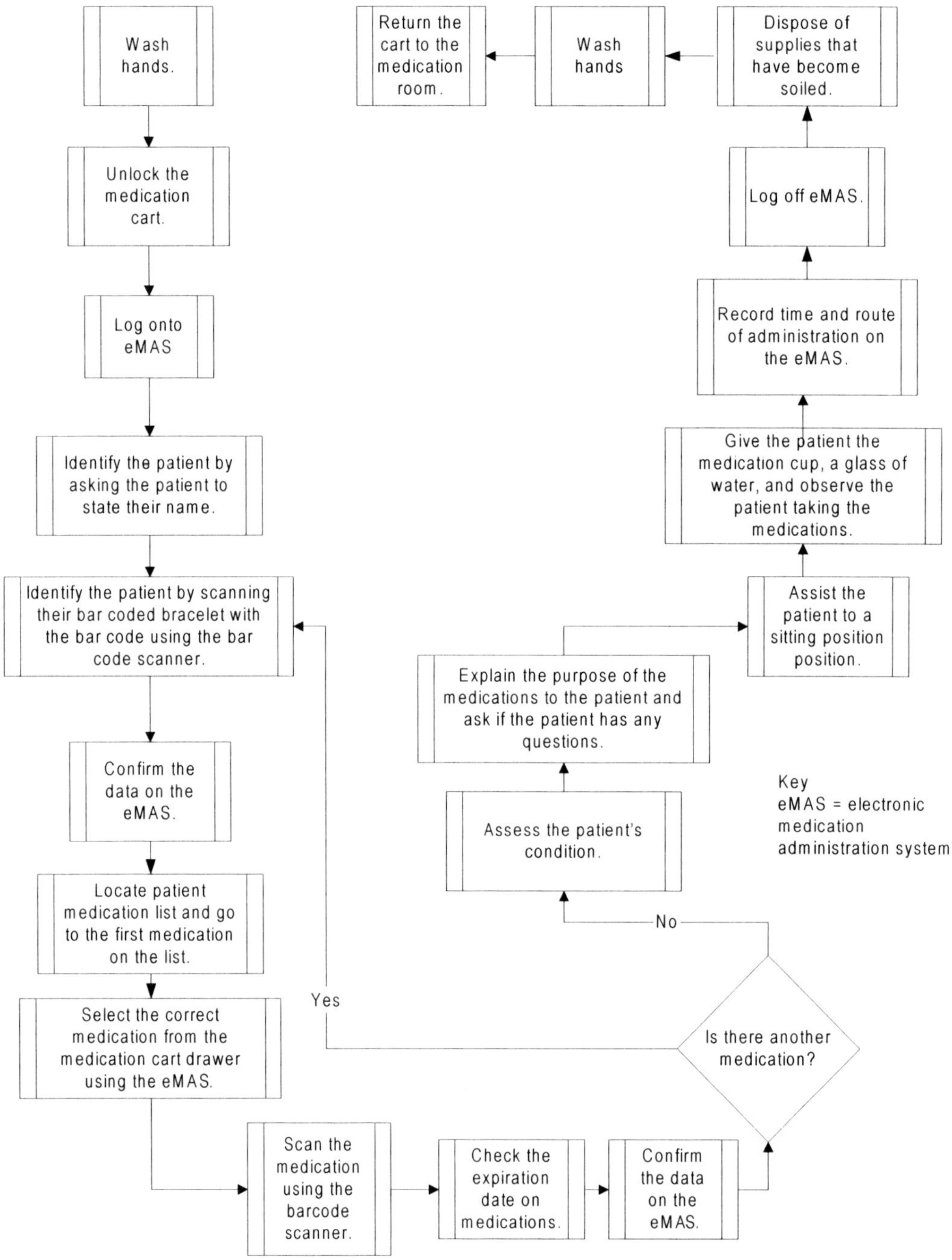

(Altman, 2004). During the simulation one can add complexity to the routine nature of administering a single oral medication, by adding more oral, IV, IM and/or S/C medications during one medication administration event involving one patient. Essentially, the nurse administering the medications must locate and pour the medication, scan the patient identification bracelet, and scan each of the oral medications, IV, IM and/or possibly S/C medications in a fixed sequence. This requires first searching the system for the first medication, scanning the bar code on the medication bag, scanning the patient's identification, pouring the medication and then repeating this process over and over again until each medication is administered. Such a rigid workflow revealed (during the video analysis of the simulation data) that integrating a medication administration system with others technologies (such as bar coding) could potentially increase the complexity of work associated with locating, preparing and administering medications to patients under certain conditions (e.g. multiple medications under time-constrained conditions). This may increase the nurses' cognitive load during medication administration. According to cognitive theory people have a difficult time processing more than five to seven pieces of information at one time (Miller, 1956). In addition, the new workflow may also decrease the nurses' ability to navigate the social interactions that accompany medication administration (i.e. interactions between the nurse, a physician and/or the patient).

As illustrated above, the mapping of nurse workflows and work processes using flow diagrams based on observations obtained from simulations of work activities is necessary to determine if redesign involving technology simplifies and/or improves nurse workflows or if it leads to increased social and cognitive work complexity, cognitive load and unintended consequences. In the example described above, cumbersome workflows were identified and as a consequence the system was modified to allow for more flexible user interaction with the system in their work environment (Kushniruk et al., 2006).

In summary, health technologies/information systems can be used to alter nurses' work. The integration of new health technologies/information systems could lead to the simplification and redesign of the way nurses' work is undertaken. The integration of cognitive, social and technical aspects of work into cognitive-socio-technical work has moved incremental automation of specific nursing tasks using technology/information systems into more fundamental redesign of nurses' work involving technology. With the move towards redesign there is a need to determine if the implications of integrating cognitive-socio-technical work using technology in typical work situations simplifies nurses' work or increases its complexity. Simulations offer an opportunity to effectively determine the impact of the technology/health information system on nurse users. One of the most important benefits of using a simulation based approach is the ability of the nurse informaticians to evaluate the impact of a technology/information system prior to its introduction into a real world environment. This allows nurse informaticians to evaluate the effects of redesign upon work and make changes aimed a simplifying nurses' work prior to implementation to prevent costs incurred and associated with re-implementation. In addition to this, nurse informaticians can evaluate their choice of technology/information system during the SDLC and procurement (Borycki & Kushniruk, 2005; Kushniruk et al., 2004). Again, preventing costs associated with re-implementation.

SUMMARY

In summary socio-cognitive-technical fit is an important aspect of designing, procuring, assessing and testing health information systems and their associated devices prior to implementation in the clinical environment. Methods for analyzing workflow and conducting simulations of user behavior can be used to assess and improve the fit of systems to users. More specifically, we discussed some of the methods that we have developed to identify work and workflow problems (i.e. unintended consequences) as health information systems and their associated devices are designed, developed, procured, purchased and implemented by applying assessment and testing techniques from the simulation literature to nursing and health informatics. We have provided an overview of approaches to socio-cognitive-technical fit and the context for our current work involving simulations to assess and test the impact of redesign of work and workflows in clinical settings.

FUTURE DIRECTIONS

Recent research has revealed there are significant socio-technical and cognitive implications for nurses associated with introducing new health information systems and/or an emerging technologies for the purposes of streamlining nurses' work and workflows. Over the past several years, nurse informaticians have used health information systems to make incremental improvements to nurses' work. With the emergence of the Internet and wireless technologies, new types of devices have offered nurse informaticians the opportunity to radically redesign the ways in which nurses' work is done. In some cases the redesign of health professional work (i.e. physician and nurse work) has led to intended consequences. In other cases unintended consequences have emerged. In the next few years, nurse informaticians will need to develop a comprehensive strategy towards evaluating new health technologies/information systems and to assess and test these systems and to determine their effects upon nurses' work and workflows. Assessment and testing will allow nurse informaticians to determine the impact that new software and/or hardware will have upon aspects of nurses' work. Ideally, such assessment and testing should take place within the context of simulations before a health information system and its associated devices are implemented in real world clinical settings. Future work is needed to further develop and refine simulation-based methods and to begin to incorporate their application in the widespread implementation of technologies/information systems in health care settings (i.e. hospital and home care). Furthermore, if such assessment and testing becomes commonplace, nurse informaticians will be able to develop a body of knowledge that will lead to the development of evidence-based guidelines for information system designers, developers and implementers to use when designing and developing such systems. Ultimately, it is expected that this will lead to improvements in nursing practice and reductions in the costs associated with implementing new technologies/information systems.

REFERENCES

Altman, G. (2004). *Delmar's fundamental and advanced nursing skills* (2nd ed.). Toronto: Thompson Delmar Learning.

Anderson, J. G., & Aydin, C. E. (2005). *Evaluating the organizational impact of healthcare information systems* (2nd ed.). New York: Springer.

Ash, J. S., Sittig, D. F., Dykstra, R. H., Guappone, K., Carpenter, J. D., & Seshadri, V. (2007). Categorizing the unintended sociotechnical consequences of computerized provider order entry. *International Journal of Medical Informatics, 76*(1), 21-7.

Avison, D., & Wood-Harper, T. (1990). Multiview methodology. Oxford: Blackwell Scientific Publishers.

Berg, M. (1999a). Patient care information systems and health care work: A sociotechnical approach. *International Journal of Medical Informatics, 55*(2), 87-101.

Berg, M. (1999b). Accumulating and according: Occasions for information technology in medical work. *Computer Supported Cooperative Work, 8*, 373-401.

Berg, M., Langenberg, C., Berg, I., & Kwakkernaat, J. (1998). Considerations for sociotechnical design: Experiences with an electronic patient record in a clinical context. *International Journal of Medical Informatics, 52*(1), 243-251.

Borycki, E. M., & Kushniruk, A. W. (2006). Identifying and preventing technology-induced error using simulations: Application of usability engineering techniques. *Healthcare Quarterly, 8*, 99-105.

Borycki, E. M., Kushniruk, A. W., Kuwata, S., & Kannry, J. (2006). Use of simulation in the study of clinician workflow. *AMIA Annual Symposium*, 61-65.

Borycki, E. M., & Lemieux-Charles, L. (2008). *Does a hybrid electronic-paper record environment impact upon health professional information seeking?* Conference Proceedings for Medical Informatics Europe, Goteborg, Sweden., May 26-28.

Checkland, P. B. (1981). *Systems thinking, systems practice.* Chinchester: John Wiley.

Checkland, P. B., & Scholes, J. (1990). *Soft systems methodology in action.* Chinchester: John Wiley and Sons.

Eason, K. D. (1988). *Information technology and organizational change.* London: Taylor & Francis.

Eason, K.D., & Harker, S. (1989). *An open systems approach to task analysis.* Internal Report, HUSAT Research Centre, Loughborough University of Technology.

Friedman, C. P., & Wyatt, J. C. (1997). *Evaluation methods in medical informatics.* New York: Springer.

Gaba, D. M. (2000). Structural and organizational issues in patient safety: A comparison of health care to other high-hazard industries. *California Management Review, 43*(1), 83-102.

Hammer, M., & Champy, J. (1993). *Reengineering the corporation.* New York: HarperBusiness.

Issenberg, S. B., McGaghie, W. C., Petrusa, E. R., Gordon, D. L., & Scalese, R. J. (2005). Features and uses of high-fidelity medical simulations that lead to effective learning: A BEME systematic review. *Medical Teacher, 27*(1), 10-28.

Kaner, C., Falk, J., & Nguyen, H. Q. (1999). *Testing computer software* (2nd ed.). New York: Wiley.

Koppel, R., Metlay, J. P., Cohen, A., Abaluck, B., Localio, A. R., Kimmel, S. E., & Strom, B. L. (2005). Role of computerized physician order entry systems in facilitating medication errors. *JAMA, 293*(10), 1197-1203.

Kushniruk, A. W., Patel, V. L., & Cimino, J. J. (1997). Usability testing in medical informatics: Cognitive approaches to evaluation of information systems and user interfaces. In *Proceedings of the 1997 AMIA Annual Fall Symposium: The Emergence of 'Internetable' Health Care, Systems that Really Work, 21,* 218-222). Philadelphia: Hanley and Belfus.

Kushniruk, A. (2002). Evaluation in the design of health information systems: Application of approaches emerging from usability engineering. *Computers in Biology and Medicine, 32*(3), 141-149.

Kushniruk, A. W., & Patel, V. L. (2004). Cognitive and usability engineering methods for the evaluation of clinical information systems. *Journal of Biomedical Informatics, 37*, 56-76.

Kushniruk, A., Triola, M., Stein, B., Borycki, E., & Kannry, J. (2004). The relationship of usability to medical error: An evaluation of errors associated with usability problems in the use of a handheld application for prescribing medications.

In M. A. Musen, C. P. Friedman & J. M. Teich (Eds.), *AMIA/MedInfo 2004 Symposium: Building High Performance Health Care Organizations, 28*, 1073-1076. San Francisco: American Medical Informatics Association.

Kushniruk, A. W., Borycki, E., Kuwata, S., & Kannry, J. (2006). Predicting changes in workflow resulting from healthcare information systems: Ensuring the safety of healthcare. *Healthcare Quarterly, 9*, 114-118.

Kuwata, S., Kushniruk, A., Borycki, E., & Watanabe, H. (2006). Using simulation methods to analyze and predict changes in workflow and potential problems in the use of a bar coding medication order entry system. *AMIA Annual Symposium*, 994.

Lapointe, L., & Rivard, S. (2006). Getting physicians to accept new information technology: Insights from case studies. *CMAJ, 174*(11), 1573-1578.

Lauesen, S. (2007). *Guide to requirements SL-07.* Lauesen Publishing.

Lemieux-Charles, L., & McGuire, W. L. (2006). What do we know about health care team effectiveness? A review of the literature. *Medical Care Research and Review, 63*(3), 263-300.

Massaro, T. A. (1993). Introducing physician order entry at a major academic medical centre: Impact on organizational culture and behaviour. *Academic Medicine, 68*(1), 20-30.

Miller, G. A. (1956). The magic number seven plus or minus two: Some limits of our capacity for information processing. *Psychological Review, 63*(2), 87-87.

McLaughlin, C. P., & Kaluzny, A. D. (2006). *Continuous quality improvement in health care: Theory, implementations and applications* (3rd ed.). Toronto: Jones and Bartlett.

Orlikowski, W. J. (1992). The duality of technology: Rethinking the concept of technology in organizations. *Organizational Science, 3*(3), 398-427.

Patel, V. L., Kushniruk, A. W., Yang, S., & Yale, J-F. (2001). Impact of a computer-based patient record system on data collection, knowledge organization, and reasoning. *JAMIA, 7*(6), 569-585.

Patton, R. (2001). *Software testing.* SAMS: Indianapolis, Indiana.

Patterson, E. S., Rogers, M. L., Chapman, R. J., & Render, M. L. (2002). Improving patient safety by identifying side effects from introducing bar coding in medication administration. *JAMIA, 9*, 540-553.

Preece, J., Sharp, H., Benyon, D., Holland, S., & Carey, T. (1994). *Human-computer interaction.* Toronto: Addison-Wesley.

Satzinger, J. W., & Orvik, T. U. (2001). *The object-oriented approach.* Thompson Learning: Canada.

Shortell, S. M., & Kaluzny, A. D. (2006). *Health care management: Organizational design and behaviour* (5th ed.). New York: Thompson.

Shortliffe, E. H., & Cimino, J. J. (2006). *Biomedical informatics: Computer applications in health care and biomedicine.* New York: Springer Verlag.

Trist, E. L., & Bamforth, K. W. (1951). Some social and psychological consequences of the longwall method of coal getting. *Human Relations, 4*, 3-38.

Wilson, B. (1984). *Systems: Concepts, methodologies and applications.* Chinchester: Wiley.

Zuboff, S. (1988). *In the age of the smart machine: The future of work and power.* BasicBooks: United State of America.

KEY TERMS

Cognitive-Socio-Technical: A workers understanding of the social interactions that occur between individuals and the technology they work with in order to complete work tasks.

Cognitive Work: The human activity of processing information for the purpose of completing work.

Intended Consequences: Those outcomes of information systems and their associated technological devices that were expected to occur following their implementation.

Socio-Technical: The social interactions that occur between individuals and the technology they work with in order to complete work tasks.

Unintended Consequences: Those outcomes of information systems and their associated technological devices that: (a) did not occur but were expected to occur and (b) those outcomes that occurred that were not originally conceived of when the technology designers designed and developed the system and/or device (e.g. programmers and analysts).

Chapter XI
Socio-Technical Structures, 4Ps and Hodges' Model

Peter Jones
NHS Community Mental Health Nursing Older Adults, UK

ABSTRACT

This chapter explores the potential of a conceptual framework – Hodges' model – both as a socio-technical structure and means to explore such structures of relevance to nursing informatics theory and practice. The model can be applied universally by virtue of its structure and the content which it can encompass. In apprehending this chapter, readers will be able to draw, describe and explain the scope of Hodges' model within contemporary healthcare contexts and the wider global issues presented by the 21st Century that influence and shape nursing informatics. Critically, the reader will also gain insight into how socio-technical structures can facilitate cross fertilization of clinical and informatics theory and practice; drawing attention to information as a concept that provides a bridge between socio-technical, clinical, and informatics disciplines. This chapter will review the socio-technical literature and venture definitions of socio-technical structures related to Hodges' model and advocate the need for sociopolitical-technical structures. The chapter also proposes the 4Ps as a tool to facilitate reflection upon and the construction of socio-technical structures. The adoption and significance of the hyphenated form as per "socio-technical" will also be explained.

INTRODUCTION

Data is a plural noun (Pearsall, et al., 1998). Technology has plural - compound uses. The word *technology* is somewhat unique among the family of '-ologies'. The word is applied as a noun, adjective and used in everyday conversation and media to an extent that no other -ology can match. The word refers of course, not only to the study of the technical, but a phenomenon: a ubiquitous, pervasive presence in our lives. The extent to which we take technology for granted, is evident in our missing this other meaning. How often do we refer to: *This biology is playing up* (which may well be the case!)? *Geology never lasts very long! Sociology just adds to the noise.* Maths and English [all languages] are similar in not only referring to the study of a subject area, but being applied in day-to-day life – essential forms of literacy. Depending on definitions *technology* is of course an adjunct to literacy and expression, from the caves of Lascaux to virtual reality communities. It is only 'now' that *technology* is considered as the latest – the third *ology* - to become ubiquitous.

Technology presents challenges by virtue of its ability to liberate or constrain (Cooley, 1987; Nevárez, 2008). While this can confuse and disorientate us, technology also offers opportunities for discovery and integration. Viewed through the compound eye of Hodges' model (see below), socio-technology can liberate by creating fractures of the model's axes allowing leakage, seepage of meaning. We can look upon the seepage as soap that assists conceptual hygiene, as we make sense of technology across several knowledge domains. This affords us the opportunity to break the constraints of time, distance, culture (with translation) and intra-interdisciplinary theory and practice. If however, technology is poorly managed and implemented it can again in terms of Hodges' model constrain the movement of information and meaning to just one or two knowledge domains? When allied with (clinical) language and professional practice, technology facilitates categorisation which can depersonalise and alienate human actors. Alternately, positive effects are witnessed in the social networking phenomenon with its tags and labels.

From a socio-technical perspective technologies ability to fracture is not catastrophic, but is a circumstance that carries an ecological impact. It helps us to conjoin what are usually disparate disciplines of theory, practice and policy and also highlights the need for a philosophy of technology (Scharff and Dusek, 2002) and elaborated (integrated) definitions of informatics. Elsewhere (Jones, 2008), the author discusses how Michel Serres (1995), the French philosopher, employs the ancient god *Hermes* as a trope to explain technology and communication. Hermes is well suited to this task being the philosopher of plural spaces. Hodges' model constitutes a plural - pantological space (Jones, 2008). Perhaps this plurality explains the extended significance of technology in our (clinical) language and practice. Historically, our culture is built upon layers of technology: fire, the wheel, agricultural tools, weapons through to the rapid lifecycle rate experienced today in the *technopolis* (Nevárez, 2008).

This chapter begins with a brief introduction to Hodges' model, followed by definitions of socio-technical structure. Then several key sources in the socio-technical literature are introduced leading to the formulation of socio-technical structures within Hodges' model. These are explicated by introducing the *4Ps* (e.g., process) followed by closing discussion. If a paper is afforded one gross assumption, then at this point let me suggest that nurses and the majority of other health and social care practitioners are either suspicious of ICT due to previous experiences at work, or they are pragmatic in their expectations. Pragmatic in that they recognise the inevitability that in the 21st century informatics will figure in their working lives, just as it does in their personal lives. Therefore, this paper also addresses how (nursing) informatics can be informed by a model of nursing and how health can contribute to informatics. This connection utilises Hodges' model and the concept of *information*.

Hodges' Model: A Cognitive Periplus for Life-Long Learning[1]

Developed in the UK during the early 1980s, Hodges' Health Career Model (hereafter referred to as h2cm) is a conceptual framework that is person-centred and situation based. In structure h2cm combines two axes to create four care (knowledge) domains (Figures 1 and 2). Academics and practitioners in many fields create models that help support theory and practice (Wilber, 2000). Models act as a memory jogger and guide. In health care generic models can encourage holistic practice directing the user to consider the patient as a whole person and not merely as a diagnosis derived from physical investigations? Exposure of h2cm is limited to a small (yet growing) cadre of practitioners; several published articles (Hinchcliffe[2], 1989; Adams, 1987; Jones 2004). In addition to a website (Jones, 1998) a blog and podcast were published in 2006. The most recent paper is that already mentioned which relates h2cm and the work of Michel Serres to social informatics (Jones, 2008).

The best way to explain h2cm is to review the

Figure 1.

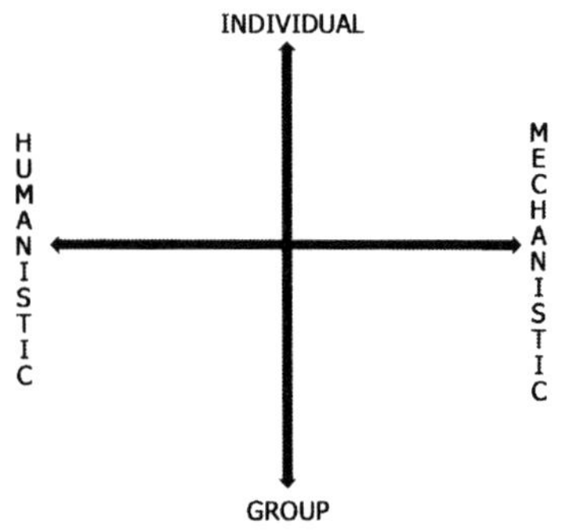

Figure 2.

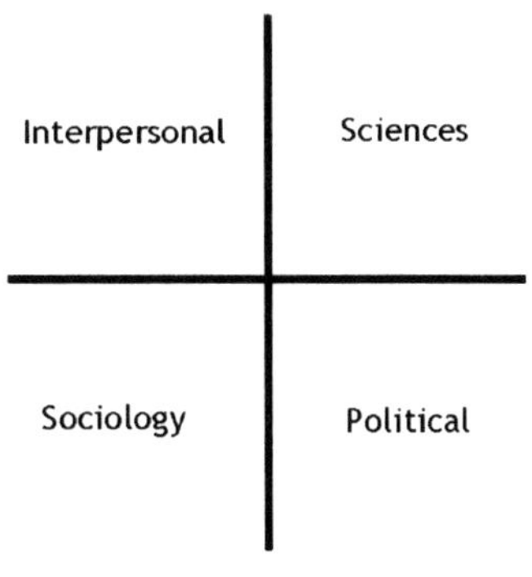

questions that Brian Hodges originally posed. To begin, who are the recipients of care? Well, first and foremost individuals of all ages, races and creed, but also groups of people, families, communities and populations. Then Hodges asked: what types of activities - tasks, duties, and treatments - do nurses carry out? They must always act professionally, but frequently according to strict rules and policies, their actions often dictated by specific treatments including drugs, investigations, and minor surgery. Nurses do many things by routine according to precise procedures, rather like the stereotypical matron with machine-like efficiency? If these actions are classed as mechanistic, they contrast with times when healthcare workers give of themselves to reassure, comfort, develop rapport and engage therapeutically. This is opposite to mechanistic tasks and is described as humanistic; what the public usually think of as the *caring* nurse. In use this framework prompts the user to consider four major subject headings or care domains of knowledge. Namely, what knowledge is needed to care for individuals - groups and undertake humanistic - mechanistic activities? Through these questions Hodges' derived the model depicted above.

Initial study of h2cm on the website has related Hodges' model to the multicontextual nature of health, informatics, consilience (Wilson, 1998), interdisciplinarity, and visualization. H2cm says nothing about the study of knowledge, but a great deal about the nature of knowledge is implied in Figures 1 and 2. This prompted two web pages devoted to the structural and theoretical assumptions of h2cm (Jones, 2000a, b.). Although the axes of h2cm are dichotomous, they also represent continua. This duality is important as an individual's mental health status for example is situated on a continuum spanning *excellent* to *extremely unwell*. There are various states in-between affected by an individual's beliefs, response to stress, coping strategies, epigenetic and other influences. H2cm was created to meet four educational and service-side objectives:

1. To produce a curriculum development tool.
2. Help ensure holistic assessment and evaluation.
3. To support reflective practice.
4. To reduce the theory-practice gap.

Since h2cm's formulation these objectives have grown in relevance. The 1980s may seem remote, but these problems are far from archaic as expansion of points 1-4 reveals. Student life is preparation for life-long learning. Curricula are under constant pressure. Despite decades of policy declarations, truly holistic care (combining physical, mental and pastoral care) remains elusive. The concept and practice of reflection swings like a metronome, one second seemingly de rigour, the next moment the subject of web based polls. H2cm can be used in interviews, outlining discussion and actions to pursue, an agenda - agreed and shared at the end of a session. The model is equally at home on paper, blackboard, flipchart and interactive whiteboard. Finally, technology is often seen as a way to make knowledge available to all practitioners; the means to bridge theory-practice gap through activities such as e-learning, governance and knowledge management.

The model's expressive power arises from its structure; a conceptual space created by diagrammatic representation of four pivotal concepts – *individual, group, humanistic* and *mechanistic*. This construct leads to a conceptual framework with generic and specific, broad and detailed capacities. The conceptual dynamics of the model can be represented as a horse and litter. The horse and its direction of travel constitutes the situation – context. Hodges' model is the litter, a framework which can carry our ideas, concepts, problems, issues (our 'sick and unwell'); plus hypotheses and solutions. The challenge follows though from the fact that health and social care is multi-contextual - multiaxial. One horse and litter is simply not enough. The horse and litter need to travel in several directions at once.

What Hodges' model encourages and provides in one context is vicarious travel. The axes within h2cm create a *conceptual space* as explored by Gärdenfors (2000). A third axis projecting through the page can represent history; be that an educational, health or other 'career'. It is ironic, that an act of partition can simultaneously represent reductionism and holism. Reductionism has a pivotal role to play, which h2cm acknowledges in the sciences domain. What h2cm can do is prompt the expert (single domain) practitioner that there are three other pages to reflect and write upon. In total with the addition of faith h2cm could also be said to represent the spiritual domain. The model's title was extended with 'Care Domains' in order to differentiate it from job and professional career website and resources.

Definitions: What do we Mean by 'Socio-Technical', 'Socio-Technical Structure' and 'Socio-Political-Technical'?

Nursing informatics can be considered as a socio-technical structure. This structure and health informatics more generally boasts not only a history, but an autobiography (Hayes and Barnett, 2008). The multi-axial nature of health has been recognised for millennia from the fundamental dichotomy of life-death to more recent pre-occupations of supply-demand, public-private and many others. There are more specific axes instantiated in terminology systems such as SNOMED CT; for example, *diseases, drugs, function, procedure* and *event* (Melton, et al.; 2006). Relating this to h2cm, a dichotomy such as subjective - objective can be defined as spanning and linking all four care domains. This may seem so general that it is useless as the basis for a meaningful definition; but a definition of *socio-technical structure* should demarcate the space it inhabits whether physical or conceptual (psychophysical). Being situated in application h2cm informs novices and experts alike of the primacy of context in health and social care (Berg and Goorman, 1999; Bricon-Souf and Newman, 2007; Westbrook, et al., 2007).

Defining these terms is difficult and what follows will not find agreement with everyone. For all that globalisation says about the world today, our appreciation of the world remains less than wholly. The world is constantly partitioned: North-South and East-West. C.P. Snow's seminal book *Two Cultures* (1959) noted the fracture within the pursuit of knowledge; with the existence of two camps the *sciences* and the *humanities* that were divorced and non-communicative. This dichotomy is symptomatic of a profound tendency for human beings to polarise, as evinced in the psychological literature through Tomkins' *Polarity theory (*Stone and Schaffner, 1997). As all students quickly realise, a key part of learning entails unpacking dichotomies, continua, axes and contexts. It could be argued that our capacity to dichotomize in situations assures the creation of socio-technical structures even if this *ticket to enlightenment* is only 'half-used' (in the socio-technical sense). After the finale many ticket stubs litter the ground. In informatics the need to tackle the skills divide provoked the quest for hybrid managers; senior personnel gifted with management acumen and information skills to deliver (socio-technical) change in the new organisation (Earl and Skyrme, 1990). The objective and subjective are clearly germane to health as Sullivan (2003) argues:

If medicine is now to aim for patient-centred outcomes, it needs a new object of study. Outcomes research is as yet undecided if this will be the patient's health or the patient's life. Each step in this direction brings medicine closer to pursuing "what really matters to patients" and also brings greater scientific, ethical and social complexity. Subjective health is more meaningful to patients than objective health measures ... p.1602

If I ask you the reader to place, first the *social* on Hodges' model followed by the *technical*, you quickly realise looking at the structure of Hodges' model that it provides an immediate high level template and prescription for assessment, planning, intervention and evaluation. The *social* obviously belongs to the humanistic left-hand side of the model, while the *technical* is to the right – the mechanistic. Hodges' model can provide a conceptual and propositional (Jones, 2008) bridge from the socio-technical to health and social care as shown in Figure 3.

Our definitions – working or otherwise - must be cognisant of history. The *socio-technical* movement began in the late 1940s, giving rise to the Tavistock Institute (Mumford, 1983; Coakes, Willis and Lloyd-Jones, 2000). After the Second World War, science and the earliest modern computers had proved themselves, but in the search for increased production and commercial advantage it became apparent that technical solutions alone do not guarantee success. If attempts to apply technology are not managed properly with the impact considered holistically, then technical solutions can become part of the problem. At the Tavistock Institute a series of field studies provided the first major contributions to the theory of socio-technical design with research in the British coal industry (Mumford, 1983).

Definitions: 'Socio-Technical'

From the outset it is important to differentiate between *socio-technical* as applied within the informatics contexts of information systems design, software development plus project management; and definitions that operate in organisational management. So, for the purposes of this paper *socio-technical* is defined as the combination of two types of knowledge (objective and subjec-

Figure 3. "Socio–technical" in h2cm east-west

Socio-	intrapersonal	sciences	technical
	sociology	political	

tive) comprised of people, artefacts, a retinue of concepts and dynamic (chaotic?) fields of human practice notably management, finance and organisation. Whether consciously acknowledged or not, this combination may be coherent or incoherent, depending upon the structures (see below) used to integrate and manage conceptually proximate and disparate parts.

'Socio-Technical Structure'

Building on the definition of socio-technical, the structural aspect is a hybrid, an in-situ analogue-digital creation made up of physical (devices/infrastructure), concepts, human and political ingredients based on various theoretical conceptual schemas and methodologies. Socio-technical structures are multiple and composite in that they span human-machine-organisational boundaries: subject to mathematics and nebulosity. They are transient, their existence and timescales ranging across the human-machine interface, database, available network configuration, hardware and software life-cycle management, organisational and governmental longevity. Socio-technical structures are curricula for change, especially in the form of Masters in Informatics and MBA courses. The clinical-education partnership necessarily entails socio-technical structures from the research councils - Economic and Social Research Council (ESRC), Engineering and Physical Sciences Research Council (EPSRC), the JANET-NHS partnership through to group and one-to-one e-supervision. Education and training (lifelong learning and business change) act as a transport system for ideas that test the business, social, finance and infotech ideologies of the day. Socio-technical structures must also be defined economically as key drivers of creativity and innovation. The result is an amalgam comprised of humanistic and mechanistic systems, software (infrastructure), policy and social groupings.

'Socio-Political-Technical'

In formulating h2cm, Hodges' inclusion of the political domain is pivotal. In any intra-interpersonal - social scenario, politics holds sway. Not necessarily in that formal legal, party political sense, but an informal socially conveyed politics encompassing for example; power relations, gender, choice, consent and autonomy. Globally - creativity, innovation and leadership (design) are no longer relatives *twice removed* from enterprise whether social, technical or socio-technical. Hodges' model can represent through its structure the need for rules in the organisation of the many. For at least two decades the debate about technology shaping society versus society shaping technology has been ongoing (Bijker, et al., 1987): Informal and formal politics in action; as Aarts and Gorman (2007) put it "*To Err is System*". The NHS boasts a prime example in the National Programme for Information Technology managed by Connecting for Health. This ongoing programme is remarkable for its funding, ambition, the attention of the media and academia (see: http://www.nhs-it.info retrieved June 8 2008) its socio-technical impact thus far and the need for a socio-technical approach in the years to follow (Peltu, et al., 2008).

Background: Existing Socio-Technical Structures and Methods

This section scratches the pages of the socio-technical literature by introducing two seminal contributions and briefly discusses other sources. The two authors discussed are Mumford (1983) in the socio-technical sense and Giddens (1984) who is more generic socially and organisational oriented. Enid Mumford created ETHICS, a systems design methodology: *Effective Technical and Human Implementation of Computer-based Systems*. The need for ETHICS is to help manage change with three objectives. First, ETHICS stresses that the future users of computer systems, whether directly or indirectly involved should play a major part in designing these systems. User involvement is closely related to subsequent job satisfaction and efficiency gains and hence the realization of benefits. The users of systems are credited as experts; if this knowledge and experience is recognized and utilized then job satisfaction gains are likely as the users are active agents in the change process and not passive. There is an interesting correspondence here with the continuing emphasis on patients and carers being acknowledged as experts in their care assessment, management and evaluation.

The second objective focuses on the human – behavioural response to change. It is important that specific job satisfaction objectives are factored into the design from the outset and not left to chance, lost amid technical specifications and objectives. In this way potential negative change impacting the quality of work life can be anticipated and avoided or at least ameliorated. Technology has frequently been associated with deskilling and of course the loss of traditional jobs. The prospect of technical, management led change can cause consternation in the user community. If alienated, employees may be absent, seek alternate employment, and overall be less productive.

ETHICS is not restricted to the computer system; the third objective highlights the need for a new computer system to be 'surrounded by a compatible, well functioning organizational system' (Mumford, 1983). Design must be viewed globally as a whole. The technical design is just one part of a very complex design process that must also incorporate the details of human-machine interaction; what would be called gap analysis, the differences in existing processes and proposed new processes and procedures. In addition, as per objectives one and two, individual jobs and workgroup activities must be reviewed; how are existing roles and relationships altered and newly defined? What new management arrangements are needed, since middle management is rarely untouched (Pinsonneault and Kraemer, 1997)?

Giddens' structuration theory seeks to integrate structure and agency. Giddens (1984) defines structuration as "the structuring of social relations across time and space, in virtue of the duality of structure" (p.376). The duality arises from Giddens' emphasis on social action as being comprised of human agents and social structures:

The basic domain of study of the social sciences, according to the theory of structuration, is neither the experience of the individual actor, nor the existence of any form of social totality, but social practices ordered across space and time. Human social activities, like some self-reproducing items in nature, are recursive. That is to say, they are not brought into being by social actors but continually recreated by them via the very means whereby they express themselves as actors. In and through their activities agents reproduce the conditions that make these activities possible. (Giddens, p.2).

This definition allows Giddens to traverse the human individual experience through to the macro level structures of institutions and organisations. A focus purely centred on the technical ignores people as knowledgeable agents; people must not be lost amid objectivism. The links between the thought of Mumford and Giddens are clear. The items that follow are mentioned briefly, they are more specific with a technical bias focusing on IT services, customer services and project management. The complexity of software and hence software development has led to the production and ongoing refinement of tools and frameworks to assure safe, fit for purpose, reliable and efficient code on the one hand and the effective management of projects on the other, such that risk reduction ensures success as in the deployment of a new (or updated) information system.

Influential for several decades Soft Systems Methodology (SMS) (Checkland, 1981) is introduced by Lane and Oliva (1998):

SMS was developed during the 1970s by Peter Checkland and his colleagues at the University of Lancaster's Department of Systems. The methodology emerged from an action-research process that to date includes 400+ cases and still continues the evolution of the methodology. (pp.216-217)

SMS incorporates an organizational history, real world problem situation, a rich picture which includes input from the would-be improvers of the situation. This leads to descriptions of the situation described as streams of culture and tasks and issues. Two forms of analysis are applied cultural and logic-based. This analysis enables identification of differences between the models produced and the real world with proposed changes that are systematically desirable and culturally feasible. Within SMS actions to improve the situation should then follow as a final output. (Lane and Oliva, 1998, p.281).

The essential perspectives of SMS are captured in the mnemonic "CATWOE":

- Customers
- Actors
- Transformation process
- Worldview
- Owner
- Environmental constraints (Checkland and Scholes, 1999).

Atkinson's (2001) Soft Information Systems and Technologies Methodology (SISTeM) was developed from SSM and provides a contingency approach to integrated decision making and development.

Launched in 1996 PRINCE2 - PRojects IN Controlled Environments is a process-based method for effective project management. PRINCE2 is an Open Source international de facto standard used extensively by the UK Government in the public and a skill also sought in the private sector. The history of PRINCE can be traced back to 1975. According to Wikipedia *Structured Systems Analysis and Design Method* (SSADM) is a systems approach to the analysis and design of information systems. In SSADM information systems design is derived through a waterfall method and is seen as a rigorous document-led approach.

PRINCE2 and SSADM are being challenged by more socially-iterative methods of what is called Rapid Application Development (RAD) and Agile Software Development (Thomas, et al.; 2007). *IT Infrastructure Library* (ITIL) refers to a series of five volumes that describe a lifecycle framework for IT Service Management: the volumes include Service Strategy, Service Design, Service Transition, Service Operation and Continual Service Improvement. ITIL can be adapted to various business settings (e.g. telecommunications, helpdesk, information system customer services) the framework defines how Service Management is applied within an organisation and is associated with the international standard - ISO 20000. There are many other tools including the *SocioTechnical Framework*. Web links to this and other methods follow the references.

Socio-Technical Structures of h2cm and Nursing Informatics: The 4Ps

The previous discussion and citations highlight that existing socio-technical structures are employed to help realise effective information systems. The idealised objectives are systems that can facilitate fluid organisational change through the efficient utilisation (dissemination, reuse and refinement) of skills and knowledge. Essentially, this same motivation applies to h2cm, but in a caring context. The fusion of h2cm and the socio-technical depends upon either:

1. Users bring their existing socio-technical structures (as above) and deploy them through the reflective lens of h2cm, confirming a high-level role for Hodges' model or;
2. Researchers study Hodges' model and the extent to which it can support socio-technical perspectives within customary information systems environments. Novel formulations between informatics disciplines or other areas tainted (as are most) by informatics (office applications) may be revealed by this more powerful socio-technical light.

Figure 4 below extends Figure 3 through the 4Ps: PROCESS; PURPOSE; POLICY and PRACTICE each is associated with a knowledge domain. The adoption of the 4Ps arises from the combined clinical and informatics experience of the author and the significance accorded these concepts in the literature. For example, while admittedly a crude device a word search within Ure, et al. (2007) for *policy*, *practice*, *process* and *purpose* produces two, fifteen, fifteen and six occurrences respectively. The 4Ps then are the constants of the socio-technical *program* – a unique program that involves people.

PURPOSE

To be at cross-purposes is a sorry state; it variously denotes disarray, uncertainty, disorganisation and confusion. The NHS finds itself at cross-purposes; the commonly cited anecdote that 'NHS' really stands for *National Ill-Health Service* bears repeating here. Given our propensity to polarise, the profusion of dichotomies in health care and the regular cycles of re-organisation, it is strange that these two world's of disease and health promotion still wear the same uniform. This state of affairs has not gone unnoticed amid health-social care structural and policy review. PURPOSE lies at the heart of socio-technical structures as a fusion of people (as individuals and groups), skills, knowledge, function and form. Key social structures are obviously embedded in the humanistic domains.

For the individual, motivation is a primary psychological factor. Having a sense of PURPOSE is essential in terms of response to a given situation and any subsequent problems solving. People are sense making machines (Kurtz and Snowden, 2003). They need to be fed with a sense of purpose. Not programmed. Nursing should not be purely task-oriented; nursing is about people not (just) PROCESS. Purpose matters from the level of technical with local project planning and management to National engagement in informatics programmes. Whilst organisations are primarily group centred (production, payroll, sickness) planning and change must be framed in individual terms.

Figure 4. Hodges' model and the 4P's

PURPOSE	PROCESS
PRACTICE	POLICY

PRACTICE

If clinically, informatics is seen as little more than a management abacus, then the user's sense of purpose will be reduced to that of a *bean counter*. The much vaunted aim of personalised care then becomes nothing more than numbers on paper related to serious untoward incidents, the number of complaints and similar data. Tasks have been viewed pejoratively in the past within nursing, but *tasks are* an essential consequence of time and currency of description. Tasks can readily be quantified and they are a vital part of the totality of care and informatics. For staff to be motivated and have a sense of purpose, qualitative considerations must be brought into play. Care is always situated; priorities, education and training, the environment and technology and much more all affect PRACTICE. In making these distinctions this is not to divorce PURPOSE and PRACTICE from the SCIENTIFIC and POLITICAL domains. The 4Ps are interdependent. They can support or hinder the learning organisation. Effective socio-technical structures must create and respond to change; producing improvement through data-to-knowledge transformation that delivers meaning at all levels. Meaning is nothing if not disseminated. There is an acute issue in nursing, that of ensuring that user engagement:

- Actually takes place and is actively pursued by project leads and developers;
- Is recognised and valued by nursing managers;
- Provision is made by senior managers to allow clinical users time-out to engage with backfill of posts if needed;

PROCESS

Whether sequential or parallel, PROCESSES are first and foremost grounded in the SCIENCES domain. A beginner's guide to IT might include a description of *what computers do best*. Computers excel in their number crunching abilities. It is their capacity to represent, simulate and transform processes that makes them so powerful. Although PROCESS may have something to say about delivery of narrative, it seems reasonable to declare that what narrative is to the SOCIOLOGICAL domain, so PROCESS is to the SCIENTIFIC? In socio-technical structures however, health care is about PEOPLE and PROCESS. The debacle in November 2007 with the merger of HM Revenue and Customs and loss of the personal data of millions of UK citizens is a stark reminder of the dependencies between the 4Ps and PEOPLE. The advent of the nursing process, with its 4-6 iterative stages - assessment; diagnosis; planning; implementation and evaluation (Wilkinson, 2006) - saw some nurses concerned that patients were literally being 'processed'.

PROCESS in informatics now has a socio-technical home in clinical practice through role based access and control [RBAC] (El-Hassen and Fiadeiro; 2007), as deployed in the UK's National Programme for Information Technology. Now *roles* take on an extended socio-technical meaning within the organisation. Roles are also of import in gap analysis, a key activity completed in the preparation, roll-out and review of new information systems. What are the existing processes? Are there any 'show-stoppers', new processes that do not support vital tasks, for example, specific reporting requirements or referral pathway events?

It is salutary to reflect on the distance between practice and software development approaches such as *computation, coordination, configuration* [CCC] (El-Hassen and Fiadeiro; 2007); *models, views and controllers* [MVC] (Thomas, et al., 2007) and developer-analyst engagement with end-users? Given their properties and purposes as formal tools computer programming languages reside in the sciences domain. This means there is wide gap between the language and syntax of the programmer and the domain expert (nurse). Computing now includes a diverse range of so-called Domain Specific Languages (DSL). Although definitions remain a contentious point there are signs that DSLs could bring these disparate worlds closer together with increased productivity for all. The challenge remains however in that existing DSLs seem confined to computing, finance and technical applications (Olsen, 2007). Wither the business rules for nursing?

POLICY

Figure 3 showed socio-technical as a vertical bisection of h2cm. Is there a horizontal form as per Figure 5?

In the same way that the individual precedes the group as the focus within Hodges' model,

Figure 5. "Socio–technical" in h2cm: north-south

technical

interpersonal	sciences
sociology	political

socio-

so too for the *technical* which can also be said to occupy the INTRA-INTERPERSONAL and SCIENCES domains. Distributed social networks are a product of devices and other technologies that are designed and used by individual users. It follows then that the *socio* component spans the SOCIOLOGY and POLITICAL domains. This is why the construct of socio-political-technical previously mentioned is needed. PROCESS is found in the SCIENCES, but is enacted (or not!) in the humanistic domains. A further justification of the need to add politics to our socio-technical definitions could rest solely on standards: and information standards in particular. Technical standards provide the intelligent glue that holds the structures together and releases them appropriately. Standards are of course subject to evaluation and supervision, being embedded and enshrined within professional practice. Information standards are critical in assuring the quality of data and safety of the public. The realisation of health care quality information systems is an ongoing quest, as reported by Niland, et al. (2006).

So, to conclude the 4Ps we tend to think of the parts-whole debate as intimately connected with reductionist SCIENCES – PROCESSES. In attempting to grasp (sense make!) the 4Ps, perhaps there is a need to consider mereology, the study of whole-part relations across all the h2cm knowledge domains? Perhaps, a key to fully apprehending socio-technical structures is to treat them as organic and study their morphology (Bortoft, 1996)? We need new ways of seeing. Before there is a vision we need to envision – in new ways.

A World of Two Halves or Four Quarters And Enforced Relations

Figures 3, 4 and 5 maintain the two distinct socio-technical camps. A more accurate (and rather obvious) depiction is that of a subset combining both social and technical factors as in Figure 6.

To contemplate the socio-technical is to contemplate a world of knowledge, experience and thought that is so obviously divided. I have adopted the convention of the hyphen, inspired by the work of Serres (1995), plus the nexus of Hodges' model and because small things can denote large. Let us ask *the* question then: how hard does that hyphen have to work? Is the union forced and the two worlds produce seismic waves; or is the union one of ready accommodation with a regulated need to re-focus eased by artifice on both sides? Perhaps, the hyphen is not as passive as may first appear? It makes it possible insofar as Hodges model is concerned to use our imagination and travel between the *social* and the *technical*. At times it does appear we are dealing purely with a sociological agenda, at other times technical. The hyphen becomes a switch either analogue or digital seeing the technical from an analogue perspective and vice-versa; facilitating inclusion as recognised above in the socio-political-technical.

The hyphen can act like the lunar terminator (the dividing margin between night and day), waxing and waning according to context. Experienced lunar observers recognise that the terminator is where shadows are to be found, providing contrast more detail. The full moon [TECHNICAL] brings illumination for focused action, but the

Figure 6. Socio-technical as Venn diagram

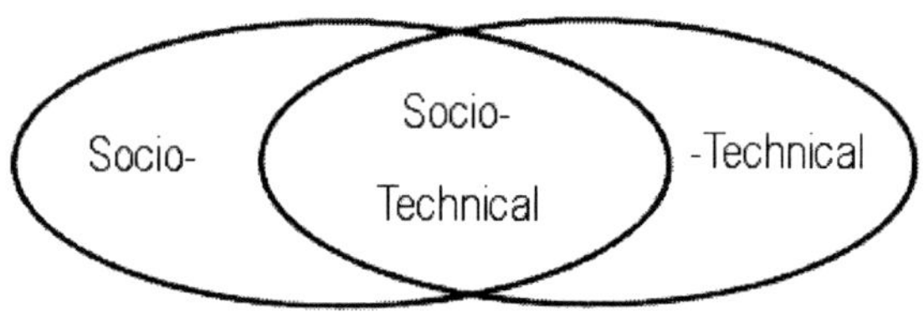

glare of Harold Wilson's 'white heat' (Cooley, 1987) can be blinding. The new moon [SOCIAL] promotes a need for collective safety, reflection and planning. The half moon (both 'quarters') relates to the socio-technical in balance; a time for connection, creativity and fusion. It may seem strange that an object of myth can feature within informatics. In truth myth must have a place in the *socio*-technical. Just as circuit boards are the substrate for technology; so myth is the substrate for society and history.

One of the problems in melding together and conceptually sustaining socio-technical structures is a lack of unifying concepts. *Information* is the concept of choice (Stamper, 1985; Jones, 1996). If *information* is not the logical choice, then it is surely *the* holistic candidate? Informatics might provide the basis for a foundation that is not only flexible, multi or non-contextual, but can also operate at the required levels of description and across them; for example, machine code – public mental health strategy; information strategy - information prescription; ontology – patient advice. Nursing informatics practitioners readily embrace the vocabulary and techniques of the informatics world. They can also utilise and champion tools developed in health care that can provide the bracing to reinforce the integrity, resilience, longevity and functionality of our socio-technical structures. A case in point is the *stress vulnerability model* of Zubin and Spring (1977), which helps to explain an individual's response to stress with reference to level of stress exposure and the person's degree of vulnerability. This model can also be used to characterise information use and information overload (as per Figure 7) plus the transformational benefits of education and training.

Closing Discussion

The market, policy makers and enthusiasts have sold informatics on the back of promised benefits. In these most commercial of times, we must ask what of value Hodges' model adds to the socio-technical debate? As the nursing literature reveals concept analysis has long been a tool of nurse theorists. Hodges' model can stimulate and augment conceptual analysis, encouraging exploration and identification of concepts and thereby highlight ill-defined or much needed conceptual cross-members to marry the social (political) and

Figure 7. Stress-vulnerability model

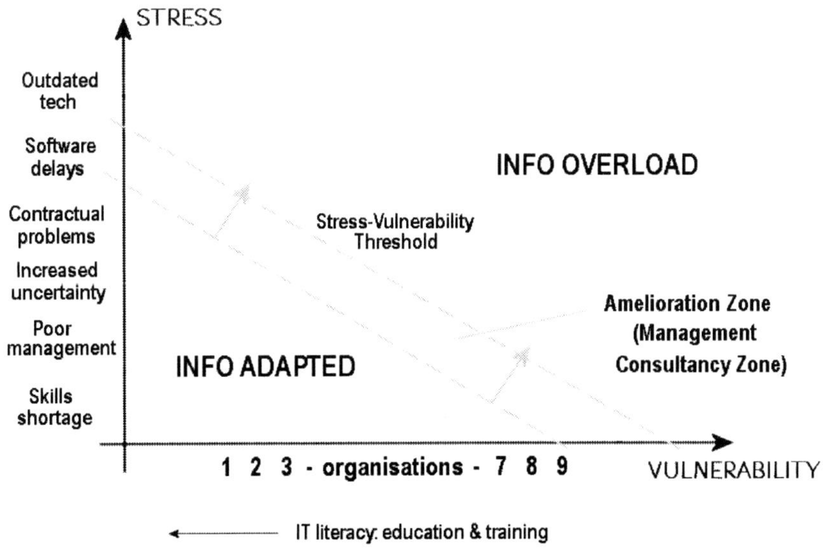

technical realms. It is no accident that *scaffolding* is a common metaphor and technique in education, engineering, cognitive science and software development. Safety first principles dictate that due care and diligence is taken as we leverage existing structures and when necessary build new ones. For all informatics practitioners and participants the issue is not just the existence and creation of socio-technical structures, but access and utilisation and how this is measured.

Nursing as a profession must constantly aspire to make a difference and effect positive change. In the decades ahead (nursing) informatics can help leverage positive change in tackling health inequalities, and addressing the ongoing revision of the new health agenda of health promotion and education. To do so though nursing informatics must also recognise its limits; it must seek out or help create new socio-technical structures through partnerships with other informatics disciplines, such as - *community, social (care), urban*, and *citizen*. Although 2 x 2 matrices are ubiquitous as a structuring device for concepts, ideas and much more, they are also much maligned: a *ready reckoner for gross assumptions*. Upon first encounter Hodges' model may be considered merely as a brainstorming tool. On the contrary, h2cm can act as a framework for weaving; a template for a socio-technical tapestry. The framework provides a lattice upon which vital conceptual connections can be displayed explicitly on its public face, or privately when the handicraft is viewed from the back – the (propositional) infrastructure.

ACKNOWLEDGMENT

I would like to express my sincere thanks to the editors for their interests and the very helpful comments from the referees on early drafts of this paper.

REFERENCES

Aarts, J., & Gorman, P. (2007). IT in Healthcare: Sociotechnical Approaches "To Err is System"; Editorial. *International Journal of Medical Informatics*, 76(Supplement 1)S1-S3.

Adams, T. (1987, February). Dementia is a Family Affair. *Community Outlook*, 7-8.

Atkinson, C. (2000). The Soft Information Systems and Technologies Methodology (SISTeM): A Contingency Approach to Integrated Decision Making and Development, In (Eds.) Altmann, G., Lamp, J., Love, P., et al. *Proceedings of IC-STM2000: International Conference on Systems Thinking in Management*, Geelong, November 8-10, 2000.

Berg, M., & Goorman, E. (1999). The contextual nature of medical information. *International Journal Medical Informatics, 56*, (1-3), 51-60.

Bijker, W. E., Hughes, T. P., & Pinch, T. J. (Eds.) (1987). *The Social Construction of Technological Systems: New Directions in the Sociology and History of Technology.* Cambridge, MA: MIT Press.

Bortoft, H. (1996). *The Wholeness of Nature: Goethe's Way of Science*. Floris Books.

Bricon-Souf, N., & Newman, C. R. (2007). Context awareness in healthcare: A review. *International Journal of Medical Informatics, 76*(1), 2 – 12.

Checkland P. (1981). *Systems Thinking, Systems Practice*. Wiley, Chichester.

Checkland, P., & Scholes, J. (1999). *Soft Systems Methodology in Action.* John Wiley.

Coakes, E., Willis, D., & Lloyd-Jones R. E. (Eds.) (2000). *The New Sociotech: Graffiti on the Long Wall*: London: Springer-Verlag.

Cooley, M. (1987). *Architect or Bee? The Human Price of Technology.* The Hogarth Press, p.117.

Earl, M. J., & Skyrme, D. J. (1990, May). Hybrid Managers: What should you do? *Computer Bulletin*, 19-21.

El-Hassen, O., & Fiadeiro, J. L. (2007). Role-based Architectural Modelling of Socio-Technical Systems. *Electronic Notes in Theoretical Computer Science,181*, 5–17.

Gärdenfors, P. (2000). *Conceptual Spaces: The Geometry of Thought*. MIT Press.

Giddens, A. (1984). *The Constitution of Society: Outline of the Theory of Structuration*. Berkeley, University of California Press.

Hayes, G., & Barnett, D. (Eds.) (2008). *UK Health Computing: Recollections and Reflections*, BCS.

Hinchcliffe, S. M. (Ed.) (1989). *Nursing Practice and Health Care*, [1st Edition only], London, Edward Arnold.

Jones, P. (1996). Humans, Information, and Science. *Journal of Advanced Nursing, 24*(3), 591-598.

Jones, P. (1998). *Hodges' Health Career Care Domains Model.* Retrieved June 8, 2008, from http://www.p-jones.demon.co.uk

Jones, P. (2000a). *Hodges' Health Career Care Domains Model, Structural Assumptions.* Retrieved June 8, 2008, from http://www.p-jones.demon.co.uk/theory.html

Jones, P. (2000b). *Hodges' Health Career Care Domains Model, Theoretical Assumptions.* Retrieved June 8, 2008, from http://www.p-jones.demon.co.uk/struct.html

Jones, P. (2004). Viewpoint: Can Informatics And Holistic Multidisciplinary Care Be Harmonised? *British Journal of Healthcare Computing & Information Management, 21*, 6, 17-18.

Jones, P. (2008). Exploring Serres' Atlas, Hodges' Knowledge Domains and the Fusion of Informatics and Cultural Horizons, In Kidd, T., Chen, I. (Eds.) *Social Information Technology Connecting Society and Cultural Issues.* IGI Global.

Kurtz, C. F., & Snowden, D. J. (2003) The new dynamics of strategy: Sense-making in a complex and complicated world. *IBM Systems Journal, 42,* 3.

Lane, D. C., & Oliva, R. (1998). The greater whole: Towards a synthesis of system dynamics and soft systems methodology. *European Journal of Operational Research, 107,* 214-235.

Melton, G. B., Parsons, S., Morrison, F. P., Rothschild, A. S., Markatou, M., & Hripcsak, G. (2006). Inter-patient distance metrics using SNOMED CT defining relationships. *Journal of Biomedical Informatics, 39,* 6, 697-705.

Mumford, E. (1983). *Designing Human Systems for New Technology - The ETHICS Method,*

Retrieved June 8 2008, from http://www.enid.u-net.com/C1book1.htm

Mumford, E. (1996). *Systems Design Ethical Tools for Ethical Change*, Macmillan.

Nevárez, J. (2008). *The Reversal of Technology.* In Kidd, T., Chen, I. (Eds.) *Social Information Technology Connecting Society and Cultural Issues.* IGI Global.

Niland, J. C., Rouse, L., & Stahl, D. C., (2006). An Informatics Blueprint for Healthcare Quality Information Systems. *Journal of the American Medical Informatics Association, 13*(4), 402–417.

Olsen, R. (2007). *Design Patterns in Ruby,* Addison-Wesley, Chapter 16.

Pearsall, J., et al. (Eds.) (1998). The New Oxford Dictionary of English, OUP. p. 468.

Peltu, M., Eason, K., & Clegg, C. (2008). How a Sociotechnical approach can help NPfIT deliver better NHS patient care, Report produced following BCS Workshop 7 February 2008. Retrieved

8 June 2008, from http://www.bcs.org/server.php?show=nav.9932

Pinsonneault, A., & Kraemer, K. L. (1997). Information Technology and Middle Management Downsizing: A Tale of Two Cities, CRITO Working Paper URB-115, 4/16/97. Retrieved June 8, 2008 from http://repositories.cdlib.org/cgi/viewcontent.cgi?article=1090&context=crito

Serres, M. (1995). *Conversations on Science, Culture, and Time*. With Latour, B., University of Michigan Press.

Scharff, R., & Dusek, V. (2002). *Philosophy of Technology: The Technological Condition - An Anthology*. Blackwell Philosophy Anthologies.

Snow, C. P. (1959). *The Two Cultures*. Cambridge University Press. Reissued 1993.

Stamper, R. K. (1985). Towards a Theory of Information: Information: Mystical Fluid or a Subject for Scientific Enquiry. *The Computer Journal*, 28, 195-199. BCS, Oxford Journals.

Stone, W. F., & Schaffner, P. E. (1997). The Tomkins Polarity Scale: Recent Developments. *Bulletin of the Tomkins Institute*, *4*, 17-22.

Sullivan, M. (2003). The New Subjective Medicine: taking the patient's point of view on health care and health, *Social Science & Medicine*, *56*(7), 1595-604.

Thomas, D., Heinemeier, D., & Breedt, L. (2007). *Agile Web Development with Rails*, Pragmatic Bookshelf; 2nd Revised edition.

Ure, J., Procter, R., Lin, Y., Hartswood, M., & Ho, K. (2007). *Aligning Technical and Human Infrastructures in the Semantic Web: A socio-technical perspective,* e-Social Science 2007 Conference, Ann Arbor, Michigan. Retrieved June 8, 2008 from http://ess.si.umich.edu/papers/paper188.pdf

Westbrook, J. I., Braithwaite, J., Georgiou, A., et al. (2007). Multimethod Evaluation of Information and Communication Technologies in Health in the Context of Wicked Problems and Sociotechnical Theory. *Journal of the American Medical Informatics Association*, *14,* 6, 746-755.

Wilber, K. (2000). *Integral Psychology: Consciousness, Spirit, Psychology, Therapy*. Shambhala Publications.

Wilkinson, J.M. (2006). *Nursing Process and Critical Thinking*, 4th Edition, Prentice Hall.

Wilson, E.O. (1998). *Consilience: The Unity of Knowledge*. Abacus.

Zubin, J., & Spring, B. (1977). Vulnerability - a new view of schizophrenia. *Journal of Abnormal Psychology*, *86*, 2, 103-124.

Socio-Technical Websites

http://www.sociotechnical.org/ (British Computer Society Sociotechnical Specialist Group)

http://www.prince2.com/what-is-prince2.asp (PRINCE2)

http://www.itil.org.uk/ (ITIL)

http://wisdom.usc.edu/stf/ (Sociotechnical Framework)

ENDNOTES

1. This brief introduction to Hodges' model has been published previously online and in print (Jones, 2008).
2. Hinchcliffe includes a chapter by Brian E Hodges (1st Edition only).

Chapter XII
Strategies for Creating Virtual Learning Communities

Beth Perry Mahler
Athabasca University, Canada

Margaret Edwards
Athabasca University, Canada

ABSTRACT

Teaching nursing online requires teachers to purposefully use strategies that facilitate the development of virtual learning communities. The chapter proposes answers to the question, "How can educators effectively teach the very social discipline of nursing in virtual classrooms?" Specific online teaching strategies including Photovoice, Virtual Reflective Centers, and Conceptual Quilting are explored. The social and socio-technical implications of teaching nursing online are considered. A final section in the chapter describes how these developments in online nursing education are changing the social and pedagogical perspectives of distance learning. Research questions that arise from this exploration are presented.

INTRODUCTION

The Internet has changed how nursing is taught. Now many universities offer nursing programs, or selected nursing courses, online. Baumlein (2003) predicted that by the year 2010 most universities would offer some of their degree programs as Web-based options. Internet based nursing education is flourishing and is making education available, accessible, and convenient for those seeking basic to advanced degrees (Mancuso-Murphy, 2007).

Nursing is a complex discipline requiring a mix of intellectual and social knowledge, psychomotor and interpersonal skills, and compassionate and professional attitudes. As many have said, including Nightingale back in 1859, nursing is an art and a science. Part of the complexity is the very interpersonal nature of nursing. Given that nursing is such an intensely human discipline it is important that all student nurses become skilled in interpersonal interaction. Whether an individual is studying to be a clinical nurse, a nurse educator, or a nurse administrator all need to become adept at human relations, equipped with relevant knowledge, skills, and attitudes. Within this context, a major question for those who teach nursing online becomes, How can nursing students develop human relationship skills, knowledge, and appropriate attitudes if they are taking courses over the Internet?

In this chapter we argue that to successfully teach nursing online, educators need to incorporate strategies that facilitate the development of interpersonal abilities. We propose that an important step in creating an online learning environment that supports the growth of interpersonal intelligence is the development of virtual learning communities. Exemplary online nurse educators develop and utilize innovative teaching strategies that help to create virtual learning communities in which interpersonal knowledge, skills, and attitudes can be honed (Perry & Edwards, 2006).

The purpose of this chapter is to explore specific online teaching strategies that facilitate the creation of virtual learning communities online. It is our belief that learning online can be a community experience if instructors are diligent and accomplished at including online teaching strategies in Internet delivered courses. Broadly the chapter addresses the question, "How can educators effectively teach the very social discipline of nursing in virtual classrooms?"

Major themes explored in the chapter include a discussion of the existing literature on the role of relationships in learning, the creation of online educational communities, and the part immediacy plays in establishing these communities. One section of the review focuses specifically on the Community of Inquiry (COI) Model (Rouke, Garrison, Anderson, & Archer, 2001) (see Figure 1). This is followed by a review of philosophical shifts that influence online community development including the shift from objectivism towards constructivism, from behaviorism towards socio-cognitive views of education, and the pedagogical shift from direct instruction to the facilitation of collaborative learning. Illustration of these themes is provided by examples of practical online teaching strategies that the authors have found promote the establishment of virtual learning community for student nurses. The strategies of Photovoice and Virtual Reflective Centers, among others, are highlighted. The concluding discussion focuses on the social and socio-technical implications of teaching the intensely human discipline of nursing online. A final section in the chapter describes how these developments in online nursing education are changing the social and pedagogical perspectives of distance learning. The chapter ends with a proposal for further research studies related to teaching nursing online.

Figure 1. (Rouke, Garrison, Anderson, & Archer, 2001)

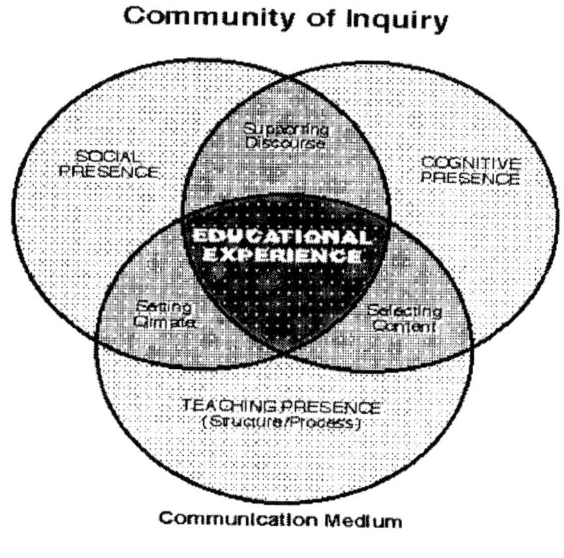

This chapter should be of interest to nurse educators and practitioners. Additionally, operating authorities in universities and health care facilities who are looking for ways to effectively use computer technology to maximize teaching and learning in nursing and health care may discover both strategies to adopt, and foundational understandings to support the evolution of their own approaches. Finally, this chapter provides a solid foundation for further research projects related to online nursing education.

BACKGROUND

To more fully understand the successful teaching of nursing using the Internet, and ways educators can create virtual learning communities online, we look first to the published scholarly literature on this and related topics. Specifically this literature review includes the role of relationships in effective online instruction, creating community in the online classroom, and philosophical shifts and the creation of community as a foundation for achieving this goal.

THE ROLE OF RELATIONSHIPS IN EFFECTIVE ONLINE INSTRUCTION

In an era of rapid technological change, online educational opportunities for health care students, including nurses, are growing at an exponential rate (Hodge, Bosse, Faulconer, & Fewell, 2006). However, not all online educational experiences are positive. Sit, Chung, Chow, and Wong (2005) analyzed students' level of satisfaction with Web-based learning. The respondents keyed in on inadequate opportunity to study with others, inadequate opportunities for discussion with faculty, and lack of peer support as learning hindrances in the online learning environment (2005). Atack and Rankin (2002) described the experiences of Registered Nurses (RNs) enrolled in a Web-based course. The RNs in their study appreciated the convenience of taking an online course but found the lack of perceived feedback from instructors a negative factor (2002). Halter, Kleiner, and Hess (2006), Hyde and Murray (2005), and Mueller (2001) all concluded studies on student satisfaction with online learning saying that technological expertise, interaction and relationships, convenience, and flexibility were important in student satisfaction with online learning. Zhang, an expert in "e-immediacy," identified the instructors' ability to stimulate frequent and consistent interactions throughout the course as most important to program effectiveness (2005). If interactions, and the resulting relationships, were absent or superficial student satisfaction with online learning waned (2005). Thurmond (2003) also cited interaction as the core element in an effective online environment.

The research reviewed to this point features a common theme; student-teacher and student-student interactions are an important element in Web-based learning from the students' perspective. Students see human to human interactions as a critical learning strategy in the online environment and lack of the opportunity for relationship hinders their learning (Atack, 2003). Sit, Chung, Chow, and Wong (2005) found that teachers in an effective online environment facilitate establishing peer support between students and also dialogue one to one with learners. Meaningful communication between instructors and students encourages participation, provides reassurance, and generally increases success in online learning (Cuellar, 2002).

The key terms in the literature on the importance of interaction in online teaching and learning seem to be "relationships" and "meaningful communication." While researchers found interactions in the online classroom are important, the interactions need to be such that they lead to the development of relationships. "Relationship" implies a connection or affinity between people (Merriam-Webster, 2007). Effective interaction that builds relationships, even when participants are separated by distance, helps to reduce feelings of isolation and facilitates effective online learning (Mancuso-Murphy, 2007).

Based on the literature we propose that developing relationships through effective interpersonal communication begins with interaction. Exemplary online teaching is interactive (Perry & Edwards, 2006). Robley, Farnsworth, Flynn, and Horne (2004) call interaction "the core of online learning" (p. 335). Interaction between students, and between the students and the instructor, helps students to learn from the experiences of others. The interaction also helps to build community in the online environment in part because of the sharing of experiences and opportunities to offer support and encouragement that come with interaction. The experience of community connectedness gives rise to students feeling valued and respected which is essential to personal and professional growth (Robley et al., 2004). Thiele (2003) contended that interaction is directly related to improved learning and concluded that there is a direct relationship between students' levels of interaction with the instructor and levels of learning in online courses.

In a direct sense, interaction and the resulting building of relationships, are linked, with one leading to the other as a positive cycle is created. As the online instructor interacts with students, and as students interact with each other, relationships are built. As relationships are established the potential for further positive interaction between participants is enhanced and community is potentially established. As the course continues, relationships grow and a sense of closeness and intimacy in the online community develops. In a way a cycle begins as meaningful interactions facilitate establishing relationships, and effective relations lead to more significant interactions. We have alluded here to the way interaction and establishing relationships are forerunners to the development of online educational communities. The follow section explains these possible links more fully.

CREATING COMMUNITY IN THE ONLINE CLASSROOM

There is a growing body of literature supporting the importance of the community construct in online courses (Liu, Magjuka, Curtis, & Lee, 2007). Why is it important that the experience of community be a component of the online environment? Some time ago a common belief was that a strong sense of community was limited to the traditional classroom; however in 2002 Rovai published a paper arguing that virtual classrooms had the potential to equally build and sustain a sense of community. Rovai defined a "learning community as a group of students who have feelings of trust and belonging, possess shared expectations, and are committed to shared educational goals" (2002, p. 12). A sense of online community is viewed "as consisting of four related dimensions: spirit, trust, interaction, and commonality of learning expectations and goals" (Rovai, 2002, p.12).

Benefits of online learning communities. As first proposed by Rovai (2002) the benefits of online learning communities are many. Research evidence suggests that the creation of an online learning community serves as the foundation for a successful learning environment (Conrad, 2002; Lee, Carter-Wells, Glaeser, Ivers, & Street, 2006). In a recent study by Lee and co-authors (2006) graduate students "commented that community involvement made them feel more committed to attaining the shared goals of the program (93%); community membership enhanced their sense of self-worth and efficacy (80%); and engagement in the community decreased their sense of isolation and increased their social support for learning (74%)" (p.18). Further, in this same study, graduate students cited a community centered approach on the part of the teacher as most essential for building community followed by a constructivist learning environment (Lee, et al., 2006). There is also confirmation that a significant positive relationship exists between sense of community and perceived cognitive learning (Rovai, 2002).

These positive outcomes support the value of learning communities in online instruction.

Challenge of creating online learning communities. While the value of online learning communities is evident, facilitating their formation is challenging. Educators who teach via the Internet face this challenge each time they teach. Rovai (2002) recognized that "the particular affective nature of forming and maintaining a sense of community online places extra demands on facilitators" (2002, p.3). Ouzts suggested that "By integrating learning activities that promote interaction, negotiation, and debate in online courses, instructors may begin to build a learning community in which students collaborate" (2006, p. 286). Rovai (2002) proposed "that instructors teaching at a distance may promote a sense of community by attending to seven factors: transactional distance, social presence, social equality, small group activities, group facilitation, teaching style and learning stage, and community size" (p.12). Supporting this Hodge et al. (2006) recommended that communities of learning can be formed by "mimicking proximity." Creating this sense of nearness requires addressing social and psychological factors, such as social space and social presence, that impact and facilitate communications (2006). It is apparent from this literature that development of learning communities is primarily instructor driven. This finding supports the importance of teacher presence in the online environment. In other words, effective online teachers need to generate immediacy.

Immediacy and Establishment of Effective Online Communities. Successful establishment of learning communities seems to depend, at least in part, on the instructor's facility to create immediacy. "Immediacy refers to communication behaviours that reduce social and psychological distance between people. Immediacy strategies include both nonverbal and verbal behaviours" (Arbough, 2001, p. 43). Likewise, Hutchins (2003) defined teacher immediacy as "behaviors that enhance closeness and nonverbal interaction with another" (p. 2).

It is only recently that immediacy in the online environment has become a focus of research studies, with the biggest challenge being how nonverbal communication can be transmitted via the Internet. Richardson and Swan (2003), Woods and Ebersole (2003), Rourke et al. (2001), Na Uban and Kimble (2004), Kreijns, Kirschner and Jochems (2002), Woods and Baker (2004) all make reference to the importance of immediacy behaviors in the virtual classroom. Although immediacy has become a popular theme in the literature on effective online instruction and the creation of virtual classroom communities rarely do studies describe how to facilitate this experience. The Community of Inquiry (COI) Model (Rouke, Garrison, Anderson, & Archer, 2001) provides some direction for online educators who seek to develop immediacy and create virtual online learning communities.

Community of Inquiry Model. The COI Model provides a framework that encompasses the concepts of relationships, communication, immediacy, and interaction discussed thus far in the literature review (Rouke, et al, 2001). It provides some clues as to how instructors who teach online can facilitate these experiences which are valued by students.

The COI model highlights three major aspects of the online learning community; social presence, cognitive presence, and teaching presence which overlap to form the educational experience of the learner (Rouke, et al, 2001). These researchers concluded that "creation of adequate levels of cognitive, social, and teaching presence is associated with high levels of deep and meaningful learning" (Archer, Garrison, Anderson, & Rourke, 2001). A COI is created online when a group of people who are strongly linked both socially and cognitively, experience learning through the leadership of a teacher (teacher presence). Social presence, or the sense of relationship, occurs among learners who project their personal qualities into the learning environment and as Rourke et al said, "become real people" (2001, p. 87). Cognitive presence, the third element of the model, is considered the extent to which learners are able to make meaning through interaction and discussion in a critical community of inquiry (Rourke, et al., 2001).

White, Roberts and Brannan (2003) wrote about ways online teachers can establish cognitive, social, and teaching presence. Specifically they recommended encouraging learner participation, using the right message so that it is received, understood, and remembered, and eliciting feedback from students as strategies to help to create a community of inquiry (White, Roberts & Brannan, 2003, p. 173). Rogers (2002) wrote about employing the "reflective cycle" and structured feedback as ways teachers could create a sense of community in the class. For Rogers the "reflective cycle" involved encouraging teachers to "attend to student learning in more rich and nuanced ways" (2002, p. 231). Rogers also stated the central role that feedback from students can play in helping teachers assess the extent of their own perceived cognitive, social, and teaching presence in the class. Knowing if students are experiencing a sense of community in the class is important for teachers who strive for this eventuality. Feedback from learners regarding lack of sense of community should propel teachers to re-strategize their approaches.

Perry and Edwards concluded that online educators who are highly successful at establishing teaching, social, and cognitive presence as outlined in the COI model create a sense of virtual community and are considered "exemplary educators" by students (2005). These researchers found that online instruction that students consider highly successful takes place when the group of learners is strongly linked to one another socially and cognitively. Further, in exemplary online educational experiences there are also social and cognitive links between the learners and the instructor facilitated by the perceptible presence of the teacher in the virtual classroom (Perry & Edwards, 2005).

In summary, the COI model helps to explain what makes some online educators very effective as they attend to the social, cognitive, and teaching presence in their online classrooms and in doing so create the sense of community that students seem to value. Understanding some fundamental philosophical shifts related to education helps to explain why the components of the COI model are important for successful creation of community in the online teaching environment.

PHILOSOPHICAL SHIFTS AND CREATION OF COMMUNITY

The movement toward offering more education online, and the focus exemplary online teachers place on the development of community, is paralleled, or perhaps fueled, by foundational philosophical shifts. These shifts are not distinct from one another and in ways are closely linked. Specifically, the shifts include movement from objectivism towards constructivism, from behaviorism towards socio-cognitive views of education, and from direct instruction to the facilitation of collaborative learning. These major philosophical swings seem to underlie much of the understanding we currently have of effective online teaching and learning and are important for considering why specific teaching strategies are successful in online education. Each shift is addressed independently in the following section; however we acknowledge the overlap and interrelationship between them.

Social Constructivism. The first trend is that of constructivism in learning. Social constructivist theory (SCT) is a dominant learning paradigm linked to Vygotsky who developed it in 1978 (Hung, 2001). SCT focuses on processes and interactions within a social context (Hung, 2001). Like constructivism theory, SCT assumes that knowledge is constructed by students, however emphasis is placed on the importance of interaction with people and social context as it influences learning. According to SCT, learning is characterized by mediation through language, discovery of differing perspectives, and achievement of shared meaning (Hung, 2001).

Tynjala stated that constructivism is a dynamic process through which students construct their own meaning and develop a personal representation of knowledge (1997). As Entwistle (1991) echoed, it is the individual's subjective perception of the educational context and process that are central to this construction. Teachers with a constructivist philosophy aim to facilitate the learners' construction of their own views about the course curriculum (Bryson & Hand, 2007).

The literature offers some guidance for instructors who seek to assist learners in the self-construction of meaning. Gerber and Scott (2007) proposed broadly that the Web itself is potentially a "tool of social constructivism" because of the potential it offers for interaction (p. 461). Interaction is recommended by Yacci (2000) as a primary method of self-construction of meaning as interaction can lead to collaborative learning. Collaborative learning can take many forms and can involve the learner collaborating with classmates, instructors, their wider personal or professional community, or with self. Petraglia (1998) noted that collaborative learning is often equated with group work. However, Petraglia cautioned, "the assumption that making students work with others replicates the natural processes of social construction demonstrates a thin appreciation for how meaning is negotiated" (Petraglia, 1998, p. 101). Shulman, Lotan, and Whitcomb (1998) said that if facilitated by an effective instructor having students work collaboratively in groups can be highly successful and lead to social construction of knowledge. The key phrase in this finding is "effective facilitation" by the instructor; suggesting an active, purposeful, and helpful role (1998). Petraglia explained that collaborative learning is a mediating theory of social constructivism because interaction is an aspect of the construction of knowledge (p. 101).

Beyond helping to explain why the experience of community is important in effective online education, SCT also provides the foundational rational for explaining why interactive teaching technologies are valuable in teaching via the Internet. Proponents of social constructivism highlight the role of social influences and community in the learning process in distance teaching (Hung, 2001). Implementing effective interactive teaching strategies in any learning environment is challenging. This is especially so in online instruction where some say asynchronous communications and the potential for disconnectedness may impede interaction and result in feelings of isolation for learners (Ambrose, 2001). The feeling of community helps to prevent disconnectedness and feelings of isolation as learners and instructors feel part of something bigger than themselves. The importance of creating community in higher education offered through distance is essential "to support collaborative learning and discourse associated with higher levels of learning" (Garrison, 2006, para 3). In an important online student satisfaction study by Ali, Hodson, Carlton and Ryan (2004) the researchers concluded that students' perceptions of online learning could be interpreted within the context of adult learning theory and were congruent with constructivism theory.

Socio-Cognitive. The second major philosophical transition is the movement from behaviorism to social-cognitive views of education. Simply put, socio-cognitive philosophy emphasizes the importance of relationships in successful teaching and learning. Scardamalia (2002) puts this phenomenon into a wider context when she considers the socio-cognitive dynamics of knowledge building discourse in the academic environment. According to Scardamalia, "the discourse of knowledge building communities results in more than sharing of knowledge; the knowledge itself is refined and transformed through the discursive practices of the community, practices that have the advancement of knowledge as their explicit goal" (p. 76). Raider-Roth (2004) examined the relational aspects of classroom environments and in doing so also emphasized the socio-cognitive view of knowledge as socially constructed. Raider-Roth proposed that the interpersonal relationships that exist within a classroom community can profoundly affect the learning and self-assessment processes that occur in this milieu (2005).

Like social constructivism, social construction of meaning through collaboration, the socio-cognitive relationships that influence learning can include relationships with peers, instructors, community, and self. It is interesting that the body of literature on effective interpersonal and therapeutic relationships also seems related to effective social-cognitive learning. Descriptions of characteristics of effective interpersonal relationships in the literature are abundant and include mutual problem solving, human respect, encouragement, and supportive affiliation (Duffy, 2007). Effective cognitive-social relationships in highly functioning classrooms, traditional or virtual, could include all of these characteristics as well. Raider-Roth (2005) emphasized the quality of trust as the "fundamental component" in teaching-learning relationships and noted that trust hinges on "(1) the teacher's capacity to be connected to the student, (2) the teacher's genuine interest in nurturing students' own ideas, (3) collaborative study on the part of teacher and student, and (4) an environment in which trust can prevail" (p. 30). Recall that Rourke et al. (2002) also singled out trust as an essential element of an effective online community.

Interactivity. The third fundamental philosophical shift is the movement from direct instruction that could be characterized as top-down, teacher focused, passive, one way instruction, to collaborative learning. An overlap between the emphasis on interactivity and the trend toward constructivism and the socio-cognitive is apparent. Collaborative learning is one means by which constructivism is enacted, but it merits further discussion here around the place interactivity plays in collaborative learning.

Interactivity is more that interaction and collaboration with other people in a virtual classroom. Interactivity "refers to features which allow mutual actions between learners, the learning environment and learning material" (Narciss, Proske, & Körndle, 2007, p. 514). These authors differentiate three dimensions of interactivity that are particularly relevant to online learning (2007). The first dimension is the "technical dimension" which includes the features of the web-based learning environment that allow learners to find, manipulate, and save information. The second, the "social dimension" includes the features of the online learning environment that facilitate social exchange with others. Finally, the "mental dimension" refers to "features of a web-based learning environment that allow learners to process the learning materials constructively, engage in learning activities actively, and take control of their learning processes" (Narciss, Proske, & Körndle, 2007, p. 514). This multidimensional view of interactivity supports our standpoint that interactivity is more than the simple human exchange such as text messaging or emailing. Interactivity, of the nature that facilitates social construction of knowledge, requires a social engagement between participants. Interactivity in which participants are truly engaged with one another can lead to the building of intimate highly functioning communities steeped in trust. A learning environment ideal for successfully teaching nursing knowledge, skills, and attitudes at a distance.

Several researchers consider interactivity in all three dimensions essential for effective online learning (Yacci, 2000; Borsook & Higginbotham-Wheat, 1991) and concluded that the natural potential for interactivity in online learning environments makes them unique and superior to classroom instruction because it provides "immediacy of response, nonsequential/nonlinear access to information, adaptability, feedback, user options, bidirectional communication channels, and interruptability" (p. 17). Baumlein's (2003) study revealed that student work is richer, more informed, and of a higher standard in online courses when high levels of meaningful interaction with classmates and course content takes place.

As explained by Rinehart (1999) collaborative learning is a process of developing new knowledge and new communities with others. Requiring students to work collaboratively in groups is a well-documented and highly recommended strategy for teaching and learning (Shulman, Lotan, & Whitcomb, 1998). Collaborative learning also supported the critical and postmodern stance, as through collaboration individuals are not as likely to compete with each other because the group effort is focused to explore a common issue (Cabrera, Nora, Crissman, & Terenzine, 2002, p. 387). The movement is toward a decentralization of the traditional power base in teacher-student relationships and a redefinition of the roles of students and teachers (ACDE, 2001). Since collaboration treats teaching and learning as interpretive acts that occur within social relationships this form of learning supports the concepts of learning communities (Bruffee 1984).

Baumlein (2003), among others, pointed out that when online learners engage in effective interaction and truly collaborate on social and intellectual levels with classmates and instructors they develop a feeling of community. Rouke et al (2000) noted that this sense of community fuels interaction and a positive sequence is established. Constructivism, socio-cognitive views of education, and the concept of collaboration in learning all set the milieu in which there is potential for the creation of effective virtual learning communities.

Putting all of this together, the goal of exemplary online educators should be the establishment of the Interaction-Interactivity-Collaboration-Community Cycle (I-I-C-C-C). (see Figure 2) The unanswered question is, What online teaching strategies are catalysts for igniting this sequence?

Summary. The social aspect of learning and the importance to students of feeling community membership are well documented in the literature. However, there is little research on the use of specific online teaching strategies in developing a sense of community conducive to a positive learning environment in online nursing courses. The next section in this chapter builds on this literature review and examines specific teaching strategies that can facilitate the creation of a sense of community in the online educational environment with a focus on the social implications and advantages of these online strategies.

Specifically the research of Perry and Edwards (2006) is featured. These investigators focused on the use of interactive teaching strategies to facilitate the development of online learning

Figure 2.

The Interaction-Interactivity-Collaboration-Community Cycle

Interactions (student to student, student with instructor, student with self)
↓
Fledgling relationships established
↓
Interactivity (Increasingly meaningful interactions)
↓
Collaboration (Enhanced depth of relationships)
↓
Community established
↓
Community fuels interaction ↕

communities in the teaching of nursing and health studies students. Several online teaching strategies including Photovoice (Perry & Edwards, 2006) and Virtual Reflective Centers (Ronaldson, 2004) are presented.

Examples of Practical Online Teaching Technologies that Promote Virtual Leaning Communities of Nurses

Photovoice

Although the way people learn is being revolutionized by technology, particularly the Internet, the literature is largely silent with regards to specific examples of effective online teaching technologies. Perry and Edwards (2006) conducted research on one online teaching strategy called "Photovoice" (Wang & Burris 1997; Woolrych, 2004) that was found to facilitate the establishment of virtual learning communities for nurses. Photovoice was originally created as a data collection technique for participatory research by Wang and Burris (1997). In the research application of Photovoice research participants were given cameras and asked to record visual images in their own communities. These visual images and accompanying stories were considered participatory means by which study participants could share their expertise (Woolrych, 2004). The originators of Photovoice considered it an action research methodology that built on the theoretical underpinnings of critical consciousness and feminist theory (Wang, Burris, & Xiang, 1996: Wang & Burris, 1997).

Perry and Edwards (2006) modified the Photovoice concept to create an interactive online teaching technology that was trialed initially in nursing and health studies courses. Photovoice as an online teaching strategy took the form of a teacher selected image that was posted each week at the start of a new unit. The photograph selected depicted a scene or subject that was relevant to the main theme to be covered in the online discussions that particular week. For example, if the topic of the upcoming week was the experience of change, then the image selected was one of a fence that was under construction with part of the fence new and freshly completed and the other part of the fence unkempt. (see Figure 3) In another example the topic of the week was vulnerability of the elderly and the image was of a sunflower trying to bloom in rather depressing surroundings (see Figure 4). Along with the image the instructor posted a focus question that students were invited to reflect on. The question referred specifically to the image and was an invitation to learners to react, or give voice, to the photo through a written conference posting. In the case of the change example the question affiliated with

Figure 3.

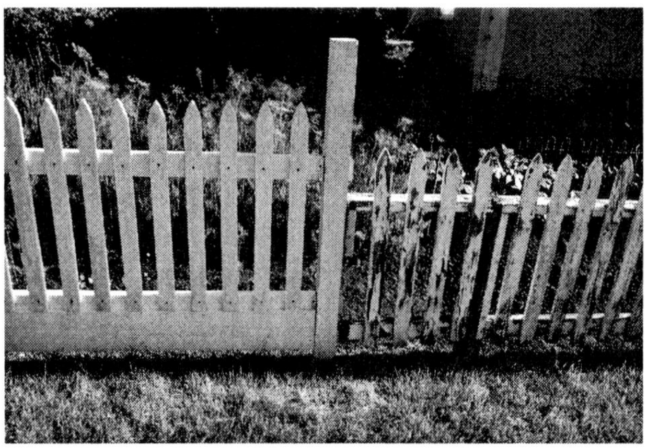

Figure 4.

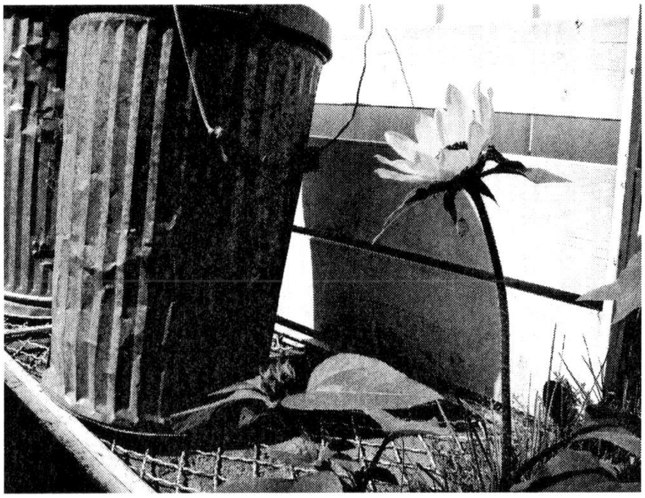

the partially completed fence was, "How can this fence that is undergoing a major renovation help you understand the experiences of people you care for who are undergoing major changes in their lives?" In the case of the vulnerable flower the affiliated question students were asked to reflect on was, "How can this flower that is struggling to bloom in less than ideal conditions help you to understand how it must feel to be vulnerable to a harsh environment?" Students were invited to post their Photovoice responses in a separate online forum. Students were told that participating in the Photovoice activity was voluntary, that no marks were attached to participation, and that they did not need to do the readings for the week prior to participating.

The course that the Photovoice teaching strategy was originally trialed in was a 13 week online course and the participants were nurses and other health care professionals. At the end of the 13 weeks of classes the instructor invited learners to contribute to an online forum set up to receive their comments about their experience with Photovoice. The survey question asked of the 40 participants was, "Photovoice was used in the course you just completed as an interactive teaching strategy. Has it served this purpose for you? What comments do you have regarding how Photovoice has contributed (or not) to your learning in this course." All participants consented to have the transcripts of their conference postings used for research purposes and comments were not solicited until after all final grades in the course had been finalized. To maintain anonymity all respondents were given pseudonyms.

Data in written form were analyzed using narrative analysis (Priest, Robert, & Woods, 2003). This was considered appropriate for this study as narrative analysis is a method by which interpretation of meaning may be made from textual data. The narratives provided by the participants were reviewed and elements of the narratives were organized into themes. In all 40 textual submissions were reviewed.

Three major themes identified from the students' responses were capturing attention, stimulating creativity, and creating community. Each theme will be discussed with examples from students' comments and integration of supporting literature.

Capturing attention. To teach effectively online, as in the traditional environment, the teacher first needs to get the attention of the learners. Creating interest in the topic to be discussed and helping learners see the relevance of the topic to them helps to capture the learners' attention. As Faulk and Ternus (2005) wrote, "educators are challenged to create interactive classes by developing learning activities that engage and involve students" (p. 527). Engaging adult learners can be challenging under optimum conditions but when students are in virtual classroom getting the learners' attention can be even more difficult. Teaching strategies that require learner participation and that focus them immediately on the topic to be addressed may be most effective in capturing attention.

The students who responded in this study claimed that because the Photovoice activity was the first instructor comment each week in the online conference it caught their attention. It was not buried in an abundance of discussion postings. Some respondents said that it was a non-threatening exercise (because it did not require pre-reading) and that it got them thinking about the topic under study. One student Jane said, "it was a great way to start discussion as there were no right or wrong answers." Caroline commented, "it set the tone for the week and set the stage for how I would think about the topic." Barb one of the students who was usually first to post in response to a Photovoice said, "It is a great way to introduce a topic, especially online, where it gets people thinking and being abstract about a topic rather than just speaking from an author's perspective." Tracey concluded, "It was a nice warm-up allowing me to be creative and search for meaning in the picture. I did not find it stressful but loads of fun." While one anonymous responded simply said, "the photo was a hook." Another student commented, "by having something to focus on... I became engaged in the topic and it opened the door to learning."

Stimulating creativity. The second theme related to the awakening of creativity that the photos promoted in the online learners. Words like "stimulated creativity" and "helped us to think outside the box" where used often when referring to the effects of Photovoice. For example Myra's comment was, "It stirs the creative juices!" Nicole wrote, "I love this idea of Photovoice and how it extends the mind and engages the creativity of learners in distance ed!" Jacqueline's comments are suggestive of *why* PV stimulated creativity as she alluded to sub-themes such as the novelty and enjoyment factors. Specifically Jacqueline commented, "PV was always different, thus making it fun to click on the electronic paperclip to unveil what was hidden behind. PV was playful." Anne-Marie also acknowledged the role of originality in learning when she wrote, "It has drawn my thoughts away from the straight forward concepts discussed in the readings and toward some alternate ways of seeing the concepts."

Jo-Ann commented, "PV proved to be a valuable tool in that what was viewed could always be tied back to articles we were required to read. It also generated a lot of discussion with the others in the class because we were curious about what other people saw in the photo. PV was a very effective method of review and learning!"

Jane's comments speak more specifically to the *results* of stimulating creativity when she commented, "PV helped me take risks." Karen commented that "PV added great colour to an otherwise colourless and flat medium of distance learning!" Anne-Marie commented, "With the combined juices flowing I think the responses to the rest of the questions were richer, less rote and more creative and the depth of dialogue between us was amazing."

Creating community. PV had a positive influence on the creation of online community by positively influencing both the teacher-learner and learner-learner relationships. Exemplary online educators convey some sense of themselves in the virtual classroom (Perry & Edwards, 2005). Pelz (2004) agrees stating online instructors must "strive for presence" in order to be effective. Since the PV images are selected by the instructor they convey to the learners who may never actually "see" their teacher some sense of their teacher's interests, biases, activities, hobbies, or passions. The selected photos portray something personal about the teacher in a very non-threatening way. The instructor is the one who chooses the "art" that embellishes the course materials. Marie commented "I almost see each photo is like a piece of artwork that one might view as a guest entering into the teacher's home. As a visitor intriguing artwork is often a conversation piece that generates reflective and stimulating discussion and lets you get to know your host on a personal level. For me PV does this in the online learning environment."

Jane likened the weekly PV to a "gift" from the instructor. Gifts are a vehicle for sharing and are part of human interaction. The perception by the learners that the PV was a gift may have introduced an element of humanness into the course. In reference to this Helene wrote, "Towards the latter part of the course I found myself wondering just what kind of present we would receive for the beginning of the upcoming unit. I viewed the image as a gift to me and I think others saw it this way too. In fact I have saved the images and I will look back on them if I am feeling discouraged."

PV also stimulated interactivity between classmates and engaged them in collaborative learning. Joyce commented, "Photovoice presented variety in a faceless virtual world. I found reading the responses of other people allowed you a moment to glance into their world demonstrating a personal view which may not have come through regular postings." Karen's comments related to the "autobiographical" nature of each persons' reactions to the photos which seemed to be one way that learners got to know each other through the PV activity. Karen said, "I was always amazed to see the array of responses, and interpretations which were somewhat autobiographical as we all identified with the picture in different ways. It provided a forum for us to get to know each other through different lenses." Jo-Ann succinctly said, "I have also really enjoyed getting to 'know' my classmates through reading their interpretations." In this way PV helped to build social connections between online learners perhaps the beginning of establishing trust. Karen said, "Sometimes on-line learning can be isolating, and just doing the readings and learning activities is not enough for that enjoyable social interaction that can be found in a classroom. Photovoice provided that to my learning environment."

Both face to face and virtual communities thrive on social and intellectual interaction. PV in this study served to stimulate intellectual interaction. For example, Karin said, "PV provided richness, or a further dimension, to what could have been quite gray and dry subject matter." Sherry wrote, "I found PV stretched my mind and challenged me to look beyond the obvious. I also found that my own personal values, philosophies and visions became more evident to me as I examined those proposed by my classmates."

The outcomes of this study also suggest that the sense of community was strengthened by enhanced learner to learner relationships. Caroline wrote, "Photovoice improved class participation and served to knit the class of learners together in a much different way. Through the power of projection, a piece of each of us was added to the Photovoice - my voice blended with a myriad of other learners." Karen acknowledged that, "The shared experiences and perspectives and other students' analysis opened my mind to new ideas. This sharing surely must be its most important use in a class environment." Caroline commented, "The diversity of views is always highlighted as we look at the PV responses and this is a good learning in itself. It reminds me of the tenants of teamwork, 'the sum is greater that the parts.' Together all the class views are much more robust than just one interpretation." Jo-Ann commented that PV "provided opportunities to view perceptions and interpretations in a safe place where all points of view have meaning. Through this exercise we learned that we all have a point of view, different perceptions, yet we share a common goal to learn and are intertwined by this common thread."

In summary, the strategy of Photovoice was a catalyst to the I-I-C-C-C. (see Figure 2) The photo and refection questions initiated interaction; student with student, student with self, and student with instructor. As learners participated in Photovoice they shared their beliefs and values about a topic through their interpretations of the images. These initial interactions led to interactivity (more meaningful interactions) as they engaged in discussion about the image with others. Collaboration (enhanced depth of relationships) resulted as participants discovered commonalities, stretched their thinking on a topic, and considered another's perspective. The class members and instructor worked together (collaborated) to come to a fuller understanding of the topic to be studied. A sense of community evolved which in turn fueled more frequent and intimate interactions regarding the Photovoice image, but also about the related themes of the course content.

Virtual Reflective Centers

Another online teaching technology that has potential for creating online community and facilitating the teaching of human interaction skills to nurses and others who are studying via the Internet is called Virtual Reflective Centers (VRC). A "Virtual Reflective Centre is a researcher-developed virtual, simulation instrument designed to promote critical thinking in traditional nursing students" (Ronaldson, 2004). Cubbon (2007) adapted the face-to-face use of VRC for use in an online health studies course. In Cubbon's application of VRCs they became in essence Internet-based role play scenarios that were developed to teach online students motivational interviewing skills (Cubbon, personal communication, 2007). Motivational interviewing is an effective strategy in facilitating behavior change, which is a core component of health promotion. Cubbon trialed VRCs with a group of online nurse practitioner students who were trying to learn the advanced interpersonal skill of motivational interviewing. During week four of a 15 week course students in Cubbon's class were assigned to either a "patient" or a "nurse practitioner" role. Student participants were briefed and given detailed information such as medical history, social history, and diagnostic results. Students in "patient" roles were given the reasons they requested an appointment with a "nurse practitioner." The "patient" contacted the "nurse practitioner" via course email and requested an appointment and the activity began. The entire interview lasted about 15 minutes and took place in real time, online, in a private chat room. Once the role-play interviews were completed, the instructor sent a list of reflective questions to the entire group for discussion in the electronic forum accessible by the entire class. The main reflection question asked participants to reflect on how they would apply this learning experience of the VRC to their practice.

There are challenges faced when teaching technologies such as VRCs are offered in real-time. For example, when students live in different time zones this can require some careful timing and selection of the activity so that no one is "in class" at an unreasonable hour. In addition it does take great organizational skill on the part of the teacher to ensure everyone understands the exercise, the processes, and has the appropriate information to make the activity meaningful.

On the positive side Cubbon (2007) found many positive outcomes from using VRC's in her online class. For example, students reported enjoying the social aspect of the activity which facilitated the experience of community building. The opportunity to engage in a collaborative learning activity students recognized was applicable to their practice (as student nurse practitioners in this case) and the meaningful interactions between classmates also facilitated teambuilding. Motivational interviewing is a very complex interpersonal skill and this online activity gave students a chance to practice it in a safe learning environment. A further advantage of the VRCs online teaching strategy is that it is inexpensive in terms of extra resources. VRCs could be used in a variety of ways in online courses. The basic process of role-playing and reflective questioning could be adapted to suit many topics.

Other Online Teaching Strategies

There are other examples of online teaching strategies that have been used by educators who are teaching nurses and health studies students online to facilitate a positive learning experience. Cuellar (2002) suggested that demonstrations through interactive simulation, hyper linking of resources in course text online, question and answer sessions promoted through bulletin boards and chat rooms, and private e-mails between students or between instructors and students were interactive teaching strategies that help to build community in the online teaching milieu. We propose that they assist in building community as they serve as catalysts to the I-I-C-C-C.

In other courses developed by Perry and Edwards teaching strategies that facilitated meaningful interaction between course participants and the evolution of effective online communities of inquiry include the use of debates. In several courses "The Great Debate" activity offers students a topic and invites them to take the side of the debate that is contrary to their own current beliefs on the topic. Over the period of a week students present their arguments, pro or con, on the debate topic in an online conference forum dedicated to their responses. In some courses the "One Minute Self-Debate" is a variation on the debating theme. In this learning activity students are instructed to consider a specific resolution. For example in a course on organizational theory the resolution is, "Be it resolved that employees of health care organizations should be held accountable for the organization's success." Then students are asked to follow the following process:

i. Agree with the resolution and write down one point for your side (the affirmative).
ii. Disagree with the resolution and write down one point for your other side (the negative).
iii. Rebut yourself. Any heated self-discussions?
iv. Share your finest point on the conference forum.

The depth of discussion that results for this debating activity is satisfying from the instructors' viewpoint and students report that they find this a learning activity that is informative and helps them to "get to know themselves and the others in their class." In this way it is an effective strategy for the development of relationships that seem to form a foundation for further meaningful interaction and establishment of community but it is also a stimulus to interaction with self.

Similar to the debating exercises another interactive teaching strategy successfully used by Perry and Edwards is the Point-Counterpoint Reflection. In this activity students are invited to consider two essentially opposite perspectives on a topic and then to select the argument that holds most closely to their belief system and present their reflections regarding why they selected a specific perspective with the class in the online conference forum. For example, in a graduate course students are given this challenge:

Consider the two perspectives related to personality in your course textbook.

i. Point - Personality traits are powerful predictors of behavior.
ii. Counterpoint – Personality traits reflect the surrounding situation.

Which argument holds most closely to your belief system and why? Present your reflection to the class.

Again the outcome of this activity, according to participants, is the formation of community and the development of further knowledge and self-understanding on the topic at hand.

One final example of a strategy used by Perry and Edward to facilitate the building of classroom community, and as a tool for bringing closure to an online learning experience, is the Conceptual Quilting (CQ) Exercise. Students who are nearing the end of an online course are given this challenge.

Become a conceptual quilt maker. Which major concepts, theories, ideas and metaphors in this course made an impression on you and are worth holding onto and incorporating into your practice? How could you array these into a quilt pattern? Design your quilt and share it with your classmates in the online conference forum. You can use clip art etc. to develop your quilt. If you are better with words than graphics just describe your quilt to us. Alternatively other "artists" may select a different medium for pulling together the pieces of this course.

Students who have participated in this conceptual quilting online teaching activity have reported that it helped them to bring effective closure to an online course in which they had developed close relationships with their virtual classmates. This aspect of community in online classrooms, the potential for feelings of loss or grief by participates who have successfully achieved a close and intimate learning community, has yet to be fully explored in the literature.

Discussion

The Socio-Technical Implications of Teaching Nursing Online. As noted in the introduction, nursing is a very human discipline. People who are exemplary nurse educators, clinicians, and administrators are skilled at the art and science of nursing. Nursing and health care courses can be taught successfully online if educators are attentive to the social-technical implications of online course development and delivery. Some online teaching strategies such as Photovoice, VRCs, online debates, and similar strategies profiled in this chapter help online learners interact and potentially form an intimate community of inquiry. In such a learning milieu trusting relationships form between classmates, and between instructors and students, allowing participants to feel supported and safe. In safe nurturing environments participants are comfortable sharing their experiences, asking questions, animating gaps in knowledge and deficiency in skills. In such learning environments learners are able to develop their creativity, engage in honest self-reflection, and engage in exchange at the psycho-emotional as well as the intellectual level. Turpin (2007) demonstrated that capitalizing on the socio-technical potential of the online teaching environment can help to open up the classroom space so that students feel empowered and learning is fueled. Online communities of inquiry encourage students to take an active role in the learning process and in the shaping of the virtual classroom space. Such virtual classrooms provide learners with a chance to explore their intellectual pursuits with a careful balance of mentoring and advice from instructors. In such virtual classrooms there is potential for learning to occurs, even in highly interpersonally intense disciplines such as nursing.

Developments in Online Education: Changing Social and Pedagogical Perspectives of Distance Learning. Recent developments in online education have changed the social and pedagogical perspectives of distance education. As educators have realized that exemplary online teaching is more than administering a passive correspondence course; teaching strategies that lead to the I-I-C-C-C have been developed and tested (Perry & Edwards, 2006). As Underhill (2006) stated, "The pedagogy underlying online learning and teaching is being reconceptualised to incorporate the opportunities being offered by the development of online educational settings. The pedagogy of constructivism and in particular socio-constructivism is underpinning much of the online learning and teaching developments currently being developed." These shifts have fueled the evolution toward online courses in which students learn in communities of inquiry. The advent of Internet-based telecommunications technology has increased the potential for interaction and collaborative work in online courses and thus changed the social and pedagogical perspective of distance learning (Dabbagh, 2004). It is argued that these foundational assumptions point to the importance of developing virtual learning communities to enhance effectiveness of online learning (Shea, Pickett, & Pelz, 2006).

To conclude this chapter we present some key essential messages for those who teach and learn online. First, interactivity is more than interaction. Interactivity connotes meaningful interpersonal exchange with other people, the course materials, or with self. Online educators can put strategies in place that necessitate interaction, but achievement of interactivity, and resulting true collaboration and collaborated learning may require active and deliberate pedagogical interventions by a skilled instructor.

Second, learning is at least in part socially constructed. Interactivity that facilitates learning can involve meaningful exchanges with classmates, instructors, with the learner's broader personal and professional community, with the course materials, and with self.

Third, course materials in a virtual learning environment are less subscribed than in traditional classrooms. The Web is a key source of course materials in online teaching situations and it is in some senses infinite.

Trust is noted by both those who write about effective interpersonal relationships and those who study the development of effective online learning communities. Nursing is a human discipline. When teaching nursing online instructors need to pay particular attention to including strategies that prompt the I-I-C-C-C in virtual classrooms. But for success with the I-I-C-C-C a foundation of trust between participants and between the students and the instructor must be established. Part of the work of the instructor is setting the stage for trust to be established and ensuring the maintenance of trust throughout the course. Ways to establish and ensure trust in the online educational community is a question for further study.

FUTURE TRENDS

Scholarly research related to effective teaching of nursing online is only just beginning. This chapter presents theoretical background and helps to unveil some research themes that require further exploration. Systematic scholarly research on these themes will help to move online nursing education forward based on evidence and sound studied principles rather than on trial and error and methods and anecdotal reports.

One theme that merits further study is the nature of effective online learning communities. As we start to understand the importance of establishing virtual communities of inquiry that are founded on trust and serve to nurture learning, there are opportunities to investigate specifically how these communities are created and sustained. Additionally, as online communities are created for a specific time they also must also eventually be disbanded. Research into effective closure of established communities of inquiry seems important as human relationships and natural human processes such as grief and loss may be experienced by community participants. What strategies can educators use to effectively create, engage, and disband online learning communities? What is the role of trust in online education? How is trust established and maintained through the duration of the course? What are the precursors for trust to be established and what are the threats to trust?

Second, there is limited research based knowledge related to the students' experience with online learning. There is little research that describes how being part of a collaborative online learning environment, and the resulting community of inquiry, is viewed by nursing students. Current literature supports incorporating interactive online teaching strategies to influence the learner and the learning environment, but we need to address the question of how learners experience this and if there are specific learner characteristics, such as learning style, that influence the learner's experience. Although one could predict that students with certain learning styles may be more positively influenced by interactive online teaching strategies, this relationship is not yet clearly documented in the literature.

Third, there is limited published research on specific online teaching strategies. One focus of ongoing research needs to be these essential components of courses. Internet course designers and instructors spend time and energy creating various strategies they believe are helpful to online learning without knowing how these strategies affect learners and learning. Photovoice, VRCs, debates and similar strategies are being developed and included in online course without being systematically evaluated for effect on student learning and on their role in establishing the communities of inquiry. Studies of selected innovative online teaching strategies, involving a wide variety of learners from different disciplines, is important for more fully understanding what approaches are effective for assisting students to construct their own knowledge, build relationships in the online class, and establish collaborative communities. Questions such as, Do specific online learning strategies engage learners in higher-order thinking (e.g., analysis, synthesis, and evaluation)? What online teaching techniques facilitate learners assimilating, applying and learning new knowledge? In what ways do online teaching techniques promote learner achievement, enhance motivation, and cause learners to learn more?

CONCLUSION

Effective education, whether traditional classroom or online, is *active and interactive* rather than *passive and isolating* (Perry & Edwards, 2005). Teachers are challenged to provide an academic environment that encourages learning through active participation (Chickering & Ehrmann, 1996). When the teaching takes place in the online environment facilitating active involvement is even more challenging. The importance of interactivity in the virtual learning environment is widely supported by research. Cherkering and Ehrmann list interactivity as one of the best practice principles of online teaching (1996). Pelz (2004) demonstrated that interactive teaching strategies move online courses away from being merely text-based correspondence classes. Creative online instructors develop an array of teaching strategies that lead to the interactivity-interaction-collaboration-community building cycle. It is possible for online educators to engage fully with the learner from a distance using teaching strategies that facilitate "human presence" in the virtual world (Pelz, 2004). In creating effective online courses it is thus thought to be important to include teaching strategies that require action on the part of the student, promote shared inquiry or interaction between facilitator and learner, all within a virtual world where participants feel connected.

Online education for nurses is a current and future reality. Teaching via distance requires inventive approaches on the part of the instructor in order to facilitate an optimum learning experience. Educators, administrators and practitioners need to take deliberate actions in order to ensure that online nursing education is effective. Given that nursing is a discipline with intrinsically high levels of human interaction, teaching nursing virtually presents an extra challenge. This chapter is a beginning point for those who currently, or will soon be, teaching and learning nursing online. The discussion of the literature related to creating online learning communities and the discussion of fundamental philosophical shifts toward student-centered interactive pedagogical models was developed. Specific strategies used by some exemplary online nursing educators were presented as examples of ways the virtual learning communities can be created to enhance effectiveness of online learning. This chapter presented an opening discussion of this topic. Ideas for further research studies related to teaching nursing online and the creation of effective virtual learning communities were offered.

ACKNOWLEDGMENT

Otto F. Mahler (photos).

REFERENCES

Ali, N. S., Hodson-Carlton, K., & Ryan, M. (2004). Students' perceptions of online learning: Implications for teaching. *Nurse Educator, 29*, 111-115.

Arbaugh, J. (2001). How instructor immediacy behaviours affect student satisfaction and learning in web-based courses. *Business Communication Quarterly, 64*(4), 42-54.

Atack, L., & Rankin, J. (2002). A descriptive study of registered nurses' experiences with Web-based learning. *Journal of Advanced Nursing, 40*, 457-465.

Atack, L. (2003). Becoming a Web-based learner: Registered nurses' experience. *Journal of Advanced Nursing, 44*, 289-297.

Australian Council of Deans of Education (ACDE). (1998). *Preparing a profession: Report of the national standards and guidelines for initial teacher education project.* Canberra: ACDE.

Baumlein, G. (2003). *Teaching strategies and student outcomes in Web-based instruction in nursing: A case study of expert nurse educators.* Unpublished doctoral dissertation. The University of Akron, Ohio.

Borsook, T. K., & Higginbotham-Wheat, N. (1991). Interactivity: What is it and what can it do for computer-based instruction? *Educational Technology, 37*(5), 11-17.

Bruffee, K. (1984). *Collaborative learning: Higher education, interdependence, and the authority of knowledge.* Baltimore, MD: The Johns Hopkins University.

Bryson, C., & Hand, L. (2007). The role of engagement in inspiring teaching and learning. *Innovations in Education and Teaching International, 44*(4), 349-363.

Chen, M. (1995). A methodology for characterizing computer-based learning environments. *Instructional Science, 23*(1), 183-220.

Chickering, A., & Ehrmann, S. (1996). Implementing the seven principles: technology as lever. *AAHE Bulletin*, 3-6.

Conrad, D. (2002). Deep in the hearts of learners: Insights into the nature of online community. *Journal of Distance Education, 17*(1).

Cubbon, J. (2007). Personal communication November, 12, 2007.

Cuellar, N. (2002). The transition from classroom to online teaching. *Nursing Forum, 37*(3), 5-14.

Dabbagh, N. (2004). Distance learning: Emerging pedagogical issues and learning designs. *The Quarterly Review of Distance Education, 5*(1), 37-49.

Duffy, J. (2007). Dimensions of caring: Psychometric evaluation of the caring assessment tool. *Advances in Nursing Science, 30*(3), 235-245.

Elbaz, F. (1991). Research on teacher's knowledge: The evolution of a discourse. *Journal of Curriculum Studies, 23*, 1-19.

Entwistle, N. (1991) Approaches to learning and perceptions of the learning environment-introduction to the special issue, *Higher Education, 22*, 201-204.

Garrison, D. R. (2006). *Online community of inquiry review: Social, cognitive, and teaching presence issues.* Unpublished manuscript, University of Calgary. Retrieved November 20, 2007 from http://www.communitiesofinquiry.com/documents/Community%20of%20Inquiry%20Issues.pdf

Gerber, S., & Scott, L. (2007). Designing a learning curriculum and technology's role **in it.** *Educational Technology, Research and Development, 55*(5), 461-479.

Halter, M. J., Kleiner, C., & Hess, R.F. (2006). The experience of nursing students in an online doctoral program in nursing: A phenomenological study. *International Journal of Nursing Studies, 43*, 99-105.

Hodge, E., Bosse, M.J., Faulconer, J., & Fewell, M. (2006). Mimicking proximity: The role of distance education in forming communities of learning. *International Journal of Instructional Technology and Distance Learning.* Retrieved November 19, 2007 from http://www.itdl.org/Journal/Dec_06/article01.htm

Hung, D. (2001). Theories of learning and computer-mediated instructional technologies. *Education Media International, 38*(4), 281-287.

Hutchins, H. (2003). Instructional immediacy and the seven principles: Strategies for facilitating online course. *Online Journal of Distance Learning Administration,* 4(3), 1-11.

Hyde, A., & Murray, (2005). Nurses' experiences of distance education programmes. *Journal of Advanced Nursing, 49*, 87-95.

Kreijns, K., Kirschner, P., & Jochems, W. (2002). The sociability of computer-supported collaborative learning environments. *Educational Technology and Society, 5*(1), 8-22.

Lee, J., Carter-Wells, J., Glaeser, B., Ivers, K., & Street, C. (2006). Facilitating the development of a learning community in an online graduate program. *The Quarterly Review of Distance Education, 7*(1), 13-33.

Liu, X., Magjuka, R. J., Bonk, C. J., & Lee, S. (2007). Does sense of community matter? An examination of participants' perception of building learning communities in online courses. *The Quarterly Review of Distance Education, 8*(1), 9-24.

Mancuso-Murphy, J. (2007). Distance education in nursing: An integrated review of online nursing students' experiences with technology-delivered instruction. *Journal of Nursing Education, 46*(6), 252-261.

Merriam-Webster online dictionary. (2007). Retrieved November 18, 2007 from http://dictionary.reference.com/browse/relationship

Mueller, C. (2001). Masters in nursing students' experiences as a member of a virtual classroom on the Internet. *Dissertation Abstracts International, 62*(08), 3557B.

Narciss, S., Proske, A., & Körndle, H. (2007). Interactivity and learners' achievement in Web-based learning. *Journal of Interactive Learning Research, 18(*4), 511-532.

Nightingale, F. (1992). *Notes on nursing: What it is, and what it is not.* London: Harris. (original work published in 1959)

Ouzts, K. (2006). Sense of community in online courses. *The Quarterly Review of Distance Education, 7*(3), 285-296. Retrieved November 2, 2007 from http://0-web.ebscohost.com.aupac.lib.athabascau.ca/ehost/pdf?vid=3&hid=104&sid=b8254076-4ede-4f7c-9949-46a8720b2147%40sessionmgr107

Pelz, B. (2004). Three principles of effective online pedagogy. *Journal of Asynchronous Learning Networks, 8*(3), 33-46.

Perry, B., & Edwards, M. (2006). Exemplary educators: Creating a community of inquiry online. *International Experience in Open, Distance and Flexible Education Collection of Papers* from the Open and Distance Learning Association of Australia (ODLAA) conference proceedings.

Perry, B., & Edwards, M. (2005). Exemplary online educators: Creating a community of inquiry. *Turkish Online Journal of Distance Education, 6(2),* Retrieved October 6, 2007 from http://tojde.anadolu.edu.tr/tojde18/articles/article6.htm.

Petraglia, J. (1998). The real world on a short leash: The (mis)application of constructivism to the design of educational technology. *Educational Technology Research and Development, 46*(3), 53-65.

Priest, H., Roberts, P., & Woods, L. (2003). An overview of three different approaches to the interpretation of qualitative data. Part 1: Theoretical issues. *Nurse Researcher, 10*(1), 30-43. Retrieved November 3, 2007 from http://www.nursing-standard.co.uk/nurseresearcher-archive/nr_archive/nrv10n1-2002/nrv10n1p4351.pdf

Raider-Roth, M. (2004). Taking the time to think: A portrait of reflection. *Teaching and Learning, 18*(5), 79-97.

Raider-Roth, M. (2005). *Trusting what you know: The high stakes of classroom relationships.* San Francisco: Jossey-Bass.

Richardson, J., & Swan, K. (2003). Examining social presence in online courses in relation to students' perceived learning and satisfaction. *Journal of Asynchronous Learning Networks,*7(1), 68-88. Retrieved October 5, 2007 from http://www.sloan-c.org/publications/jaln/v7n1/pdf/v7n1_richardson.pdf

Rinehart, J. (1999). Turning theory into theorizing: Collaborative learning in a sociological theory course. *Teaching Sociology, 27*(3), 216-233.

Robley, L., Farnsworth, B., Flynn, J., & Horne, C. (2004). This new house: Building knowledge through online learning. *Journal of Professional Nursing, 20*, 333-343.

Rogers, C. (2002). Seeing student learning: Teach change and the role of reflection. *Harvard Educational Review, 72*(2), 230-255.

Ronaldson, S. (2004). Untangling critical thinking in educational cyberspace. Unpublished doctoral dissertation. The University of British Columbia, Canada.

Rourke, G., Garrison, D., Anderson, T., & Archer, W. (2000). Critical inquiry in a text-based environment: Computer conferencing in higher education. *The Internet and Higher Education, 2*(2-3), 87-105.

Rourke, G, Garrison, D., Anderson, T., & Archer, W. (2001). Critical thinking, cognitive presence, and computer conferencing in distance education. *American Journal of Distance Education, 15*(1).

Rovai, A. (2002). Building sense of community at a distance. *International Review of Research in Open and Distance Learning, 3*(1). Retrieved October 4, 2007 from http://www.irrodl.org/index.php/irrodl/article/viewFile/79/153

Scardamalia, M. (2002). Collective cognitive responsibility for the advancement of knowledge. In B. Smith (Ed.), *Liberal education in a knowledge society* (pp. 76-98). Chicago: Open Court.

Shea, P., Pickett, A., & Pelz, W. (2003). A follow-up investigation of "teaching presence" in the SUNY learning network. *Journal of Asynchronous Learning Networks*, 7(2), 61-80. Retrieved November 7, 2007 from http://www.aln.org/publications/jaln/v7n2/pdf/v7n2_shea.pdf

Shulman, J., Lotan, J., & Whitcomb, J. (1998). *Groupwork in diverse classrooms: A casebook for educators*. New York: Teachers College.

Sit, J. Chung, J., Chow, C., & Wong, T. (2005). Experiences of online learning: Students' perspective. *Nurse Education Today, 25*, 140-147.

Slagter van Tryon, P.J. & Bishop, M.J. (2006). Identifying "E-mmediacy" strategies for web-based instruction: A Delphi study. *The Quarterly Review of Distance Education, 7*(1), 49-62.

Thiele, J. (2003). Learning patterns of online students. *Journal of Nursing Education, 42*, 364-366.

Thurmond, V.A. (2003). Defining interaction and strategies to enhance interactions in web-based courses. *Nurse Educator, 28*, 237-241.

Turpin, C. (2007). Feminist praxis online teaching and the urban campus. *Feminist Teacher: A Journal of the Practices, Theories, and Scholarship of Feminist Teaching, 18*(1), 9-27.

Tynjala, P. (1997) Developing education students' conceptions of the learning process in different learning environments, *Learning and Instruction, 7*, 277-292.

Underhill, A. (2006). Theories of learning and their implications for on-line assessment. *Turkish Online Journal of Distance Education, 7*(1), 165-174.

Wang, C., Burris, M., & Xiang, Y. (1996). Chinese village women as visual anthropologists: A participatory approach to reaching policymakers. *Sac Sci Med, 42*, 1391-1400.

Wang, C., & Burris, M. (1997). Photovoice: Concept, methodology, and use for participatory needs assessment. *Health Education Behavior, 24*, 369-387.

White, A., Roberts, V., & Brannan, J. (2003). Returning nurses to the workforce: Developing an online refresher course. *The Journal of Continuing Education in Nursing, 34*, 59-64.

Woods, R. & Baker, J. (2004). Interaction and immediacy in online learning. *International Review of Research in Open and Distance Learning.* Retrieved November 2, 2007 from http://www.irrodl.org/content/v5.2/woods-baker.html.

Woolrych, R. (2004). Empowering images: Using Photovoice with tenants with special needs. *Housing, Care and Support, 7*(1), 31-36.

Yacci, M. (2000). Interactivity demystified: A structural definition. *Educational Technology, 40*(4), 5-16.

Zhang, D. (2005). Interactive multimedia-based E-learning: A study of effectiveness. *The American Journal of Distance Education, 19*(3), 149-162.

KEY TERMS

Community of Inquiry Model: Highlights three major aspects of the online learning community; social presence, cognitive presence, and social teaching which overlap to form the educational experience of the learner (Rouke, et al, 2001).

Conceptual Quilting: An online teaching activity in which learners create a virtual quilt of themes, ideas, or experiences from the course that they found most personally meaningful. It assists in bringing effective closure to an online course.

Immediacy: Refers to communication behaviours that reduce social and psychological distance between people. Immediacy strategies include both nonverbal and verbal behaviours (Arbough, 2001, p. 43).

Learning Community: A group of students who have feelings of trust and belonging, possess shared expectations, and are committed to shared educational goals" (Rovai, 2002, p. 12).

Photovoice: Action research methodology that built on the theoretical underpinnings of critical consciousness and feminist theory (Wang, Burris, & Xiang, 1996: Wang & Burris, 1997).

Relationship: Relationship implies a connection or affinity between people (Merriam-Webster, 2007).

Sense of Community: Consists of four related dimensions: spirit, trust, interaction, and commonality of learning expectations and goals" (Rovai, 2002, p.12).

Virtual Reflective Centre: A virtual, simulation instrument designed to promote critical thinking in traditional nursing students" (Ronaldson, 2004).

Chapter XIII
The Impact of Technology in Organizational Communication

Roberta Cuel
University of Trento, Italy

Roberta Ferrario
Laboratory for Applied Ontology (ISTC-CNR), Italy

ABSTRACT

In this chapter a case study is presented, in which the ethnomethodological approach is used to analyze the impact of the implementation of an information system, called Sispes, on organizational communication processes in the residence for elderly Giovanelli (Italy). Sispes is a Web-based platform which sustains communication processes and knowledge management according to a customized workflow management system. Adopting structuration theories in the analysis of the case study, and taking inspiration from the philosophical tradition, especially in epistemology and in the analytic philosophy of law, an innovative perspective is adopted, which specifically acknowledges the role played by the communication processes in shaping both the attitudes of the involved actors and the social reality in which they are immersed. According to this perspective, three types of communication processes are presented, namely the normative, descriptive and constructive approach. These latter are then applied to a concrete case study.

INTRODUCTION

It is commonly known that the introduction of any technology system in an organizational reality causes some relevant changes in internal processes and in the workers' attitude to share knowledge. This chapter investigates the evolution of communication processes within the organization and the impact of the use of information systems (ISs from hereafter) on knowledge management assets. In order to overcome some problems deriving from the adoption of classical theories on organizational communication processes, a new approach based on a philosophical analysis is introduced, that distinguishes communication processes into three main categories: normative, descriptive and constructive. These latter allow the analysis both of the attitudes of the involved actors and of the social reality in which they are immersed[1]. By applying this new vision to the analysis of the impact of technology on communication processes within a small firm in Italy, the residence for elderly Giovanelli, the chapter investigates how the introduction of an IS, named Sispes, has affected the information strategy of the firm, the workers' attitude to share information and knowledge, and some communication processes. Finally, the chapter shows that the proposed normative, descriptive an constructive approaches allow to better understand the communication processes' dynamics. In the two following sections, some background literature (e.g. theories on technological impact and on communication processes within organizations) is presented. In the main part of the chapter, theories on communication processes and a case study are described. Finally, some future trends and final remarks are discussed.

BACKGROUND

In the last decades, organizations had to deal with dynamic markets, characterized by specialization of work, outsourcing processes, just in time and distributed production, etc. In this scenario the continuous innovation in technology solutions and its contradicting empirical effects on organizations have maintained a strong interest for researchers who try to develop new and more complete theoretical models.

Even if non profit organizations (such as cooperative and social based firms) are working in a more stable environment, the turbulent network of stakeholders influence them. In this scenario, public or private residences for elderly are not an exception, they become part of inter-organizational or informal networks, opening their virtual value chain to other companies, outsourcing their non core services and, finally, specializing their core activities such as nursing, medical, and physiotherapeutic services (see for instance Child, 1972; Child and Faulkner, 1998; Cook, 1977; Lowndes and Skelcher, 1998; Murray, 1997; Vangen and Huxham, 2003). This allows residences for elderly to offer a good quality service, improving the guests' welfare. In order to do that, they have to coordinate a constellation of specialized units, some of which are part of the organization (administration, R&D, etc.) while others refer to different companies (such as restaurant, cleaning, transportation and logistic services).

In order to stimulate coordination in a complex environment, innovative Information and Communication Technologies (ICT) solutions are implemented and communication processes are continuously reengineered. The following paragraphs describe some organizational coordination and communication processes, and how ICT, information or knowledge management systems might sustain these processes. Finally, it is argued that these latter are not neutral assets in organizations, but are strictly related to pre-existing coordination processes and types of production.

Organizational Coordination and Communication Processes

The importance of coordination and communication processes has constantly increased at any level of the organization: technical, managerial and institutional (Parsons, 1951). This very complex organizational issue can be studied in accordance with contingency theories, which consider the organization as dependent on the complexity and the dynamicity of the environment in which the firms operate (Emery and Trist, 1960; Lawrence e Lorsch, 1967; Ashby, 1967; Mintzberg, 1983) and on the types of production technology adopted within the organization. For instance, through an empirical analysis of English production firms, Woodward (1965) has discovered that coordination and communication processes might change according to the kind of model of production (called "technology" in the organizational literature) developed within the firm. Also, Thompson (1967) has extended her analysis, depicting the following models:

- Long linked technologies: they imply a serial interdependency among single production phases. These are scientifically analyzed and organized, and communication processes have to maintain the efficiency of production phases.
- Mediated technologies: they allow people to communicate in order to share opinions, negotiate, and achieve common agreement. Technology has the role of mediator among individuals, and its infrastructure should be very easy to understand and use, thus comprehensible and standardized.
- Intensive technologies: workers have to use various communication channels, according to their emerging needs. The aim is to achieve new and innovative shared opinions, ideas, information, and desires in a non-predefined way, typically developed by teamworks or communities of practice.

Taking also into consideration some important studies on knowledge management[2] (KM from hereafter) and IS, coordination and communication processes might be related with the information and KM strategies adopted within the organization. In particular, Davenport et al., (1998) describe four different models, which represent both the way in which information should be organized and the way in which communication processes should be designed:

- Information anarchy: every worker manages her/his personal information and networks of communication channels. The dimension of the communication network depends on the ability and attitude of each single agent to manage relationships and communicate with colleagues, customers, suppliers, etc.
- Information hierarchy: workers adapt their communication processes to communication channels that are scientifically organized, typically by the management. Usually these are vertical channels, which enable the twofold processes of top down and bottom up communication.
- Information feudalism: workers share knowledge within each single unit, teamwork, or community. Communication channels are organized and managed within each single group and there is no official communication channel across units.
- Information federalism: the personalized and informal communication channels, developed within each single unit, are placed side by side with the formal communication processes managed across the firm.

Galbraith (1973) argues that complexity, information asymmetry, uncertainty, and strong interdependencies among units force organizations to elaborate information, and to coordinate their activities. Thus, in a complex organization the four models of information strategy are often mixed together in order to satisfy all the organizational needs. Together, the information strategy and the technical complexity of production determine the structural complexity of the firm, and change the types of communication processes.

Information and Knowledge Management Systems

For long time, a huge amount of organizational resources, in terms of time and money, have been invested in ICT solutions such as very traditional

ISs or more innovative KM systems, which aim at effectively and efficiently managing communication processes within and across organizational units. Disregarding the contingency theories described above, practitioners have for long time considered that ISs are neutral assets within the firm, and can be implemented to deterministically direct and change human coordination and communication actions. For instance, ICT, IS and KM systems facilitate synchronous and asynchronous communication processes when there is no physical proximity (Sarbaugh-Thompson and Feldman, 1998), enable knowledge sharing among organizational units, simplify some managerial decision processes, and support the electronic data interchange among firms.

The typical KM architecture, described by Davenport and Prusak (1997), is a centralized system, composed by the following elements which enable various communication processes:

- The enterprise knowledge portal, which provides a unique access point to corporate knowledge, with personalized services. This is often a web-based interface which guarantees, through authentication processes, the creation of personalized channels of communication within the firm;
- Groupware applications, as chats, forums, discussion groups, e-mails, etc., which enable social interactions within workgroups and across organizational units. The high level of informal communication, that technology can sustain, contributes to make the newcomer feel as a central member of the organization;
- Workflow management systems, that allow users to model communication and production processes.

Different components of KM and IS solutions can sustain a particular information strategy model and a type of production technology rather than another; for instance, workflow management systems may support information hierarchy and long linked technologies, while groupware applications usually favor feudalism in information strategy and intensive production technology. Practitioners usually don't take into account the organizational complexity and the unpredictability of the effects of an ICT solution.

Phenomenological and Structuration Theories

The considerations underlined above determined the inclusion in the research of more phenomenological approaches, focusing on the relations among social actors, organizations (in particular the system of communication and coordination processes), and technologies. Along these lines, Weick (1979; 1996) sees the organization as a system taking in equivocal information from its environment (enactment), trying to make sense out of that information (selection), and using in the future what was learned in the past (retention). Organizations evolve as they make sense of themselves and their environment. He argues that technologies are stochastic systems implemented in a very complex environment, thus it is impossible to foresee their positive or negative effects. Thus communication is a key process because of its role in the sense-making processes people use.

Also, the structuration theories, based on (Giddens, 1984), show that technologies and social structures are strongly related and interdependent (Orlikowski, 1991; Orlikowski & Gash, 1994; Orlikowski & Robey, 1991). According to these theories, there are strong relationships and interdependences among human actions, institutional roles (the *de facto* organizational model) and the technology architecture of IS or KM systems in use within the company. In particular, the design of technology should be strongly influenced by the institutional roles and organizational properties. Its introduction forces people to try to understand the processes designed in the system, and often to change their traditional activities. If people adopt the new processes, they introduce new activities, new beliefs, new expectations that in the long term might change the organizational structure of the firm. On the other side, if the traditional activities are too different from those embedded within the system, people tend to desert IS and KM systems, and continue to work as they did before, retaining a stable environment. One of the critical factors of these processes is the interpretative flexibility that exists. In other words, the choice of changing channel of communication or of not adopting the new ICT system very strongly depends from the capability of workers to understand it. Often workers interpret and adopt technology in a way that is not predictable beforehand and might use the same technology in different processes and for different aims.

To conclude, from what said, it derives that on one hand the effectiveness of IS and KM systems introduced within a firm is dependent on the information strategy of the firm and the type of production technology that has been developed; on the other hand, the design of these technologies is in its turn affected by the organizational structure, and at the same time by the users. The effects of these interdependencies cannot be clearly foreseen, as they depend on the ability of workers to understand the technology and to adopt/adapt it for their business needs.

COMMUNICATION PROCESSES

As explained in previous paragraphs, communication has nowadays become one of the most important assets in organizations. This is because organizations cannot be considered just as "containers" of individuals with common aims, but have to be regarded as evolving social contexts in which real persons face various situations and problems (see for instance Foresto, 2004; Klein, 1998; Malizia, 1993). Thus, communication is the means they possess in order to understand and adapt to the dynamics of these changing environments.

Classical Organizational Communication Theories

The discipline that studies the relations between communicative processes and organizational settings is called "organizational communication"; it has the twofold purpose of:

- Understanding how communicational processes shape organizations and
- Understanding how organizational life influences the form and content of communicative acts of the individuals who interact within it.

Putnam et al. (1996) singles out three fundamental questions that organizational communication tries to answer:

- Do communicational processes depend from the type of the organization or, vice versa, the latter depends on communicational processes?
- Do communicational fluxes follow the direction of the organizational hierarchy or these fluxes influence the structure and the workflows of the organization?
- Is communication a central element in the creation of the identity of an organization or it is merely a functional instrument?

Considered the relevant role of technology in communication processes, it is reasonable to add another relevant question to the analysis.

- Are communication processes affected by the channel of communication, in particular by technology?

Organizational communication includes both internal processes of communication (among the members of the organization itself) and communication towards the outside (how the organization presents itself and exchanges information with external stakeholders). In this chapter only the internal dimension of organizational communication is analyzed.

The literature in this discipline has classified communication according to different criteria that we will try to sum up very briefly:

- Level of formality;
- Direction of informational fluxes;
- Content of the messages;
- Function that it performs;
- Purpose that it has.

The first typology distinguishes between formal communication with its rigidity, precision and authority, which follows predefined patterns and informal communication, which is flexible, personal and is free from etiquettes (Stohl and Redding, 1987). Alternative ways to describe informal communication are coordination by feedback (March & Simon, 1958) or by clan mechanisms (Ouchi, 1980).

The typology based on informational fluxes is more articulated, as it includes vertical communication (both top-down, from the top management to the basis and bottom-up, from the basis to the top management), horizontal (between individuals who occupy the same positions in the hierarchy), and transversal (or cross-channel, which is similar to the horizontal one in character but involves wider parts of the organization, namely members working for different units). Very traditional works explored these types of information fluxes, for more details see (Simpson, 1959; Welch, 1980; Penley, 1982).

The typology based on the content of the messages singles out political messages (relative to strategies, correct behaviors etc.) basic messages (information for the well functioning of the organization) and messages related to the image (definition of the style of the organization) (Tanis, 2008; Watzlawick, et al., 1967).

The typology based on the function of the communication sees the properly functional communication as the one in charge of guaranteeing the correct functioning of the organizational "machinery", the informative communication as the one in charge of the visibility of the enterprise, with its products and services, the creative communication as the one ensuring the promotion of changes and progress and, finally, the formative communication as the one with the function of establishing a sense of belonging through presentations, meetings, parties etc. (Goffman, 1974).

The last typology, based on the purposes, includes messages to inform, create involvement, and sell products and services. Companies must communicate with their present and potential customers, casting into the role of communicator and promoter (Prandelli and Verona, 2006).

Why these Classifications are not Fit to our Target

The typologies just presented overlap in many respects and this is not by chance; one thing that they definitely have in common is that they describe the communication processes as they take place inside an organization. They accomplish this aim starting from different perspectives and targeting various aspects but, despite the questions listed in the analysis in (Putnam et al. 1996), they focus much more on communication itself than on the interaction of this latter with the organizational reality and its actors. As the main objective of this work is to understand the changes in the complex interrelations between communication processes, organizational structure, and technologies, we find the solutions offered by the classical theories of organizational communication unsatisfactory.

In other terms, our aim is to analyze whether the changes into the communication processes induced by the implementation of an IS for the management of data (developed according to a managerial information strategy and coherent with the technology of production of the firm) give as output the creation of new objects and practices or contribute to create a new organizational reality. The traditional classifications present different aspects of the communication processes, but most of the times these are simultaneously present in organizational life and are intermingled, thus they are not able to properly explain these dynamics. In order to analyze these changes we will propose a new classification anchored in the philosophical tradition. The rationale of our proposal is that of characterizing the different "attitudes" that social actors, inside an organization, can enact with respect to communication processes. Finally, this new classification reflects the need to understand the interdependences among organizational structure, actors, and ISs, typically described by structuration theories.

Our Proposal of Classification

Our proposal is rooted in the philosophical tradition, especially in epistemology and in the analytic philosophy of law. In the latter ambit, a sharp distinction between normative and descriptive discourse has traditionally been traced (Villa, 1999). This same distinction can be translated in more general terms by the epistemological conception of normativism and descriptivism conceived as different kinds of epistemological analyses. In both traditions a third element, namely contructivism, has lately been added, which presents new peculiar features (see Piaget 1967; Vygotsky 1978).

We will rely on these previously proposed classifications and apply them to the study of communication processes, thus indicating three different types of communication; the typology is meant to specifically address the role played by the communication processes in shaping both the attitude of the involved social actors and the social reality in which they are immersed. Under this perspective, the effects of the communication on the organizational reality become the real focus of the analysis. These three types of communication processes are: normative, descriptive and constructive.

Normative Processes

The communication is unidirectional, namely directed from the "top" (the management) of the organization down to the workers and it possesses some peculiar features, as being constituted by formal rules that are meant to be clear, precise and rigid. In this case the purpose of communication is that of giving a list of requirements to be met; in a sense it is presupposed that the knowledge about what is right is possessed only by the top management, which becomes a sort of guide for the other members of the organizations. In the normative vision, the function of communication is that of giving directions and prescriptions and transmitting an evaluation scale (Villa 1984; Wrenn 2001). Communication is seen as the carrier of the judgment on what is right or wrong, good or bad.

Descriptive Processes

Communication processes are bidirectional; instead of imposing rules aimed at the ideal functioning of the organization, the management tries to understand which are the real processes at stake inside the organization and the communication has the purpose to gather information from workers so that their condition could be improved in order to allow them to work more effectively. In this case, communication doesn't have the purpose of transmitting values, but rather of drawing a faithful description of the organizational reality "as it is" (Rorty 1980). Thus, according to this vision, interpretations should ideally be avoided in favor of a neutral and objective rendering of "how things really are".

Constructive Processes

Communication processes are informal, "horizontally and transversally oriented" processes in which participants negotiate the meaning of the content of communications, thus they cooperate in the building of socially constructed concepts that are used inside the organization. This results in what has been called "sense-making" (Weick, 1979; Weick, 1996; Weick and Roberts, 1993), the social construction of organizational reality, which includes the creation of common values and of a sense of identity and of belonging to the organization itself.

The assumption behind this conception of communication is that reality (and organizational reality in particular) is not detached from the individuals who perceive it, thus knowledge of this reality is not neutrally given (and transmissible), but is always filtered by the interpretative schemas of subjects. These interpretative schemas are continually reshaped as individuals interact with other individuals, thus creating new concepts and other social products (von Glasersfeld 1987; von Glasersfeld 1999; Watzlawick 1984; Raskin 2002). In this sense, communication is not merely an exchange of information, but is rather the creation of new ways of experiencing the reality and from these new social entities can emerge.

To sum up, the advantage of the classification that is proposed is that it directly indicates what a communication process does to a social environment: the name of each type of communication process already concisely explains its aim. In the normativistic case the communication aims at regulating social interactions, in the descriptivistic case it aims at illustrating the contents of such interactions and, finally, in the constructivist case communication reshapes the social environment.

Advantages and Drawbacks of the Three Approaches

After having explained the advantages of the classification we are proposing, we will now sketch the advantages and drawbacks of the three types of approaches to communication that the classification indicates, in order to understand what to expect when passing from one type of communication to the other.

Normativistic communication has the advantage to be controllable and precise but, on the other hand, it is very rigid and this can prevent the spontaneous emergence of initiatives from the bottom of the organization.

Descriptivistic communication enjoys the advantages of its being bidirectional, in the sense that information comes from more sources and this, for sure, enhances participation from the bottom and the possibility for the top management to sense the mood of the whole organization. On the other hand, it is based on a debatable assumption, namely that it is possible to exchange information which is neutral with respect to values. Therefore, even though in this case the top management takes into account the feedbacks from the basis, it can happen that the basis is not satisfied in the end because the requests that they are allowed to express have to follow predefined patterns that are biased on the top management's vision, even if the latter pretends to be neutral.

Finally, constructivistic communication has the advantage of being free from imposed patterns, its content and form are completely determined by the actors involved in the communication process; in this way, new and unpredictable results can emerge, leaving room for creativity and spontaneity.

On the other hand, in this case, communication can be very fuzzy and uncontrollable and it can be more difficult for the top management to extract the results of these processes, as they are often not readily available.

What can be induced from this brief analysis is that, roughly speaking, normativistic communication is fitter to environments in which there is a strong and well defined hierarchy and the job mostly consists in well consolidated practices and the actors at the lowest levels of the organization have mainly to execute predefined routines. Descriptivistic communication is instead desirable in those settings in which the structure of the organization is flatter and the jobs of all the actors involve a higher degree of autonomy. Constructivistic communication appears to be very effective in scenarios where many different independent units coexist and thus it is very hard to have a global vision that encounters the needs of all. Since in these settings communication must cross the boundaries of specific work units, it is difficult to find "a language that everyone can understand", while it seems more plausible that the consensus on how to communicate and the understanding of what is being communicated must be negotiated, given the heterogeneity of competences and capabilities.

THE CASE STUDY

The analysis carried out in the residence for elderly Giovanelli is part of a wider project[3], in collaboration with Spes Trento[4] and the department of computer and management sciences of the University of Trento. The researchers have spent 4 months in the residence Giovanelli, in order to help the director of the residence to introduce Sispes, and help licensed practical nurses (LPNs), physiotherapists, social assistants and sanitary assistants to understand the technology, adopt it, and use it in the most effective way.

Description of the Company

The residence Giovanelli, founded in 1729 as a hospital for elderly, is located in Tesero, in the province of Trento, Northern Italy. Nowadays, the residence is a public institution of assistance and charity. Currently, the residence guarantees some core services such as sanitary attendance, nursing, medical, physiotherapeutic, entertainment, and often religious services. The labor force is of approximately 50 employees, plus a variable number of volunteers.

The professional roles are divided in five units: the administrative office, the assistance and sanitary unit, the entertainment unit, and the technical services division.

The administrative office has to manage three main activities. The first one concerns all the bureaucratic and administrative activities that are related to the guests. For instance, to guarantee contacts between the residence and guests' relatives, help guests to obtain certifications from the public government (such as residential certification, identity card, etc.), organize the documents to ask for public funds, evaluate new requests of guest staying, manage the general and analytical accounting, etc. The second group of activities is focused on the relationships with public stakeholders, such as the Province of Trento, which finances all the public residences for elderly in Trentino, and other public institutions that take care of security, privacy of the healthcare procedures, human resources administration, etc. The third group of activities concerns the economic and financing programming, the management of the residence's patrimony and all the economic aspects of outsourcing processes such as collaborations with practitioners and specialists.

The social assistance operators, who have direct contact with the guests and are in closer contact with their more or less explicit needs, constitute the assistance unit.

The sanitary unit has to guarantee the sanitary, medical, and pharmaceutical services that guests need. The three major roles in this unit are the physician of general medicine, LPNs - including the nurses' coordinator -, and the physiotherapists. The physician has to guarantee the basic medical assistance to the guests, maintain a good relation with relatives, and cooperate with other workers in order to provide a good quality service. The LPNs are professionals that enact the therapies suggested by the physician, and the nurses' coordinator has to coordinate the nurses' turnover, the activities carried out in the residence, and has to control the distribution of medicines. Finally, the physiotherapists have the goal to improve the life and welfare of the guests, through the most effective physical and psychological rehabilitation.

The entertainment unit has to guarantee a good level of social life to guests, paying also attention to their relations with relatives and cultural or religious local associations. It is constituted by animators who usually organize recreational events, such as newspaper readings, birthday parties, visits in tourism destinations, etc.

Finally, the technical services division has the aim to guarantee some services such as laundry, restaurant, and instruments and furniture maintenance.

Description of the Technology

The technology introduced in the residence for elderly Giovanelli is Sispes, an IS created by Spes Trento. It is a web-based system, which manages most of the information flows among socio-assistance, sanitary, entertainment, and administrative units.

It is composed by an enterprise knowledge portal, which provides the unique access point to corporate knowledge. Information can be obtained and added only through an authentication process. It includes also a groupware application, which enables workers to share documents, start forums, leave messages, and manage a group agenda. Finally, it provides a complex system of workflow and document management that allows users to add and retrieve information from the corporate archives.

The main characteristic of Sispes is that it is focused on the residence's guests and all the information is managed according to this perspective. Thus, all information, autonomously managed by each single unit, is not shaped according to the theme or the topic of interest of the group, but rather according to the guest's needs. Therefore, physicians, nurses, animators, and administrative offices collectively contribute to the management of guests' information, according to some predefined channels of communication. Each contributor accedes to the IS through an authentication process, sees the most relevant links to document management systems related to her/his activity, and can add information which she/he is responsible for.

Figure 1 shows how workers can access the enterprise knowledge portal in order to add their information.

One of the most important services provided by Sispes is the creation of guests' integrated folders, which report on all the information about each single guest. An example is depicted in Figure 2. The data, provided by each single integrated folder, refer to the fundamental information of the guest (such as age, gender, relatives' phone numbers, etc.) and on her/his state of well-being and health.

Methodology of Analysis

In this work we have adopted the ethnographic approach. Ethnography is mainly based on the active participation of the observer inside the firm, with the aim to get a detailed understanding of the circumstances, the strategies and the relationships of the subjects being studied (Spradley, 1979). In the first phase of our analysis, an investigator spent four months working in the administrative offices of the residence Giovanelli, helping workers to understand the technology, adopt it, and use it in the most effective way. In doing that, he has analyzed how the implementation of Sispes affects both technical processes and the social attitude of communication. Even though, in most cases, four months are not enough to deeply understand the organizational culture, the hidden power of

Figure 1. The Sispes enterprise knowledge portal

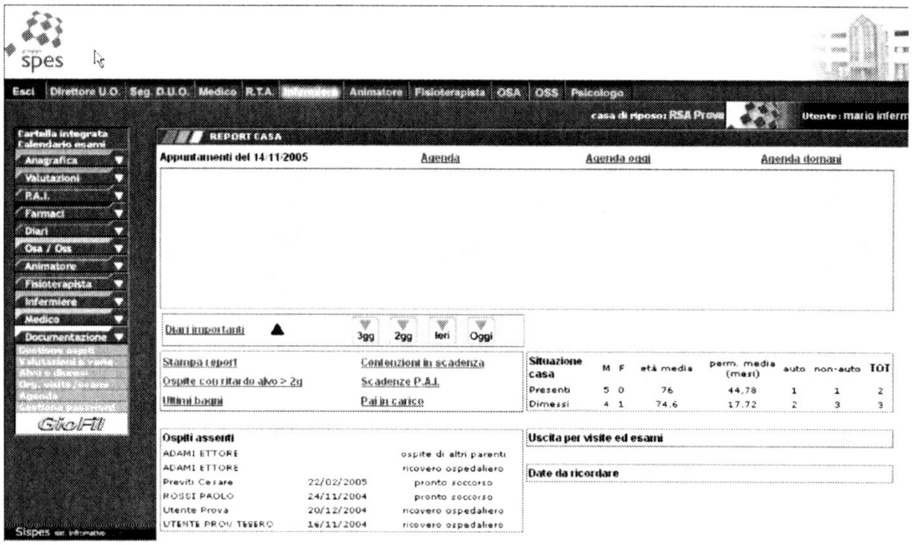

workers' relations, and some of the tacit aspects of communication, in this case this experience was complemented by official documents of the firm and a series of qualitative interviews to the 15 key employees of the firm. They play various roles within the firm and utilize different services supported by the technology platform.

The second phase of our analysis has been made two years after the first implementation of Sispes, and was motivated by the fact that, in the first phase, workers might have been biased by the introduction of an innovative solution or might have needed time to get used and to deeply understand the IS. We interviewed 8 key employees, maintaining the same structure and method of analysis of the first phase. Workers spent from 40 to 60 minutes, presenting from their points of view the effects of Sispes on the communication processes and on their attitude to share knowledge.

Figure 2. An example of a guest's integrated folder

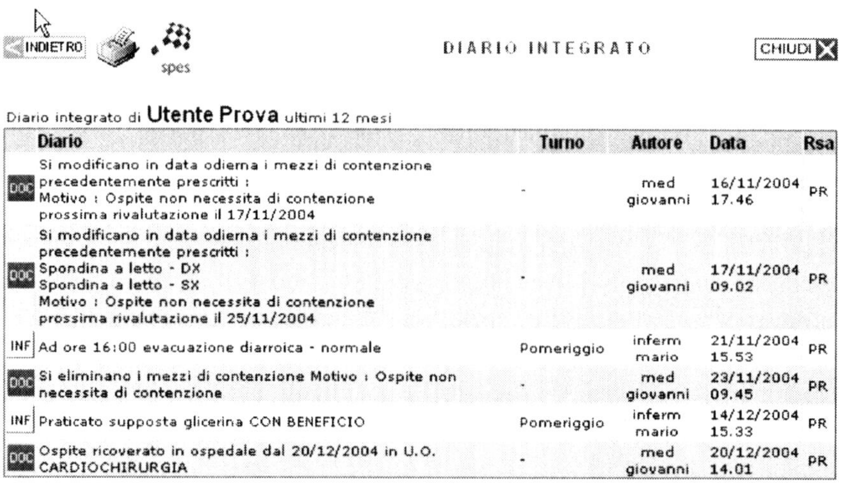

All the documents, the interviews and the direct observations made by the investigator have been deeply analyzed using the analytic induction method to systematically examine similarities among various knowledge bases in order to prove how communication processes evolve in an organization (Ragin, 1994; Taylor and Bogdan, 1998).

RESULTS OF THE CASE STUDY

In this section, we will highlight the changes determined at a communicational level by the introduction of the system Sispes in the residence for elderly Giovanelli. We will also evaluate the impact of these changes on the work environment and on the services provided to the guests.

Before Sispes

We will start with a brief presentation of the ante-Sispes situation, namely of the ways in which communication used to be carried out in the residence. For the sake of simplicity, we could group these communication processes in two categories: informal and formal.

Informal Communication

With respect to the informal communication, we could single out two subcategories: completely unstructured, like occasional conversations and gossips, and semi-structured.

Unstructured informal communication, as is very common in many work settings, played a very important role prior to the introduction of Sispes, especially due to the lack of official occasions for contact among people belonging to different units (for instance nurses and animators). Informal communication had in this sense the purpose of filling the gap determined by the absence of formal communication and information procedures involving all the people working with the same guest but at different times or under different perspectives. Under another respect, we could say that it substituted the processes needed by the intensive production technology of the residence.

Nevertheless, informal communication often carries with it undesired consequences, like malicious gossips, negative moods, competition among different units that should cooperate instead and the like and all this can sometimes degenerate, thus creating a (socially) unhealthy environment. This adds to the reasons why not too much of the "burden" of information about professional matters should rely on completely unstructured informal communication.

A partial solution to the problem of the informative gap mentioned above was given in the residence Giovanelli by semi-structured communication, as in the case of the so-called "Guest's diary"[5]. This used to be a paper diary in which LPNs wrote notes about the stay of guests; what could be written in these notes varies between particularly relevant information on what happened in the last turn of work to very ordinary and general information about the guest. Since there were no precise rules to determine the content and the format of these notes, very often they needed to be explained during formal meetings by the LPNs who wrote them.

In many cases, these explanations could not wait for the scheduled formal meetings, as for instance when seemingly relevant information was graphically unreadable or when relevant information was submerged and lost in the mass of other – maybe not so relevant - notes. In these and similar cases what intervened was again unstructured informal communication.

Formal Communication

On the other hand, formal communication used to be (and for the most still is) exchanged through four kinds of formal meetings: consignation meetings, meetings for the Individual Assistance Plan

(IAP from hereafter), meetings of the LPNs and meetings of the units.

- Consignation meetings are held on a daily basis, at the time of the change of turn, with the participation of the LPN who finishes the turn, the one who begins the new turn and the representative of the social assistance operators (SAOs from hereafter). They are aimed at informing about the variations in the conditions of the guests that could have taken place during the previous turn.
- IAP meetings[6] are technical meetings among physicians, LPNs, physiotherapists, animators and the representative of the SAOs, in which interventions and goals to be achieved in every assistance domain are discussed. The result of these meetings is written in the IAP file-card, which is then hung to the guest's bed. These meetings are not held on a regular basis, their frequency depends on the guest's conditions, but they have to be scheduled at least once every six months.
- LPNs meetings are held once in a month, with the participation of all LPNs and - often - of the Administrative Director; organizational aspects are discussed.
- Meetings of the units are organized once every two months, and specific problems of each particular unit are discussed. The participation to these meetings is obviously restricted to the members of the relative unit.

This is, roughly speaking, the communicative scenario in which Sispes was introduced in November 2004.

After the Implementation of Sispes

After the implementation of Sispes in the residence for elderly Giovanelli many changes in communicative processes took place, some at a general and widespread level, others in very detailed procedures. We will start by describing what has been changed as a general attitude, then we will give a pair of illuminating examples of specific practices that have been modified and, finally, we will try to give an interpretation of these changes in the light of the paradigm previously introduced.

Generally speaking, first of all, for what concerns professional matters, information used to be mainly transmitted during regularly scheduled formal meetings, where the representatives of the different teams normatively gave instructions on what to do. Nowadays, even these formal meetings are based on reports printed out from Sispes. In these reports information coming from all Sispes users is contained; this means that members of teams who didn't have the occasion to share information before the introduction of Sispes are now allowed to communicate in this virtual space. The result of this global process is the writing of an "integrated folder" that enables the collaboration of the different teams for the creation of a "holistic profile of the guest", taking into account sanitary, physical, social and sometimes even spiritual needs at the same time. Before Sispes, goals to be achieved and rules to be followed in order to reach the guests' well-being were pre-imposed by people occupying the highest positions into the hierarchy of the residence. Now the sharing of data, information, ideas and opinions across different units results in a capitalization of specialized knowledge and capabilities and the profile of guests (with relative problems and needs) emerges from this cooperative exchange.

There are others, maybe less striking effects of Sispes that is anyway worth considering. A first aspect is linked to the initial difficulties connected with its introduction; most workers were not that used with information technologies, some of them were not even familiar with computers at all, indeed.

This novelty encouraged people to talk to each other in order to learn to use Sispes more effectively. As one of the interviewed people put it:

For a certain period some of my colleagues and I couldn't talk of anything else. Sometimes it happened that we met a bit earlier than the beginning of the turn in order to try to learn together how to use it. Some colleagues were more "expert" in the daily journal, some others on the guest's diary, so we tried to unify our strengths.[7]

A second aspect is the rigor that the use of Sispes and computers in general brought to work practices. This manifests itself in many respects: the creation of a new, more organized archive (that adds to the paper archive), the use of e-mail for communications, which has the double advantage of being immediate but written (so permanent, in a sense), the execution of the various activities following specific workflows and practices, thus gaining in accuracy and precision.

Finally, a tool that enables workers to at least have an idea of what is going on in the whole organization makes them more aware of the role they play, of the usefulness of their work, of their contribution to the global results of the enterprise. This can give motivations to the workers by providing a sense of belonging and participation in the organization. This was also observed in a modification in the behavior of some workers of the residence Giovanelli.

How these changes were instantiated is maybe better explainable by giving a couple of examples.

The first example is the guest's diary; as already explained, this is a sort of repository of records of the events occurred during a turn and it is read at the consignation meeting. Before Sispes a lot of initiative was left to the person filling a diary, who could more or less decide, based on her/his judgment what and how to write. Sispes, instead, presents the users with forms containing predefined fields and menus; this on the one hand contributes to structure information, to make it more precise and more easily readable and accessible, even though, on the other hand, it introduces some rigidity that sometimes annoys the user.

The second example is given by the IAP meetings; they used to be started by a general update where everyone communicated with the others about all the information she/he could gather under her/his domain of competence and only after that people could begin discussing about the future plans. Nowadays this phase has become nearly useless, as people already come to the meeting with reports printed from Sispes where information from all available sources (even cross-units) is contained. Given this, much more time is left to brainstorming about the planning of the activities related to the guest's stay. Coming to the meeting already with an idea of the overall situation allows people to be more concrete and more focused on what has to be changed and what has to be improved and, instead of providing many scattered services to the guests, it is easier to perform a joint action targeted to the general well-being of the guests.

To sum up, it is certainly possible to argue that the everyday use of Sispes has improved both the communication and the management of data and information but, more importantly, the common interface has given the opportunity to people coming from different units and teams to have an easy access to information produced by varied and heterogeneous sources. This interface supports a many-to-many communication channel, which makes visible and available different viewpoints on the same subject matter. It is from these varied viewpoints that new knowledge can emerge, as it is well shown by this testimony:

One of the functionalities that I really appreciate in Sispes is that it gives me the opportunity to see the guest under different points of view. For instance, once it happened that I noticed a guest who looked depressed and with Sispes I could see whether the animators got the same impression.

The visibility and availability of information encourages the discussion and thus the same information can be elaborated many times with the final result of socially constructing new knowledge. Furthermore, with Sispes it is now possible for members of different teams to jointly draw a global profile of the guests.

Finally, and more importantly, it could be said that the creation of a new holistic view of guests due to the introduction of Sispes contributes to elicit synergies among different teams whose effects are more valuable than those obtained by the sum of the activities conducted separately by the very same teams.

What happened in the residence Giovanelli is a typical example of transition of an organization from mainly descriptive and normative communication processes to more constructive communication practices. This transition has especially been made possible thanks to the introduction of a new technology, i.e. of the Sispes system. In order to validate this opinion, the following relevant remarks have been collected during the second phase of analysis:

The holistic vision of guest's information is very important. Consider when a physiotherapist changes the wheelchair of a guest, or when a physician modifies the medical treatment. I can access all this information just by reading the daily diary of the elder. This allows us to discuss on the reasons of these choices (often during the consignation meeting), thus increasing workers' consciousness and responsibility and improving the quality of our service.

While before the implementation of Sispes communication was mainly aimed at informing, with the purpose of performing a decisional process on the interventions to execute on guests, and the information "traveled" within the boarders of each working area, with Sispes cross-unit communication is no more limited to the formal meetings imposed by the top management, but becomes an everyday practice, linked to the use of Sispes. This practice contributes to the creation of a new global perspective on the treatment of guests, which can be renegotiated every time that new information is added to Sispes. As a confirmation of this statement, let's consider the testimony of a physician:

Before the adoption of Sispes, social assistants didn't share all their information with us, they were afraid of discussing this with us. Now they are aware that their knowledge is very important to us and we discuss daily the consequences of our decisions. Consider that they are the only ones who see the body of a guest naked, therefore only they can see pressure sores, or test the reactions to a particular therapy.

As we hope to have demonstrated, the constructivistic approach enhances, at least in a setting with these features (namely composed by heterogeneous units) the unpredictable creation of knowledge from social exchanges. It is exactly this unpredictability that prevents the acquisition of this knowledge through traditional normatively or descriptively oriented procedures. There is a part of knowledge, which is so intrinsic in work practices that it cannot be imposed or transmitted by the top management, it can only emerge from "experience on the field"; it is this kind of knowledge which is the special target of constructivistic approaches.

FUTURE TRENDS AND CONCLUSION

In this work a new approach for the classification of communication processes has been proposed. The approach provides a line of interpretation that allows the joint analysis of communication processes and of the organizational reality in which they take place.

While the chapter is mainly focused on the relations between communication processes and IS and ICT applications, the satisfying results encourage the application of this theoretical apparatus also to the study of the relations between communication practices and production technologies.

Once the results of this analysis will be available, it should be possible to associate to each type of production technology the communication approach that suits it better.

With respect to the case study, an interesting observation could be made: surprisingly, the very methodology that was used, namely ethnography, enhanced a particular kind of communication, which was probably already there even if latent: the constructivistic attitude. In other terms, the presence of the investigator during the phase of implementation of the technology encouraged people to cooperate and contribute to the understanding and the effective use of the application by the whole organization. What emerged in the process of interviewing people was that the lack in communication among members of different units was strongly perceived. They didn't actually work together, but their work was strongly interconnected and they shared the target - the guest - a sensible one indeed. The experience of the interviews unveiled a hidden and implicit need: that of having a consolidated practice for sharing and communicating information at all levels of the organization.

In the setting just described, the most important effect of the transition from normative and descriptive communication practices to constructive ones has been the building of a global perspective on guests, which strongly ameliorated the services offered to them and, consequently, their overall condition.

In this sense it can be said that a change in the communicational attitudes led to a change in the firm's worldview, which in turn led to a change in the work practices. The way in which services are delivered to guests has changed as a consequence of a new " internal" communicational attitude.

At a more abstract level, the analysis of this case study has taught that technology is in fact a major social actor, as it modifies pre-existing practices, like in the case of meetings (where the reports of Sispes often give the directions of the discussion) and gives new possibilities, like that of inferring new information from statistical results extracted from the data stored in Sispes.

A final remark on the future directions that the project can take is in order. So far, the main focus has been on the influence of information technology on communicative practices and social issues, but the opposite is also very interesting and under the scope of the project. This case study has already shown that people often use the very same tools for very different and sometimes unforeseen tasks and this can suggest to software designers new applications of these tools. Furthermore, it is especially when these tools are already in use, that users find bugs and weaknesses. For instance, some users found Sispes too rigid when they had to insert data whose category they could not find in the proposed menus; in these cases they were forced to use one of the predefined choices, but this made it more difficult to retrieve these data afterwards. All the criticisms emerged from the interviews should definitely be used as guidelines to improve the software and eventually to personalize it in accordance with specific needs. From a theoretical standpoint, this could result in the study of the influence of the underlying social and communicational setting on the reshaping of the ICT tools.

ACKNOWLEDGMENT

The authors gratefully thank Tiziano Amistadi for his precious help, especially in the case study; the interviews have been conducted in the scope of his thesis. We also thank Luca Nicolelli for allowing us to analyze the processes within the residence Giovanelli, and SPES Trento Cooperativa Sociale for funding the project "InConSPES".

REFERENCES

Ashby, W. R. (1967). Self-Regulation and Requisite Variety. In F. E. Emery (Ed.), *System Thinking.* Penguin: Harmondsworth.

Child, J. (1972). Organization Structure and Strategies of Control: A Replication of the Aston Study. *Administrative Science Quarterly, 17,* 163 – 77.

Child, J., & Faulkner, D. (1998). *Strategies of Cooperation: Managing Alliances, Networks and Joint Ventures.* Oxford: Oxford University Press.

Cook, K. (1977). Exchange and Power in Networks of Interorganizational Relations. *Sociological Quarterly, 18,* 62 – 82.

Davenport, T. H., & Prusak, L. (1997). Working Knowledge: How Organizations Manage What They Know, *Harvard Business School.* Boston: HBS Press.

Davenport, T. H., Long, D. W. D., & Beers, M. C. (1998). Successful Knowledge Management Projects. *Sloan Management Review, 39*(2).

Emery, F. E., & Trist, E. L. (1960). Socio-technical Systems. *Management Sciences Models and Techniques, 2.*

Foresto C. (2004). *La comunicazione organizzativa: spunti di riflessione, appunti di lavoro, resoconto di un'esperienza alla Michelin Italia.* Milano: Centro Studi Logos.

Galbraith, J. R. (1973). *Designing Complex Organizations.* Reading, MA: Addison-Wesley.

Giddens, A. (1984). *The Constitution of Society.* Berkeley, CA: University of California Press.

Goffman, E. (1974). *Frame analysis: An essay on the organization of experience.* London: Harper and Row.

Harris, K., Fleming, M., Hunter, R., Rosser, B., & Cushman, A. (1998). *The Knowledge Management Scenario: Trends and Directions for 1998-2003.* Technical report, Gartner Group.

Klein G. B. (1998). Osservare e valutare la comunicazione nelle organizzazioni. *Rassegna Italiana di Valutazione.* 10.

Lawrence, P., & Lorsch, J. W. (1967). *Organizations and environment.* Boston: Division of Research, Graduate School of Business Administration, Harvard University.

Lowndes, V., & Skelcher, C. (1998). The Dynamics of Multi-Organizational Partnerships: An Analysis of Changing Modes of Governance. *Public Administration, 76,* 313 – 33.

Malizia, P. (1993). *Parola e sistema: saggio su comunicazione ed organizzazione.* Roma: Bulzoni Editore.

March, J. G., & Simon, H. A. (1958). *Organizations.* New York: John Wiley & Son.

Mintzberg, H. (1983). An emerging strategy of 'direct' research. In Van Maanen J. (Ed.), *Qualitative methodology.* Beverly Hills, CA: Sage.

Murray, V. (1997). Interorganizational Collaboration in the Non-Profit Sector. In Shafritz J. M. (Ed.), *International Encyclopaedia of Public Policy and Administration,* 2. Boulder, CO: Westview Press, 192 – 6.

Orlikowski W. J. (1991). Integrated information environment or matrix of control? The contradictory implications of information technology. *Accounting, Management, and Information Technology, 1*(1), 9 – 42.

Orlikowski, W. J., & Gash, D. C. (1994). Technological Frames: Making Sense of Information Technology in Organization. *ACM Transactions on Information Systems, 12*(2), 174-207.

Orlikowski, W. J., & Robey, D. (1991). Information Technology and the Structuring of Organizations. *Information Systems Research, 2*(2).

Ouchi, W. G. (1980) Markets, Bureaucracies, and Clans. *Administrative Science Quarterly, 25*(1), 129 – 141.

Parsons T. (1951). *The Social System.* Glencoe, IL: Free Press.

Penley, L. E. (1982). An investigation of the information processing framework of organizational communication. *Human Communication Research, 8*(4), 348-365.

Piaget, J. (1967). *Logique et Connaissance scientifique*. Paris: Gallimard.

Prandelli, E., & Verona, G. (2006). *Marketing in rete 2nd ed - Oltre Internet verso il nuovo Marketing.* Milano: McGraw-Hill.

Putnam, L. L., Phillips, N., & Chapman, P. (1996). Metaphors of Communication and Organization. In Clegg, S. R., Hardy, C. & Nord W. (Eds.), *Handbook of Organizational Studies.* London: Sage.

Ragin, C. C. (1994). *Constructing Social Research: The Unity and Diversity of Method,* Pine Forge Press.

Raskin J. D. (2002). Constructivism in psychology: Personal construct psychology, radical constructivism, and social constructionism. In Raskin J. D. and Bridges S. K. (Eds.), *Studies in meaning: Exploring constructivist psychology.* New York: Pace University Press, 1 – 25.

Rorty R. (1980). *Philosophy and the Mirror of Nature.* Princeton: Princeton UniversityPress.

Sarbaugh-Thompson M., & Feldman, M. S. (1998). Electronic Mail and Organizational Communication. *Organization Science, 9*(6), 685 – 698.

Simpson, R. L. (1959). Vertical and Horizontal Communication in Formal Organizations. *Administrative Science Quarterly, 4*(2), 188 – 196.

Spradley, J. P. (1979). *The Ethnographic Interview.* New York: Holt, Rinehart, Winston.

Stohl, C. & Redding W. C. (1987). Messages and Message Exchange Processes. In Jablin, F., Putnam, L., Roberts, K. & Porter, L. (Eds.) *Handbook of Organizational Communication: An Interdisciplinary Perspective.* Newbury Park, CA: Sage, 451 – 502.

Tanis, M. (2008). Organizational Identification and the Communication of Identity: Effects of Message Characteristics. Paper presented at the annual meeting of the *International Communication Association,* New York City, NY Retrieved 2008-04-22 from http://www.allacademic.com/meta/p14490_index.html.

Taylor, S. J., & Bogdan, R. (1998). *Introduction to Qualitative Research Methods.* New York: John Wiley & Sons.

Thompson J. D. (1967). *Organizations in Action.* New York: Mac Graw Hill.

Vangen, S., & Huxham, C. (2003). Nurturing Collaborative Relations: Building Trust in Interorganizational Collaboration. *Journal of Applied Behavioral Science, 39*(1), 5-31.

Villa, V. (1984). *Teorie della scienza giuridica e teorie delle scienze naturali: modelli ed analogie.* Milano: Giuffrè.

Villa, V. (1999). *Costruttivismo e teorie del diritto.* Torino: Giappichelli.

von Glasersfeld, E. (1987). *The construction of knowledge: Contributions to conceptual semantics.* Seaside, CA: Intersystems Publications.

von Glasersfeld, E. (1999). How do we mean? A constructivist sketch of semantics. *Cybernetics and Human Knowing, 6* (1), 9 – 16.

Vygotsky, L. S. (1978). *Mind and society: The development of higher mental processes.* Cambridge, MA: Harvard University Press.

Watzlawick, P., Beavin, J. H., & Jackson, D. D. (1967). *Pragmatics of Human Communication.* New York: W.W. Norton & Co Inc.

Watzlawick, P. (1984). *Invented Reality: How Do We Know What We Believe We Know? (Contributions to constructivism).* New York: W.W. Norton & Co Inc.

Weick, K. E. (1979). *The social psychology of organizing* (2nd ed.). NY: McGraw-Hill, Inc.

Weick, K. E. (1996). *Sensemaking in organizations.* Newbury Park, CA: Sage.

Weick, K. E., & Roberts K. H. (1993). Collective mind in Organizations: Heedful interrelating on Flight Decks. *Administrative Science Quarterly, 38*, 357 – 381.

Welch, R. L. (1980). Vertical and Horizontal Communication in Economic Processes. *The Review of Economic Studies, 47*(4), 733 – 746.

Woodward, J. (1965). *Industrial Organization: Theory And Practice.* London: Oxford University Press.

Wrenn, C. B. (2001). *Truth and the normativity of naturalistic epistemology.* PhD Thesis, from http://bama.ua.edu/~cwrenn/work/DissBody.pdf

KEY TERMS

Constructivistic Communication: Communication that, even if often not purportedly, constructs new knowledge, which is internalized by the participants to the communication. Not only the information that the participants possess is transmitted, but new knowledge can also emerge.

Descriptivistic Communication: Communication conducted with a descriptive style, i.e. with the purpose of describing reality as it is and how things actually are. "Descriptive" can be applied to theories, statements, beliefs, etc.

The Enterprise Knowledge Portal: Is the evolution of an information system which has a knowledge management goal. It combines the enterprise information portal functionalities with knowledge management features, capturing explicit and tacit knowledge, integrating access to expertise, supporting reasoning functionalities, serving as a centre of experiential learning, and optimizing decisions.

Ethnography: Derives from Greek (ethnos = people and graphein = writing) is a genre of writing that uses fieldwork to provide a descriptive study of human societies. Ethnography presents the results of a holistic research method founded on the idea that a system's properties cannot necessarily be accurately understood independently of each other.

Knowledge Management: Comprises a set of theories and practices used by both researchers in business and computer science studies and practitioners to identify, unveil, create, organize, represent, and distribute knowledge within and across companies.

Normativistic Communication: Communication conducted with a normative style, i.e. with the purpose of communicating how things ought to be and what is right or wrong. The adjective "normative" can also be applied to theories, statements, beliefs, etc.

Structuration Theories: Firstly proposed by Anthony Giddens (1984), they are an attempt to reconcile theoretical dichotomies of social systems such as agency/structure, subjective/objective, and micro/macro perspectives. Agency refers to the capacity of individual humans to act independently and to make their own free choices. Structure refers to those factors such as social class, religion, gender, ethnicity, customs etc. which seem to limit or influence the opportunities that individuals have. The approach does not focus on the individual actor or societal totality "but social practices ordered across space and time".

ENDNOTES

1. This analysis practices includes the modification of existing practices, the creation of new ones, the modification and creation of concepts and even of physical objects, as we will illustrate later on.
2. Knowledge management is a discipline that promotes an integrated approach to the creation, organization, access, and use of an enterprise's information assets. These assets include structured databases, textual information such as policy and procedure documents and, most importantly, the tacit knowledge and expertise of individual employees (Harris et al., 1998).
3. This is a three years research project, called INterdipendences and CONnections with SPES (InConSPES). In particular, Spes Trento intends to value workers' knowledge and conduct innovation within the organization, through a series of knowledge management actions. These are (i) the analysis of communication processes within the firm; (ii) the study of the co-dependences among technologies and organizations (both humans and processes); (iii) the state of workers' welfare; (iv) the guests' healthiness; (v) the identification of rates of knowledge performances.
4. Spes Trento Cooperativa Sociale is a company that manages 5 residences for elderly in the area of Trentino (Italy).
5. We will return later in this paragraph on this practice, since it is one of the best examples of the changes brought about by Sispes.
6. IAP meetings are another meaningful example of the changes introduced with Sispes, as we will see below.
7. All the interviews are translated from Italian.

Chapter XIV
The Roles of a Nurse in Telemedical Consultations

Boris A. Kobrinsky
Moscow Research Institute for Paediatrics and Children's Surgery, Russia

Nikolay V. Matveev
Moscow Research Institute for Paediatrics and Children's Surgery, Russia

ABSTRACT

Telemedicine, or distant medical consultations using communication via electronic networks, is gradually becoming a standard of medical care delivery in distant areas worldwide, including both the most developed and the developing countries. For instance, in 2007, telemedical centres existed in 55% of the Russian regions (on average, about 4 centres in each region). In most of the cases, nurses are actively involved in the organization of various types of distant consultation. Main types of telemedical services include: (1) emergency consultations of patients by telephone, (2) telemedical consultations using videoconferences or store-and-forward systems, and (3) home telecare systems. Possible roles of nurses in different types of telemedical consultations are discussed.

INTRODUCTION

According to the definition of nursing suggested by The International Council of Nurses (ICN), nursing includes "the promotion of health, prevention of illness, and the care of ill, disabled and dying people" [1]. ICN also underlines that the scope of nursing practice is "dynamic and responsive to health needs, development of knowledge, and technological advances" [2].

The development of so-called telemedicine can be referred to as one of such technological advances that might cause significant changes in the scope of nursing practice in the nearest future.

Telemedicine is a term which was coined only several decades ago. A number of somewhat contradictory definitions have been suggested for this term [3], but generally most of the authors now agree that the term 'telemedicine' represents *medical care provided to patients at a distance by using electronic means of communication.*

Some authors prefer to use the broader term *telehealth*, which mostly refers to administrative and educational use of telecommunications in healthcare [4].

The aim of this chapter is to demonstrate some examples of nurses' roles in contemporary telemedicine and to discuss in brief what could be the nurses' roles in telemedicine of the nearest future.

BACKGROUND

The first ideas of telemedicine were probably suggested at the beginning of the 20th century by Willem Einthoven, who made attempts to transfer electrocardiograms by telephone lines [5]. Later on, in the 1930s, radio communication was used to provide medical advice aboard ships and planes [6].

Distant medical consultants became important in the 1960s, when the Soviet Union and U.S. launched their space programmes [7] and it was necessary to have some control over the astronauts' health. For a long time, telemedicine remained 'an expensive toy', as it was based on rather unique expensive technologies (e.g. satellite communications) suitable until the 1990s mostly for astronauts and military applications.

Wide introduction of personal computers and, even more important, the Internet, made telemedicine much more 'democratic'. Since the 1990s, simple telemedical equipment can be installed virtually at any clinic. Using electronic mail, a doctor could request a 'second opinion' from a distant specialist who might have better expertise for a specific case. Such communication was convenient, fast and reasonably priced.

Later on, video cameras, digital photo cameras, and scanners were successfully used to record important information about a patient in digital form. Such information could be sent to a distant consultant via electronic networks. At the same time, thousands of videoconferencing systems were installed worldwide, so that by the end of the 20th century, almost every large clinic had the possibility to organize live video connection with a number of other clinics throughout the world. Many clinics installed videoconferencing units which made intra-hospital telemedicine possible [8]. Also, a number of experiments have been done to install telemedical equipment at patient's home, so that patients could ask for medical advice without leaving their homes [9].

Now telemedicine provides a convenient means of communication between a patient (or a medical worker, representing his interests, e.g. a nurse or GP) and a highly qualified medical consultant, usually a specialist in a particular field. Normally, advice of such a consultant might not be available for a patient without special travel.

Such travel may not be feasible due to the following reasons:

1. A long time is required for such travel
2. Excessive cost of travel (compared to the cost of telemedical consultation)
3. Travel is not suitable for a patient due to the severity of his state
4. Travel is inconvenient for a patient, e.g. for a businessman with a tight schedule

Telemedicine is known to be most effective for those areas of medicine that do not require close personal interaction between a patient and a physician. In the case of teleradiology or telepathology, a consultant reviews only a radiography image or an image of some microscopic preparation; the consultant's actions do not differ much from what a physician does during regular consultation. There are virtually no differences in reviewing an x-ray image at a computer display—only the image originates from a next-door hospital room or from a hospital in a distant country.

Teledermatology is another area where distant consultations have proved its efficacy, mainly because in most of the cases dermatological diagnosis could be based mainly on still images which are rather easy to transfer via electronic networks [10].

Step by step, year by year, telemedicine has evolved from an experimental area into a widely recognized high technology medical application. For instance, in June 2008, PubMed provided as many as 10,015 hits using keyword 'telemedicine', with the first two titles dated 1974, 840 titles dated 2007, and 305 titles during the first five months of 2008.

At the moment, telemedical technologies are used most frequently in the U.S., followed by other developed countries: EU countries, Australia, Japan, etc. [11]. Nevertheless, a number of developing countries have successfully implemented their own telemedical projects, often in close collaboration with medical centres of the developed countries [12]. Russia and other ex-USSR countries are probably between the two poles, as they have highly-qualified specialists in spheres of both medicine and telecommunications, while the level of funding allocated for medical research, was inadequate. However, telemedicine is widely spread now, for instance, in Russia, where there exist telemedical centres at 55% of Russian regions, as it was demonstrated by the results of a survey organized by Federal Agency for High-Technology Medical Care of The Russian Federation in 2007. On average, there are two telemedical centres (TMC) in a regional centre, and two TMC in district hospitals outside of a regional centre in each region of Russia. Typically, regional level telemedical centres are located at large regional hospitals, where they can serve a number of departments which may be easily connected with leading Russian medical institutions of federal level (in Moscow, St. Petersburg, or other cities). District level TMCs usually communicate with regional hospitals only, sometimes using them as relays if any communication with federal level institutions is needed. Only five regions of Russia reported the number of existing TMC over 10 (Irkutsk region - 11, Altay Republic and Nizhny Novgorod region - 12, Arkhangelsk region - 24, Penza region - 30).

Possible roles of nurses are various, which reflects, first, a variety of possible roles of nurses in healthcare and, second, a variety of models of telemedicine.

Generally, a nurse can be referred to as a 'mediator' between a patient and a medical doctor. A nurse can provide necessary help to a patient in 'standard' situations requiring medical care; if the situation does not look 'standard', a nurse refers a patient to a physician. In case of referrals, it is usually a nurse's responsibility to assess the severity of a case and refer a patient to an appropriate specialist.

Nurses, assisting to physicians, perform the initial analysis of the patients' complaints and requests. It should be taken into account, nevertheless, that the role of a nurse in different countries may differ. The role of a nurse in the U.S., Canada, EU, etc., is generally more significant, while in Russia and some other countries the level of responsibility of nurses is somewhat lower. Some differences are due to a specific profile of the department where a nurse works (e.g. paediatrics, obstetrics, surgery, etc.)

Modern development of information and telemedical technologies brought additional specific features into the work of the nurses. The nurses' activity becomes especially specific in the cases of application for distant medical care in situation of emergency.

We may list several models of distant provision of medical care by nurses (a) providing certain information to a patient by phone, having performed a query using a specially developed algorithm; (b) analysis of health data obtained using automated patient's query (e.g. via Internet); and (c) preparation, transmission, and initial analysis of health information in telemedical consultations.

MEDICAL ADVICE BY TELEPHONE

Systems providing telephone advice to patients are rather widely spread throughout the world as this is probably the most budget-friendly way to provide care to distant patients without investing too much into equipment, broadband communication lines, etc. Nowadays, such an approach is widely used in many countries, e.g. Australia, where a significant part of the population has free access to telephone triage systems operated by nurses and in New Zealand all the residents may use telephone advice and symptom triage lines 24 hours per day [13]. Besides those two countries, it was shown that telephone triage was effective in the U.S., Canada, Sweden [14-17].

In Russia such systems have been used since 1970, providing telephone advice in the area of pediatrics. It was nurses who answered the calls of parents at a specially created call-centre in Leningrad. Special forms and algorithms (graphically represented as schemes) were created to allow the nurses working in such a centre efficient symptoms triage. Distant evaluation of dangerous conditions in children (suggested by Gubler E.V. [18]) was possible using the method of quantitative evaluation of the risk (so called risk assessment scale) and most probable type of disease.

Algorithms and formalized medical records were targeted for the patients not only at home but also in small hospitals, where no emergency / intensive care units were available.

Phone calls were received by a nurse of a call-centre. According to the patient's complaints and age, a proper algorithm (graphical scheme) had to be chosen; alternative solutions were either treatment at home, according to the nurse's advices, or hospitalization. If hospitalization was not required, the patient could be visited by a nurse, a physician, or phone advice may be given (see Figure 1). Various combinations (e.g. telephone advice followed by a doctor's visit) might also take place. It was shown that the use of algorithms accelerated the process of decision-making, decreased the number of errors and decreased the workload on personnel. In other words, the system promoted minimization of costs without any deterioration of medical care quality.

Telemedical Centre (TMC) is a unit (department) of a medical centre of any level (primary, secondary, tertiary) which is equipped to provide electronic communication and transfer of medical information to/from other centre(s).

At a medical centre of the primary level it is usually a nurse who conducts telemedical consultations, obtaining primary information from a patient, evaluating the obtained data and, if needed, transferring the patient's data in digital form to TMC of the next (secondary) level.

Therefore, the roles of a nurse at a telemedical centre of primary level could be decribed as:

1. Communication with a patient seeking an advice.
2. Evaluation of the patient's problem (using communication with a local or distant physician, using a computerized system if available). Evaluation concerns:
    a. What a possible diagnosis is.
    b. How urgent the problem is (life-threatening, potentially life-threatening, non life-threatening situation).
    c. If urgent care is needed, how this care could be provided (by patient himself, his relatives or other people in the neighborhood, or ambulance car/plane/helicopter should be used).
    d. If hospitalization is needed, to which hospital (department) the patient should be transported, how such hospitalization can be organized (e.g., a preliminary request might be required to be

Figure 1. Main decisions made by a nurse of a call-centre

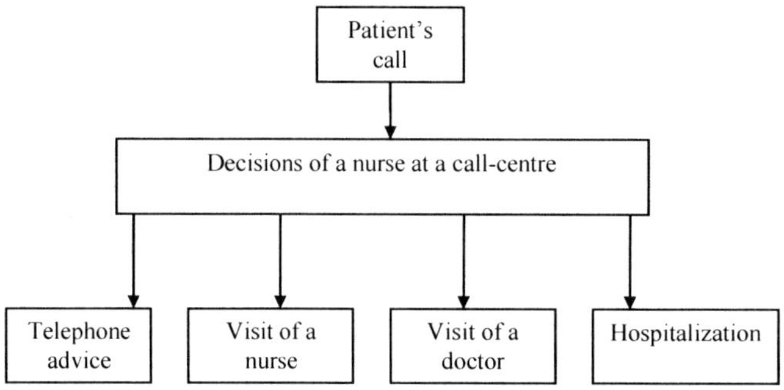

sent to a hospital or a specific department).

e. If hospitalization is not indicated, which advice could be given to a patient or his relatives.

f. How follow-up of the patient's condition might be organized.

3. When evaluation is over, adequate actions should be ordered (providing an advice, hospitalization, etc.).

Correct evaluation of a patient's condition is the key point. Therefore, the decision making personnel are expected to be the most experienced specialists. It is important that such personnel would have fast and convenient access to high-qualified physicians and reference data (or preferably, to a specially developed computerized decision-support systems [18, 19]).

Nevertheless, in some cases, nurses working with such computerized systems perceive them as a source of hindering.

Computer programs usually require the data to be input in a standardized way, while callers may vary greatly in their ability to communicate their symptoms effectively and coherently [20]. Thus, it is important to ascertain how nurses can best tailor their communication to meet the needs of individual patients [21], as well as to meet the requirements of the software they use. In other words, it is a nurse's task to translate patient's complaints into computer language.

Evaluation of the existing software demonstrated that it might not be fully adapted to real-life situations nurses face when they need pedagogical, psychological, and ethical knowledge and awareness [20]. Therefore, creation of better software for decision support systems in telenursing is one of the most challenging problems in contemporary medical informatics. On the other hand, since ideal software systems are not yet ready, it is the nurses who are to provide efficient communication with patients, so that the efficacy of telenursing systems as a whole will depend mostly on the nurses – their knowledge, their experience, and their willingness to help a patient in need.

THE WORK OF A NURSE IN THE SYSTEM OF TELEMEDICINE CONSULTATIONS

In the system of telemedical consultations, a nurse may play various roles related to primary analysis, preparation, and transmission of patient-related information. In fact, in TMC which requests an external consultation, a nurse may play either the major role (e.g. primary medical centres in countryside) or may assist a doctor to prepare patient's data.

In TMC of a secondary or tertiary medical centre, where patients with more complicated conditions are consulted, a nurse usually plays the role of coordinator, while main decisions are made by highly-qualified physicians.

In a primary medical centre, a nurse prepares a special form of request for telemedical consultation, extracting information from patient's medical records in electronic form, compiling the data of investigation, and, if needed, collecting proper medical images, etc.

Therefore, a nurse is responsible for representation of all the data in a proper form and sequence (usually TMC of different levels have to come to an agreement on what are the requirements for medical data exchange before telemedical service is established). The responsibility for facilitation of all communication between a patient and doctor is also on the nurse; submiting a request, confirming the time and conditions of a consultation, informing all participants of any obstacles, receiving the conclusion/recommendation, etc. Similar functions are laid upon nurses when telemedical services are organized to support the medical personnel in emergency situations (e.g. the staff of a field hospital in the affected area) [22].

Thus, a nurse of a medical centre requesting telemedical consultations performs the following:

1. Initial communication with a remote consultant.
2. Preparation of textual data on a patient.
3. Preparation (acquisition) of graphical/video information.
4. Submission of the electronic document to a consulting medical centre and negotiation on the time of the consultation.

In a consulting telemedical centre, a nurse performs the following:

1. Receives and registers requests.
2. Obtains approval of a doctor to participate in a consultation.
3. Confirms the time of videoconferences or time of response in case of store-and-forward consultations.
4. Controls the time of consultations to a distant centre having requested the consultation.
5. Assists a doctor during a consultation.
6. Sends the final conclusion as a result of consultation.

A nurse is also responsible for the registration of the consultation's results in a special journal.

The sequence of actions of a nurse organizing a telemedical consultation is schematically represented in Figure 2.

In a Telemedical Centre of Moscow Research Institute for Paediatrics and Children's Surgery, all the course of videoconsultations is to be recorded onto a hard disk (previously it was recorded on videotape). Such a measure may provide necessary evidence if a TMC is unsatisfied with a consultation. A nurse is also responsible for such a recording.

If an urgent consultation is requested (meaning that a response must be provided in 10-15 minutes after request), a nurse has to decide which consultants are needed and calls the physicians of proper specialties. If the consultation is not urgent, the nurse must check the availability of all supporting documents and transfer them to a consultant. If the patients' data are not properly presented (do not satisfy the established requirements), a nurse requests additional information on the patient. If the profile of the consulting centre does not correspond to the patient's condition, a nurse issues a message of rejection (if possible, the initial request might be transferred to a proper telemedical centre). If a multipoint videoconference is requested, a nurse has to inform other TMCs on the need of their participation [23].

In Russia, there are no specific requirements to a nurse involved in telemedical consultations.

Figure 2. Schematic presentation of electronic documents exchange in telemedical consultation

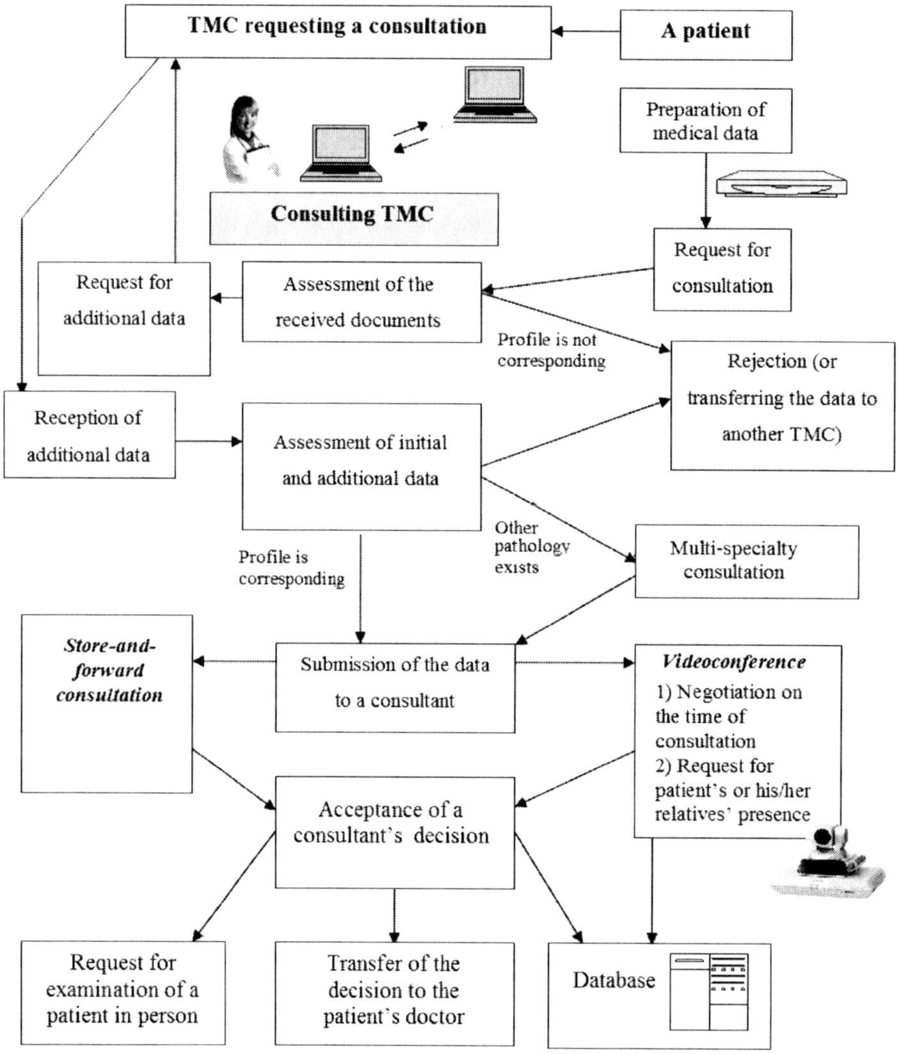

In other countries, a nurse must meet a number of requirements to participate in telemedical programs. For instance, the TelEmergency program run by the University of Mississippi Medical Centre, requires that a nurse practitioner (NP) meets the following criteria [24]:

1. Master's degree in nursing from an accredited institution.
2. Nationally certified and/or recertified FNP.
3. Evidence of current unrestricted license to practice in the United States and eligibility for licensure in Mississippi.
4. One complete year of clinical experience as an NP preferred
5. Documentation of current Advanced Cardiac Life Support, Pediatric Advanced Life Support, and Basic Cardiac Life Support.
6. Prefer second certification as acute care NP.

7. Must be willing to register for the acute care post-master's program if not dually certified
8. Completion of the Mississippi Nurse's Association Controlled Substance Workshop and obtain DEA certificate prior to staffing hospitals.
9. Complete application/requirements to attend the educational program for "Nurse Practitioners in the Emergency Department Setting'.
10. Meet privileges and credentialing requirements at the employing rural hospital

The listed requirements sound more than reasonable, though there is doubt if it is feasible to find enough personnel satisfying all the mentioned requirements given the shortage of nurses in most countries [25]

All actions of the nurses should be conducted in accordance with approved regulations which may differ from country to country and even from hospital to hospital. For instance, local regulations of Moscow Research Institute for Paediatrics and Children's Surgery propose certain sequence of the personnel actions [23]. All communication with other telemedical centres are to be performed using standard forms of documentation, certain requirements to textual, graphical and video information. A special form has been designed including a form of consultation request, internal information of telemedical centre, and the results of the consultation (doctors' conclusions).

The nurses use such forms in their work. They have to check electronic messages on the mail server of TMC (at least every 10 min), and, if needed, download the patient's information from a web server(s) or FTP-server.

A number of software programs have been developed to support the organization of telemedical consultations. For instance, there are systems such as Computerized Physician Order Entry [26, 27], which can facilitate the work of nurses, providing electronic documents exchange. Other software products might be used in specific cases, for instance, in teledermatology nurses may use special software 'TransImage' to enhance colour reproduction of digital skin images for higher diagnostic accuracy [28].

When a telemedical consultation is over, all the information concerning a patient is to be entered by a nurse into a TMC database, while the final conclusion of a consultant should be sent to the TMC which had requested the consultation.

Some authors believe that a telemedical consultation should be initiated not by a TMC, but a patient himself, who may apply for a consultation (e.g. from patient's personal home computer).

We believe that in such a case, a consultant may be unsure of the quality and reliability of the information provided by a patient. In many cases, the patient, not being a medical specialist, may either underestimate or overestimate symptoms, so that a consulting doctor may be led to a wrong conclusion. That is why we prefer to establish telemedical communication only between medical personnel (between a nurse and a doctor or between two or more doctors).

If direct communication with a patient is needed, it may mean that a decision is made rather not about accurate diagnosis but about urgency of medical care to be provided. Another option of direct communication with a patient is home telecare, when a patient usually suffers from a known chronic disease.

HOME TELECARE

Home telecare is an application of telemedical technologies to provide medical care to a patient at home, without any qualified medical personnel around. The systems of telecare are usually installed if a patient suffers from a known chronic disease (e.g. diabetes mellitus). One of the main aims of telecare systems is to evaluate initial signs of urgent conditions (e.g. coma in diabetic patients).

Special attention is now paid to the creation of such communicative relationships with the patients, which would reflect the patient's preferences [29].

A majority of home telecare systems (excluding few systems for fully automated monitoring of physiological parameters) is fully or at least partially based on involvement of nurses. Nurses participate in the following activities:

1. Posthospital monitoring of the patients who have undergone surgery or other procedures.
2. Monitoring of pregnancy.
3. Monitoring of newborn children.
4. Medical and psychological care for aged or disabled persons.
5. Control over the compliance with the prescribed medications dosage, etc.

Using the Internet as a media for data transfer, a nurse controls the information on a patient's parameters accumulating in a medical centre database (Figure 3). If a nurse recognizes dangerous signs, she transfers the information to a doctor's computer and then the doctor makes the final decision on importance of the found changes.

It is estimated that over 1.5 million telecare sessions are conducted in the U.S. annually. Using telecare technologies, a nurse who normally visits 5-6 patients, can provide medical care for 15-25 patients.

Development of home telecare is continuing. Analysis of the first results allows making certain conclusions and formulating new problems. The problems of telenursing include three interrelated dimensions [30]:

1. Related to a patient.
2. Related to knowledge and the level of responsibility of a nurse.
3. Related to organization of the distant care.

It should be mentioned that all of the above-listed aspects may be connected to any communication solutions (phone, email, videoconferencing). Creation of new, more portable devices for assessment of human functions and transmission of the results poses an additional problem for a nurse to supervise gadgets, control the correctness of their application and reliability of their data to prevent artifacts able to impede the process of diagnosis and treatment.

Generally speaking, home telecare has opened new possibilities for a nurse who can and should exercise initial control over the patients' parameters in the following cases:

1. Critical conditions (monitoring vital signs, e.g. in arrhythmias).
2. Chronic diseases (e.g. ischemic heart disease, etc.).
3. Monitoring the state of children (e.g., newborns).
4. Nurse's control over self-conducted rehabilitation.

Figure 3. A system for monitoring the physiological parameters via Internet

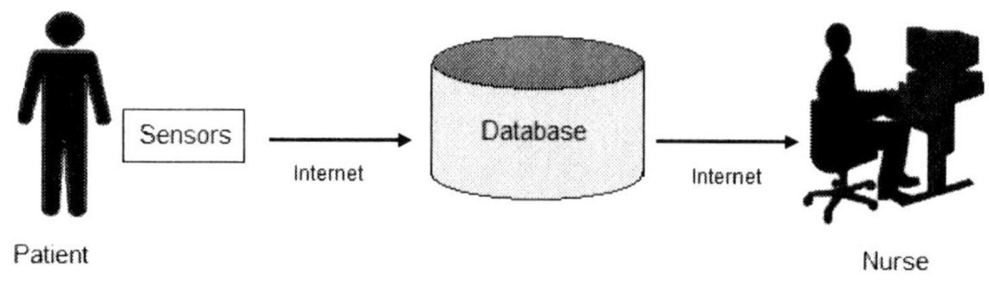

TELENURSING IN THE FUTURE

Reviewing all possible types of medical consultations at a distance, we can conclude that the role of nurses in such consultations is significant as nurses provide an important link in communication between a patient and a physician at a distance. It is always important that such a link be an efficient and reliable one.

Some authors have stated that telemedicine has historically been used primarily by physicians, while now it demonstrates its growing potential for nurse-led medical centres [31]. We would not like to oppose "physicians' telemedicine" to "nurses' telemedicine"; to a certain extent it is as absurd as trying to oppose "physicians' medicine" to "nurses' medicine". Both physicians and nurses are links of the same chain and they should not be artificially separated.

Generally, telemedicine is an embodiment of knowledge transfer between one who knows more about a specific health condition, and one who knows less about it but has to help a patient with this condition. The more the difference of knowledge levels, the more demanded the knowledge transfer is. It can be compared to electricity, where the potential difference creates electric current. Our own experience demonstrates that in the cases when a less experienced physician had to be consulted by a more experienced doctor, the former often was not fully psychologically satisfied with such 'doctor-to-doctor' consultations, presumably demonstrating his "low level of knowledge". This might be a possible reason for failures of some telemedical systems in Russia and abroad, partially due to such seeming "inequality" between a doctor applying for a consultation and a doctor providing it. At the same time, 'nurse-to-doctor' telemedical consultations may seldom pose such a danger, as nurses and doctors are two different occupations by definition, and nurses often apply for advice from a doctor in everyday practice, not only during telemedical consultations. However, there is a danger that wider introduction of "nurse-to-nurse" consultations in the future may cause the same psychological problems as present "doctor-to-doctor" consultations.

New information technologies are becoming more and more spread, even in healthcare systems of the developing countries. The experience of Western countries demonstrates how new technologies are implemented, starting from single pilot projects, later evolving into full-scale commercial or governmentally funded systems, which often leads to the changes in paradigms and business rules in healthcare. One of the recent developments is introduction of handheld computers in the practice of nursing [32]. Such technology might provide a nurse by the patient's bed with any additional information on demand, including consultation of a specialist at a distance.

Therefore, it is important that the nurses be ready for significant changes of nursing practice due to new technologies which are to be implemented wider and wider in the nearest future. Proper education of nurses is one of the main ways to be prepared to modern challenges of information technologies implementation in healthcare [33]. The example of the United States, where the issues of healthcare informatics are on the national agenda, as it was stated by National Institutes of Health, is one of the most inspirational [34].

Now we can expect an increasing need for education of the nurses in areas of telemedicine and medical informatics in general. Special curricula have already been developed in some telemedical centres (in the USA, Russia, and some other countries). We may hope that in the nearest decade the courses of telemedicine and telecare will be included into most curricula of nursing education.

REFERENCES

1. The International Council of Nurses. The ICN Definition of Nursing. Retrieved June 16, 2008, from http://www.icn.ch/definition.htm

2. The International Council of Nurses (2004). Scope of Nursing Practice. Retrieved June 16, 2008, from http://www.icn.ch/psscope.htm

3. Beolchi L. (Ed.) (2003). *Telemedicine Glossary (5th ed.)*. Brussels: The European Commission, Information Society Directorate-Generale.

4. Hager M.H. (2006). Centres for MediCare & MedicAid Services Telehealth Coverage of MNT—What ADA Members Need to Know. *J Am Diet Assoc. 4*(106), 513-6.

5. Coiera E. (1997). *Guide to medical informatics, the Internet and telemedicine*. Chapman and Hall Medical.

6. Parrish M. (1997). Medical advice is available for ships at sea. *BMJ. 315*(7114), 1020.

7. Doarn C. R., Lavrentyev V.A., Orlov O.I., Nicogossian A.E., Grigoriev A.I., Ferguson E.W., & Merrell R.C. (2003). Evolution of telemedicine in Russia: the influence of the space program on modern telemedicine programs. *Telemed J E Health. 9*(1):103-9.

8. Schneider A., Wilhelm D., Bohn U., Wichert A., & Feussner H. An evaluation of a surgical telepresence system for an intrahospital local area. (2005). *J Telemed Telecare. 11*(8): 408-413.

9. Clemensen J., Larsen B., Kirkevold M., Ejskjær N. (2007). Telemedical teamwork between home and hospital: A synergetic triangle emerges. In Westbrook J.I., Coiera E.W., Callen J.L., & Aarts J. (Eds.) *Information Technology in Health Care 2007 - Proceedings of the 3rd International Conference on Information Technology in Health Care: Socio-technical Approaches. Studies in Health Technology and Informatics. 130*, 81-89.

10. Eedy D.J., & Wootton R. (2001). Teledermatology: a review. Br J Dermatol. 144(4), 696-707.

11. Wootton R., & Craig J. (eds.). (1999). *Introduction to telemedicine*. London, UK: Royal Society of Medicine Press Ltd.

12. Wootton R. (2008). Telemedicine support for the developing world. *J Telemed Telecare. 14*(3), 109-14.

13. St George I., Cullen M., Gardiner L., & Karabatsos G. (2008). Universal telenursing triage in Australia and New Zealand - A new primary health service. *Aust Fam Physician. 37*(6), 476-9.

14. Barber J.W., King W.D., Monroe K.W., & Nichols M.H. (2000). Evaluation of emergency department referrals by telephone triage. *Pediatrics. 105*(4 Pt 1), 819–21.

15. ight P.A., Hupcey J.E., & Clark M.B. (2005). Nursing telephone triage and its influence on parents' choicc of care for febrile children. *J Pediatr Nurs. 20*(6), 424–9.

16. Hogenbirk J.C., Pong R.W., & Lemieux S.K. (2005). Impact of telephone triage on medical service use: implications for rural and remote areas. *J Agric Saf Health. 11*(2), 229-37.

17. Marklund B., Ström M., Månsson J., Borgquist L., Baigi A., & Fridlund B. (2007). Computersupported telephone nurse triage: an evaluation of medical quality and costs. *J Nurs Manag. 15*(2),180–7.

18. Gubler E.V. (1990). *Informatics in pathology, clinical medicine, and paediatrics*. Leningrad: Meditsina. [in Russian]

19. Goldberg S.I., Mahanek A.O., & Novikov I.D. Dispatcher-consultative systems. Main characteristics and an example of realization. (1991). *Vest. Vsesoyuzn. Obsh. Informat. I Vych. Tech,. 1*, 46-52 [in Russian].

20. Holmström I. (2007). Decision aid software programs in telenursing: not used as intended? Experiences of Swedish telenurses. *Nursing and Health Sciences, 9*(1), 23–28.

21. Swenson S., Zettler P., & Lo B. (2006). "She gave it her best shot right away". Patient experiences of biomedical and patient-centred communication. *Patient Educ Couns. 61*(2), 200–211.

22. Ehrlich A.I., Kobrinsky B.A., Petlakh V.I., Rozinov V.M., & Shabanov V.E. (2007). Telemedicine for a Children's Field Hospital in Chechnya, *J Telemed Telecare, 13*(1), 4-6.

23. Kobrinskiy B.A., Matveev N.V. (2006). Teleconsultations at the Moscow Research Institute for Paediatrics and Children's Surgery. In *The 6th International Conference on Successes and Failures in Telehealth* (pp.193-194). Brisbane, Australia.

24. Henderson K. (2006). TelEmergency: distance emergency care in rural emergency departments using nurse practitioners. *J Emerg Nurs. 32* (5), 388-93.

25. Mendes, I.A.C., & Marziale, M.H.(2008). Shortage of qualified health workers: a call to action for nurses. *Rev Latino-Am Enfermagem. 2* (16), 173-4.

26. Doolan D.F., Bates D.W. (2002). Computerized physician order entry system in hospitals: mandates and incentives. *Health Affairs. 21* (4), 180-188.

27. Kuperman G.L., Gibson R.F. (2003). Computer physician order entry: benefits, costs and issues. *Ann Intern Med. 139* (16), 31-39.

28. Matveev N.V. Automatic color correction of digital skin images in teledermatology. (2006). *J Telemed and Telecare. 12* (Suppl. 3), 62-63.

29. Swenson S., Zettler P., & Lo B. (2006). "She gave it her best shot right away". Patient experiences of biomedical and patient-centred communication. *Pat Educ Couns. 61* (2), 200–211.

30. Wahlberg A, Cedersund E, & Wredling R. (2005). Bases for assessments made by telephone advice nurses. *J Telemed Telecare. 11* (8), 403–407.

31. Reed K. Telemedicine: Benefits to Advanced Practice Nursing and the Communities They Serve. *J Am Acad Nurse Pract. 17*(5), 176-80.

32. Thompson B.W. (2005). The Transforming Effect of Handheld Computers on Nursing Practice. *Nurse Admin Q. 29*(40, 308-314.

33. McNeil B.J., Elfrink V., Beyea S.C., Pierce S.T., & Bickford C.J. (2006). Computer Literacy Study: Report of Qualitative Findings. *J Prof Nurs. 22* (1), 52–9.

34. Romano C. (2006). Informatics is on the national agenda and nurses need to be informed and involved. *Nurs Outlook. 54*(5), 303-5.

KEY TERMS

Home Telecare: An application of telemedical technologies to provide medical care to a patient staying at home, without any qualified medical personnel around.

Intra-Hospital Telemedicine: A telemedical system providing intra-hospital exchange of patient-oriented medical information.

Telecare: Administrative and educational use of telecommunications in healthcare .

Telemedicine: Medical care provided to patients at a distance by using electronic means of communication.

Teleradiology, Telepathology, Teledermatology: Applications of telemedical technologies respectively in radiology, pathology, dermatology.

Chapter XV
The Role of EBM and Nursing Informatics in Rural Australia

Daniel Carbone
University of Melbourne, Australia

ABSTRACT

The purpose of this chapter is to broadly discuss the need for enhanced evidence-based medicine (EBM) by nurses in the context of rural Australia and the role that nursing informatics and an informed strategy could facilitate in making such need a feasible reality. First, the introduction highlights current time gaps between health discoveries and eventual practice and the potential for information technology to positively affect this gap. Then, the need for nurses to take an active role in evidence-based medicine in rural settings is argued. The link between information literacy and evidence-based medicine is consequently presented and gaps in knowledge regarding nursing informatics training are highlighted. Concluding with the argument that to achieve evidence-based research and eventual use, there needs to be a purposeful health informatics learning strategy that recognises the role of computer and information literacy.

INTRODUCTION

Patient health outcomes in health settings are dependant on the ability of these institutions to ensure appropriate, up-to-date clinical practice. The creation of this up-to-date practice is commonly known as evidence base medicine (EBM) and it integrates a number of components and even today is not without controversy. For example, according to Sackett (1996), it requires a bottom-up approach that integrates the best external evidence with individual clinical expertise and patient-choice, it cannot result in slavish, cook-book approaches to individual patient care. External clinical evidence can inform, but can never replace, individual clinical expertise, and it is this expertise that decides whether the external evidence applies to the individual patient at all and, if so, how it should be integrated into a clinical decision (Sackett D.L. et al., 1996). Conversely, Stuart (2001) suggests that the most desirable basis to substantiate clinical practice is the evidence of well-established research findings and that developing evidence-based medicine involves defining the clinical question, finding the evidence, analysing the evidence, using the evidence, and evaluating the outcome (Stuart, 2001). Regardless of the point of view taken to EBM (clinician or research centred prevalence) there is an accepted need to find, analyse and evaluate the existing up-to-date research findings.

However, there are significant time gaps in the application of research findings into clinical practice. Using the results of a number of published studies, Balas and Boren estimated that it takes an average of 17 years to turn 14% of original research findings into changes in care that benefit patients (Balas & Boren, 2000). The current gap from research to practice has highlighted the relative ineffectiveness of traditional methods such as continuing medical education and journal publications for disseminating new medical information (Mold & Peterson, 2005).

The beginning of the 21st century has seen a surge in interest and enthusiasm for health care information technology based on its ability to demonstrate improvements in the quality, safety, and cost-efficiency of health care (Hersh, 2006; Nagykaldi & Mold, 2007). From a technological point of view, there is consensus that Information technology can support the implementation of clinical research findings in practice settings; e.g. the availability of on-line web based information is a clear example. At the most optimistic extreme, Goldstein et al (2004) suggest that technology can address the quality gap in health care by providing automated decision support to clinicians that integrates guideline knowledge with electronic patient data to present real-time and patient-specific recommendations. However, technologic developments are not sufficient to bring the value of computer and information technologies to health care systems (B. Kaplan, Brennan, Dowling, Friedman, & Peel, 2001); Goldstein also concedes that technical success in implementing decision support systems may not translate directly into system use by clinicians. Reporting that extensive clinician use of the system was associated with explicit attention to the organizational context at the time of development, deployment, and maintenance of the system (Goldstein MK et al., 2004). The difficulties in adoption, barriers and attitudes of clinicians towards computerisation and use of information systems for health research has been well documented (Janes et al., 2005; Littlejohns, Wyatt, & Garvican, 2003; Lorenzi, 2004; Walsh SH, 2004; Westbrook, Gosling, & Coiera, 2004; Winkelman, 2003; Wolf, 2001).

Nonetheless, there is a commonsense link between health informatics skills and evidence based research (EBR) to support EMB; however, the argument presented so far assumes that there are enough clinicians (with the clinical expertise) in rural settings with enough informatics skills to engage in purposeful evidence-based medicine (EBM).

The purpose of this chapter is to discuss broadly the need for enhanced evidence-based medicine by nurses in the context of rural Australia and more specifically the role that nursing informatics could play in making such need a potential reality. The perspective in this chapter is supported by applied action research outcomes in nursing informatics and education strategies currently in progress in rural Australia and marrying it to the existing literature. Ultimately, it aims at informing decision makers or those in a position to influence decisions and informatics educators of some of the informatics issues faced by nursing staff that might hinder or enable the use of evidence-based medicine in the Australian rural context.

BACKGROUND

The divide between rural and urban healthcare issues (determinants of health, health status, access to services, morbidity, mortality, etc) where the health status of rural people is inferior to that of people living in metropolitan areas have been widely identified both in Australia and other parts of the world (AIHW, 2007; American Medical Student Association, 2007; Center for Rural Health Practice, 2004; Dickinson, 2002; Dixon & Welch, 2000; Hall, Owings, & Shinogle, 2006; Johnson, Brems, Warner, & Roberts, 2005; Jordan, Roderick, Martin, & Barnett, 2004; Morgans, Archer, Walker, & Thuma, 2005; Nagarajan, 2004).

Added to this situation, the Australian Productivity Commission concedes that there is a general shortage of General Practitioner (GP - Doctors) workforce, with these shortages being more acute in rural and remote areas (AIHW, 2007; ANU, 2006). This situation is exacerbated by an older GP population that will not only retire soon but that are working increasingly less (AMA, 2004). To make matters worse, many small rural and remote hospitals do not have full time practitioners, but Visiting Medical Officers (VMOs), visiting private Doctors already overworked and overstressed contracted on a needs basis (AMA, 2007). One of the potential solutions suggested in rural settings is to tackle the impending crisis is the greater utilisation of nurses in leading clinical roles to relieve the pressure on overstretched GPs.

Conversely, there are mounting issues relating to nursing workforce that affect this paradigm as well. For example in Australia, there has been a great deal of discussion about the educational preparation required for rural nursing practice and the statistics are not promising; with 90% being female and older in rural and remote areas (average: 44 years) and working longer hours that in the cities (AIHW, 2007); with the majority of rural nurses, not having postgraduate qualifications and facing significant barriers in obtaining them (National nursing and nursing education taskforce, 2005; Victorian Centre for Nursing Practice Research, 2001).

It should be apparent so far that this is not about an argument for labour substitution —nurses for doctors, which has been raging for a while with supporters and detractors of the concept (ANU, 2006; Gutkin, 2008; Miranda Laurant, 2000; M. Laurant et al., 2007; Richardson & Maynard, 1995; Sibbald, Laurant, & Reeves, 2006; Weller, 2006). Regardless of the controversies, preferences or personal opinions, the argument in this paper is that the use of nurses in place of or in support of Doctors in this rural context might not be a choice but a necessity.

However, for rural nurses to be able to fill the gap, and be central to the delivery of health services in rural settings, rural nursing education hinges on ensuring that they have the confidence, knowledge and skills to deliver safe, appropriate and effective care and that nursing informatics education might have a greater role to play.

THE LINK BETWEEN NURSING INFORMATICS AND EVIDENCE BASED RESEARCH

We know that evidence-based medicine has a research component that involves defining the clinical question, finding the evidence, analysing the evidence, using the evidence, and evaluating the outcome (Ivanitskaya, O'Boyle, & Casey, 2006; Saranto & H., 1997). We also know that predictors of research utilization include attitude toward research, awareness of information based on research, and involvement in research activities (S. Kaplan, Rosenfeld, & Haber, 2003; National nursing and nursing education taskforce, 2005). In summary, it becomes self evident that the main skills needed are a mixture of information literacy (finding, analysing, evaluating) and research literacy (methods, techniques, participation) these skills, being to a large extent, technology intensive in particular the electronic environments; where for example, the use of the Internet in relatively isolated rural contexts, could help support some of the information literacy tasks mentioned earlier.

Nonetheless, even in non-rural areas, the literature tells us that nurse research activity is very low. In a study by Tanner and Hale (2002) at Derby City General Hospital, in the UK found that out of 1574 nurses, only 2.1%) (N=34) were "research-active"; and that only 14 of those had at least one publication (Tanner & Hale, 2002). Evidence from another systematic literature review puts the percentage at a 15% (Shirey, 2006); while in a study of 106 nurses from various practice areas in six rural counties of a south-western state in the United States revealed that only 20.8% of the participants stated they were currently involved in research utilization (Olade, 2004). Nevertheless, the current literature agrees that increasing competency in information literacy in nursing is the foundation for evidence-based practice (EBP) and provides nursing professionals with the skills to be literate consumers of information in an electronic environment (Jacobs, Rosenfeld, & Haber, 2003; McCormick et al., 2007; McNeil, Elfrink, Beyea, Pierce, & Bickford, 2006; Smedley, 2005).

This proposition is not a new or far-fetched idea, there is growing evidence that technology like telemedicine can mediate to support nurses perform clinical tasks when clinicians are not available (Hegney et al., 2007).

Is Information Literacy the Answer or are we Putting the Horse Before the Cart?

While the previous argument that information literacy is central to developing instructional strategies for evidence based research and use may be common sense, the author's own applied research across a number of rural health providers in rural Australia confirms that we might be getting ahead of ourselves. Current survey studies and field observations into information literacy readiness reveal that the majority of rural nurses currently lack the basic computer skills to engage in "information literacy" (Carbone, Sharkey, & Scully, 2007; Hegney et al., 2007). This is not a new discovery, but one that somehow gets "overlooked" when the push for use of technology is sought.

Furthermore, recent studies indicate that, while nursing students have an overall positive attitude toward technology, they also reported their formal education levels in the use of technology applications are low (Edirippulige S, Smith A, Beattie H, Davies E, & R., 2007; Hegney et al., 2007; Lynch, 2006; Maag, 2006). Other studies also corroborated that nurses with expertise in computer use had a more favourable attitude toward the use of computer records than those with less expertise (Hegney et al., 2007; Schwirian, Malone, Stone, Nunley, & Francisco, 1989; Smith K, Smith V, Krugman M, & K, 2005). In addition, and more worrying, a study by Ornes and Gassert (2007) found that nursing students received limited informatics exposure and may not be adequately prepared to use information technology (Ornes & Gassert, 2007). The concept that current freshmen student possess adequate knowledge of both computer concepts and computer literacy skills has also been found incorrect in other disciplines (Dørup, 2004; Wallace & Clariana, 2005).

Taking a Step Back

In 2000, Elfink et al found that little was known about how to design instructional strategies for integrating information technology into clinical nursing education (Elfrink VL et al., 2000); a similar study found little agreement about specific computer-focused competencies necessary for nurses (Hobbs, 2002). What is known, is that informatics training, technology applications, and professional identities are closely tied to the activities of the health professionals they serve (Masys, Brennan, Ozbolt, Corn, & Shortliffe, 2000). For example, Hobbs (2002) and Schwirian et al (1989) found that there was consensus that the computer-competent nurse possesses general knowledge and an understanding of computer technology, coupled with a positive attitude toward computers and software (Schwirian et al., 1989). This concept was further expanded on in a study of computerisation in clinical practice in a British General Hospital, where it was found that although nurses' computer-related attitudes generally were positive, significant differences were found in relation to age, length of service as a trained nurse, job title, type of nursing unit, and length of service at the study hospital (Simpson & Kenrick, 1997). In addition, Hobbs suggested that a competent nurse is skilful in computer hardware and software use and able to grasp how such technology benefits nursing and the overall healthcare environment (Hobbs, 2002). A German study also found that computer knowledge and previous acceptance of nursing process are significant predictors of final user acceptance (Ammenwerth, Mansmann, Iller, & Eichstädter, 2003). Conversely, a local study set out to measure nurses' attitudes toward computers in an Australian setting, testing 71 first-year nursing students and 99 nurses employed in a local hospital, found three aspect of concern for nurse: (1) Computers and Patient Care, (2) Computer Anxiety and (3) Patient Confidentiality and Computers (Jayasuriya & Caputi, 1996).

In summary, there is a need to take a step back in approaches to instructional design, to take into account the future needs of nurse clinicians to incorporate the right *computer literacy* foundations, to then build their *information literacy* allowing them to perform *evidence based research* competently and increase their use of evidence based medicine in future clinical practice in rural settings.

CONCLUSION

Health outcomes depend on having a clinical workforce that is engaged in the latest evidence based practice. A chronic workforce shortage of clinicians is a clear barrier to these goals. In rural settings, there are less and older clinicians and the issues are compounded by inferior health status and outcomes compared to that of city counterparts; Moreover, in rural health settings; and while there are no prospect of workforce improvement in the short term, there appears to be a greater role to be played by nurse clinicians that are evidence based practice skilled to fill the ever growing gaps in care delivery. Currently achieving EBP is at best a long term proposition. However, the use of information technology coupled with evidence based research is seen as a feasible way to support the use of EBM. However, EBP nurse clinicians must be not just information literate but also computer literate.

The intent of this chapter was to argue for an informed approach to the introduction of evidence based medicine that is cognisant of computer and information literacy issues that affect its development and therefore its ultimate effectiveness.

REFERENCES

AIHW. (2007). *Australia's Health 2006*. Camberra: Australian Institute of Health and Welfare.

AMA. (2004). Out-of-Hours Primary Medical Care.

AMA. (2007). *Rural doctors have their say on key solutions to improve rural health care delivery*: Australian Medical Association.

American Medical Student Association. (2007). Health Care Delivery: Rural vs. Urban Communities. Retrieved April 9, 2007, from http://www.amsa.org/programs/gpit/ruralurban.cfm

Ammenwerth, E., Mansmann, U., Iller, C., & Eichstädter, R. (2003). Factors Affecting and Affected by User Acceptance of Computer-based Nursing Documentation: Results of a Two-year Study. *Journal of the American Medical Informatics Association, 10*(1), 69-84.

ANU. (2006). *Responding to the primary health-care workforce shortage*: Australian National University.

Balas, E. A., & Boren, S. A. (2000). Managing clinical knowledge for health care improvement. In *Yearbook of Medical Informatics 2000: Patient-Centered Systems* (pp. 65-70). Stuttgart, Germany: Schattauer.

Carbone, D., Sharkey, L., & Scully, A. (2007). Building research capacity in a small rural hospital: Benchmarking computer literacy levels. *Paper presented at the Sydney GP & PHC Research Conference: Working Together*, Sydney.

Center for Rural Health Practice. (2004). *Bridging the Health Divide: The Rural Public Health Research Agenda*: University of Pittsburgh.

Dickinson, J. (2002). General Practice. *MJA, 176*(1), 17.

Dixon, J., & Welch, N. (2000). Researching the Rural-Metropolitan Health Differential Using the 'Social Determinants of Health'. *Australian Journal of Rural Health, 8*(5).

Dørup, J. (2004). Experience and Attitudes towards Information Technology among First-Year Medical Students in Denmark: Longitudinal Questionnaire Survey. *Journal Medical Internet Research, 6*(1), 10.

Edirippulige, S., Smith, A., Beattie, H., Davies, E., & R., W. (2007). Pre-registration nurses: An investigation of knowledge, experience, and comprehension of E-Health. *Australian Journal of Advanced Nursing, 25*(2), 78-83.

Elfrink, V. L., Davis, L. S., Fitzwater, E., Castleman, J., Burley, J., Gorney-Moreno, M. J., et al. (2000). A comparison of teaching strategies for integrating information technology into clinical nursing education. *Nurse Educator, 25*(3), 136-144.

Goldstein, M. K., Coleman, R. W., Tu, S. W., Shankar, R D., O'Connor, M. J., Musen, M. A., et al. (2004). Translating research into practice: Organizational issues in implementing automated decision support for hypertension in three medical centers. *Journal of the American Medical Informatics Association, 11*(5), 368-376.

Gutkin, C. (2008). Family physician shortages Are nurses the answer? *Can Fam Physician, 54*(3), 480

Hall, M. J., Owings, M. F., & Shinogle, J. A. (2006). Inpatient Care in Rural Hospitals at the Beginning of the 21st Century. *The Journal of Rural Health, 22*(4), 331–338.

Hegney, D., Buikstra, E., Eley, R., Fallon, T., Gilmore, V., & Soar, J. (2007). *Nurses and information technology: Final Report*: Australian Nursing Federation and Australian Government Department of Health and Ageing.

Hersh, W. (2006). Who are the Informaticians? What We Know and Should Know. *Journal of the American Medical Informatics Association, 13*, 166-170.

Hobbs, S. D. (2002). Measuring Nurses' Computer Competency: An Analysis of Published Instruments. *Computer Informatics Nursing, 20*(2), 63-73.

Ivanitskaya, L., O'Boyle, I., & Casey, A. (2006). Health Information Literacy and Competencies of Information Age Students: Results From the Interactive Online Research Readiness Self-Assessment (RRSA). *J Med Internet Res, 8*(2), e6.

Jacobs, S. K., Rosenfeld, P., & Haber, J. (2003). Information literacy as the foundation for evidence-based practice in graduate nursing education: a curriculum-integrated approach. *Journal of Professional Nursing, 19*(5), 320-328.

Janes, R., Arroll, B., Buetow, S., Coster, G., McCormick, R., & I., H. (2005). Few rural general practitioners use the Internet frequently in regard to patient care. *N Z Med J*(118), 1212.

Jayasuriya, R., & Caputi, P. (1996). Computer attitude and computer anxiety in nursing. Validation of an instrument using an Australian sample. *Computer Informatics Nursing, 14*(6), 340-345.

Johnson, M. E., Brems, C., Warner, T. D., & Roberts, L. W. (2005). Rural–Urban Healthcare Provider Disparities in Alaska and New Mexico. *Administration and Policy in Mental Health and Mental Health Services Research, 33*(4), 504-507.

Jordan, H., Roderick, P., Martin, D., & Barnett, S. (2004). Distance, rurality and the need for care: Access to health services in South West England. *International Journal of Health Geographics, 3*, 21.

Kaplan, B., Brennan, P. F., Dowling, A. F., Friedman, C. P., & Peel, V. (2001). Toward an Informatics Research Agenda: Key People and Organizational Issues. *Journal of the American Medical Informatics Association, 8*, 235-241.

Kaplan, S., Rosenfeld, P., & Haber, J. (2003). Information literacy as the foundation for evidence-based practice in graduate nursing education: a curriculum-integrated approach. *Journal of Professional Nursing 19*(5), 320-328.

Laurant, M. (2000). Evidence based substitution of doctors by nurses in primary care? *British Medical Journal, 320*(7241), 1078.

Laurant, M., Reeves, D., Hermens, R., Braspenning, J., Grol, R., & Sibbald, B. (2007). Substitution of doctors by nurses in primary care. *The Cochrane Database of Systematic Reviews*(1).

Littlejohns, P., Wyatt, J. C., & Garvican, L. (2003). Evaluating computerised health information systems: Hard lessons still to be learnt. *BMJ: British Medical Journa,* (326), 860-863.

Lorenzi, N. M. (2004). Beyond the gadgets: Non-technological barriers to information systems need to be overcome too. *BMJ, 328*, 1146-1147.

Lynch, K. (2006). Readiness to Communicate in a Digital World. *Issues in Informing Science and Information Technology, 3.*

Maag, M. (2006). Nursing students' attitudes toward technology: A national study. *Nurse Educator, 31*(3), 112-118.

Masys, D. R., Brennan, P. F., Ozbolt, J. G., Corn, M., & Shortliffe, E. H. (2000). Are Medical Informatics and Nursing Informatics Distinct Disciplines? The 1999 ACMI Debate. *Journal American Medical Informatics Association,* (7), 304-312.

McCormick, K. A., Delaney, C. J., Brennan, P. F., Effken, J. A., Kendrick, K., Murphy, J., et al. (2007). Guideposts to the Future-An Agenda for Nursing Informatics. *Journal of the American Medical Informatics Association, 14*, 19-24.

McNeil, B., Elfrink, V., Beyea, S., Pierce, S., & Bickford, C. (2006). Computer literacy study: report of qualitative findings. *Journal of Professional Nursing, 22*(1), 52-59.

Mold, J. W., & Peterson, K. A. (2005). Primary care practice-based research networks: Working at the interface between research and quality improvement. *Annals of Family Medicine, 3*(1), 12-20.

Morgans, A., Archer, F., Walker, T., & Thuma, E. (2005). Barriers to accessing ambulance services in rural Victoria for acute asthma: Patients' and medical professionals' perspectives. *Australian Journal of Rural Health, 13*(2), 116-120.

Nagarajan, K. V. (2004). Rural and remote community health care in Canada: beyond the Kirby Panel Report, the Romanow Report and the federal budget of 2003. *Canadian Journal of Rural Medicine, 9*(4), 245-251.

Nagykaldi, Z., & Mold, J. W. (2007). The Role of Health Information Technology in the Translation of Research into Practice: An Oklahoma Physicians Resource/Research Network (OKPRN)

Study. *The Journal of the American Board of Family Medicine, 20*(2), 188-195.

National nursing and nursing education taskforce. (2005). Maximising education pathways: Our Duty of Care - Recommendation 12. Retrieved January 5, 2008, from http://www.nnnet.gov.au/work/rec12.htm

Olade, R. (2004). Evidence-based practice and research utilization activities among rural nurses. *J Nurs Scholarsh, 36*(3), 220-225.

Ornes, L., & Gassert, C. (2007). Computer competencies in a BSN program. *J Nurs Educ, 46*(2), 75-78.

Richardson, G., & Maynard, A. (1995). Fewer doctors? More nurses? A review of the knowledge base of doctor-nurse substitution. 135. from http://ideas.repec.org/p/chy/respap/dp135.html

Sackett D.L. et al. (1996). Evidence based medicine: what it is and what it isn't. *BMJ, 312*(7023), 71-72.

Saranto, K., & H., L.-K. (1997). Computer literacy in nursing: developing the information technology syllabus in nursing education. *Journal of Advanced Nursing, 25*(2), 377-385.

Schwirian, P., Malone, J., Stone, V., Nunley, B., & Francisco, T. (1989). Computers in nursing practice. A comparison of the attitudes of nurses and nursing students. *Computer Informatics Nursing, 7*(4), 168-177.

Shirey, M. (2006). Evidence-based practice: how nurse leaders can facilitate innovation. *Nurs Adm Q, 30*(3), 252-265.

Sibbald, B., Laurant, M. G., & Reeves, D. (2006). Advanced nurse roles in UK primary care. *The Medical Journal of Australia, 185*(1), 10-12.

Simpson, G., & Kenrick, M. (1997). Nurses' Attitudes Toward Computerization in Clinical Practice in a British General Hospital. *Computers in Nursing, 15*(1), 37-42.

Smedley, A. (2005). The importance of informatics competencies in nursing: an Australian perspective. *Computer Informatics Nursing, 23*(2), 106-110.

Smith K, Smith V, Krugman M, & K, O. (2005). Evaluating the impact of computerized clinical documentation. *Computer Information Nursing, 23*(3), 132-138.

Stuart, G. W. (2001). Evidence-Based Psychiatric Nursing Practice: Rhetoric or Reality. *Journal of the American Psychiatric Nurses Association, 7*(4), 103-114.

Tanner, J., & Hale, C. (2002). Developing research capacity: Identifying and quantifying nursing research activity in the NHS. *Journal of Research in Nursing, 7*(3), 212-221.

Victorian Centre for Nursing Practice Research. (2001). *National Review of Nursing Education: Aspects of Nursing Education: The Types Of Skills And Knowledge Required To Meet The Changing Needs Of The Labour Force Involved In Nursing - Literature Review* The University of Melbourne

Wallace, P., & Clariana, R. B. (2005). Perception versus Reality—Determining Business Students' Computer Literacy Skills and Need for Instruction in Information Concepts and Technology. *Journal of Information Technology Education, 4.*

Walsh SH. (2004). The clinician's perspective on electronic health records and how they can affect patient care. *BMJ, 328*, 1184-1187.

Weller, D. P. (2006). Workforce substitution and primary care. *Medical Journal of Australia, 185*(1), 8-9.

Westbrook, J. I., Gosling, A. S., & Coiera, E. (2004). Do Clinicians Use Online Evidence to Support Patient Care? A Study of 55,000 Clinicians. *J Am Med Inform Assoc, 11*(2), 113-120.

Winkelman, W. J. (2003). Evaluating computerised health information systems: Opportunities were missed. *BMJ : British medical journal*(327), 162-163.

Wolf, E. J. (2001). Healthcare's New Tools of the Trade: How to Gain Physician Buy-in. *Healtcare Executive*(Sep/Oct), 14-16.

KEY TERMS

Computer Literacy: Is the knowledge and ability to use computers and technology efficiently. It also refers to the comfort level someone has with using computer programs and other applications that are associated with computers and knowing how computers work and operate.

Continuing Medical Education: Refers to a specific form of continuing education that helps those in the medical field maintain competence and learn about new and developing areas of their field. These activities may take place as live events, written publications, online programs, audio, video, or other electronic media.

Evidence Based Medicine (EMB): Also known as Evidence Based Practice (EBP) is the conscientious, explicit, and judicious use of current best evidence in making decisions about the care of individual patients. The practice of evidence based medicine means integrating individual clinical expertise with the best available external clinical evidence from systematic research.

Health Informatics: Also known as Medical Informatics is the intersection of information science, computer science, and health care. It deals with the resources, devices, and methods required to optimize the acquisition, storage, retrieval, and use of information in health and biomedicine. Health informatics tools include not only computers but also clinical guidelines, formal medical terminologies, and information and communication systems.

Information Literacy: To be information literate, a person must be able to recognize when information is needed and have the ability to locate, evaluate, and use effectively the needed information

Nursing Informatics: Is the multidisciplinary scientific endeavour of analysing, formalizing and modelling how nurses collect and manage data, process data into information and knowledge, make knowledge-based decisions and inferences for patient care, and use this empirical and experiential knowledge in order to broaden the scope and enhance the quality of their professional practice. It includes computer, information and research literacy.

Research Literacy: The ability to understand and use the IT-based tools relevant to the work of today's researcher and scholar.

Chapter XVI
Use of Handheld Computers in Nursing Education

Maureen Farrell
University of Ballarat, Australia

ABSTRACT

The use of mobile technologies in nursing education is rapidly increasing. Handheld computers are the most frequently used of these technologies as they can provide students with information for point of care clinical reference, such as diagnostics, medical terminology, and drug references. Integrating the management and processing of information into clinical practice is an effective learning approach for students and reflects a changing paradigm in nursing education. Traditionally, nursing programs have the tendency to separate the acquisition of academic knowledge from clinical practice, and the process of integrating academic information into the decision making processes in the clinical area has been difficult for student nurses. This chapter will provide an overview of the use of handheld computers in nursing and medical education, including a brief synopsis of current use in clinical practice. It will discuss the advantages and disadvantages of their use, barriers to implementation and future directions.

INTRODUCTION

Healthcare in the developed world is characterised by a rapidly increasing use of mobile technologies to deliver effective and quality patient care. Handheld computers or personal digital assistants (PDAs), have the potential to change how health-care is taught and delivered in the future as they have the ability to merge and integrate distinct functionalities in one device that is versatile, customizable, and portable (Baumgart, 2005). Research and anecdotal evidence suggest that

PDAs can be used in clinical practice to deliver valuable decision-making information at the patient's bedside. This significant improvement in the delivery of information results in improvements in patient safety and quality of care. PDAs provide instant access to diagnostics, references, and clinical decision support systems, as well as e-prescribing, patient information and dictating notes (Blair, 2006; Colevins, Bond & Clark, 2006; Choia et al., 2004; Fisher, Stewart, Mehta, Wax & Lapkinsky, 2003; George & Davidson, 2005; Lewis, 2001; Ruland, 2002).

Educational processes in healthcare have also become increasingly complex. Students require timely access to resources. Organisational constraints in both technology and personnel may further limit students' access to teaching resources. Having access to information at the bedside in real time with patients has the potential to improve the quality and safety of care by reducing adverse events and improving patient health outcomes; a solution to the problem of constrained resources. The National League for Nursing, the American Association of Colleges of Nursing, and the Institute of Medicine, to name a few, recommend the incorporation of technology into the curriculum of nursing education (George & Davidson, 2005). The incorporation of PDAs into daily practice by medical staff is far more advanced than in nursing, however this is changing and nurses are now adopting this technology in nursing practice and education. To encourage change in practice technology must be harnessed to revolutionise the design, delivery and evaluation of nursing education (Jeffries, 2005). Increasingly there is an educational shift to provide students with more learning opportunities to create innovative teaching practices and to promote current, accurate information retrieval systems for clinical nurses.

As learning and teaching adapts to the demands of the 21st century, both educators and students in the nursing profession are finding that the most effective learning approach integrates the management and processing of information into both their practice area and their personal growth and development. In higher education, there has been a shift from the notion of content to a focus on 'process based education' and this is occurring more rapidly in the healthcare arena and in nursing programs in particular. The focus will be increasingly on teaching students how to learn rather than what to learn. There is considerable evidence that suggests PDAs have the potential to improve nursing education and practice through connecting people, unifying the education process and enhancing learning. Patient safety is one of the most important aspects of nursing care and these devices can promote the quality and immediacy of bedside information and improve the accuracy of record keeping (Bates, 2000; Celler, Lovell, & Basilakis, 2003). This chapter will provide a review of PDA usage in nursing and medical education, including the advantages and disadvantages, barriers to implementation, and future perspectives.

PDAS IN CLINICAL PRACTICE

PDAs have been adopted by healthcare professionals (predominately physicians) in clinical practice and this adoption has led to a number of different uses including clinical decision support, education, and accessing or collecting data. The literature reveals that the information on usage is usually descriptive rather than evidence based, although some preliminary impact studies are indicating improved patient outcomes with regards to PDA usage. Specialty areas are prominent in the use of PDAs.

A trauma team used the PDAs to update daily progress notes, access laboratory values and medications. The nurses within the team also used the device to take photographic record of patients' wounds which were kept on their medical record. (Eastes, 2001; 2004). PDAs were used in the operating theatre by nurses as a tool to assist in updating, maintaining and retrieving surgical preference cards as well as accessing current treatment and medication references (McCord, 2003). Infusion therapy and infection control teams used PDAs for routine daily surveillance, time and information management and communication. The usage resulted in a significant improvement in time management as data could be entered while waiting for other tasks to be completed (Goss & Carrico, 2002).

The use of PDAs for clinical decision making was examined by Honeybourne, Sutton, and Ward (2006), who found that most healthcare professionals used the devices to support evidence-based practice and education, but with varying frequency and this depended on the skills of the user. These researchers believed the PDAs could provide a critical mass of information that was relevant, quickly accessible and in a coherent format, delivering clinical information at the point of need with a resulting benefit to patient safety (Honeybourne, Sutton & Ward, 2006).

The use of wireless PDAs to reduce medical errors by facilitating access to needed patient information and communication between clinicians (Choi et al., 2004) was also examined however studies were limited. Most of the applications used on PDAs either involved a one-time installation of information unto the device or obtained new information or updates through synchronization. One study by Tassani et al. (2007) reported on the use of PDAs in an orthopaedic wireless ward. The system patient ward note was shown and collected on the PDA but saved directly on the Hospital Information System. Medical images were shown on the device display, but also transferred to a high-resolution monitor and large amounts of data were dictated and translated by remote continuous speech recognition. There are some studies in progress examining the use of wireless PDAs by nurses in acute care hospitals to determine the impact on patient care in reducing adverse events or nursing errors (Farrell, McGrath, D'Arcy, & Abaloz, 2007).

The adoption of wireless PDAs is also dependent on the organisation or the hospital. The wireless environment has to be set up to accommodate all wireless healthcare technologies - a complex task requiring extensive planning. Hospitals worldwide are now establishing wireless networks as the capabilities have the potential to improve the quality and safety of patient care.

In summary, medicine has dominated in the use of PDAs in the clinical area and the key functionalities were clinical decision support, computerised patient records, patient surveyor tools and clinical data repository (Kuziemsky, Laul, & Leung, 2005). The evidence suggests in nursing that adoption of PDAs by nurses is higher in education and advanced practice rather than general nursing (Degroote & Doranski, 2004; McNeil, et al., 2003).

PDAS IN NURSING EDUCATION

Although the literature on the use of PDAs in nursing education is limited - most emanating from North America - there has been an increased interest in the use of handheld computers as they have the potential to transform nursing practice and the number of nursing schools or faculties adopting this technology has increased. With the increasingly complex and vast amount of information presented in nursing education, PDAs act as a valuable resource for nursing students, graduate nurses, clinicians and academics. These devices offer a powerful and portable means of managing nursing information and increasing clinical knowledge. PDAs may be used in the classroom for formal instruction and at the bedside in real time with the patients. Nurses can check drug orders and interactions and consult evidence based practice nursing guidelines. PDAs are also becoming an important component of patient care and documentation through electronic order entry and patient tracking applications.

This section will focus on common areas that emerged from the literature including general attitudes and use, formal teaching, feedback and evaluation, and clinical education. There was limited literature on how PDAs impacted on patient outcomes although a small study did reveal that patients believed PDA use could increase nurses' efficiency in data retrieval and calculation but were concerned about data accuracy and privacy. They preferred the nurses explained the reasons for PDA use and suggested more PDA functions (eg, entertainment for paediatric patients, wireless paging for clinicians), and valued nursing care over technology use (Lee, 2007). As medical educators are the most advanced in PDA use, comparisons and lessons learnt from their experience will be discussed where relevant.

General Attitudes and Use

There is no definitive literature identifying the number of nursing schools or faculty using PDAs in the education of nurses, however as stated previously, some nursing academic institutions (Table 1) are using the technology and others are following suit. Also the importance of PDA use in nursing education was identified in a nursing survey where 60 percent of the respondents reported that PDA use in nursing education was very important. (NursingPDA Listserve Survey, 2004).

Table 1. Examples of Nursing Schools using PDAs

• Duke University
• Robert Morris University
• RMIT University
• Curtin University
• Washington State
• University of Louisville
• Columbia University
• University of Tennessee
• Yale University
• The University of Texas at Austin
• Vanderbilt University
• Unitec New Zealand
• University of British Columbia
• University of Alberta
• Drexell University
• University of Virginia

A PDA use survey undertaken by Courtney, Pack and Porter (2004) showed that 40.3 percent of nurses (50 of 124) in an academic health system reported using a PDA. Types of nursing practice, gender, age, nursing experience level, initial educational preparation level, self described technology adoption level and number of coworkers with PDAS were not significantly related to PDA ownership among nurses. Practice in a research, education or advanced practice setting, higher self-rated computer literary, and self-description as an innovator/early adaptor predicted PDA ownership and use. In another study nurses initially resisted using the PDA then came around to using the device on a regular basis (Lee, 2006).

Berglund, Nilsson, Revay, Petersson and Nilsson (2007) examined nurses and students demands of function and usability in a PDA and found that they expected access to information about the patients, knowledge resources and functions for their daily work. Where PDAs have been used in nursing education the general attitude of the students has been positive and this often correlated with the level of experience and encouragement by their educators or clinicians to use the device (Farrell & Rose, 2008; Shortis, McGovern, Berry, & Farrell, 2006).

In medicine approximately 60 to 70 percent of medical students and residents use PDAs for educational purposes or patient care. Although there are no statistics available for nursing students the number for medical students is high, over 50 percent and this reflects the value of the device for student learning and delivery of patient care. Satisfaction was generally high and like nursing correlated with the level of handheld computer experience and use (Greenberg, 2004; Kho, Hendersen, Dressler & Kripaline, 2006).

Formal Teaching, Feedback and Evaluation

Handheld computers are becoming a valuable tool in the classroom setting for both teacher and the student and this is most evident in medical education (Kho et al., 2006). Nursing educators have been too slow to adopt this technology for classroom teaching, feedback and evaluation mainly due to cost, large numbers of nursing students and computer literacy of the user. Lehman (2003) reported on her own experience of using a handheld computer for keeping nursing and clinical evaluations and found that it solved the problem of having to carry text methods of record keeping and evaluation and provided an improved method of maintaining records. Farrell (2005) conducted a small pilot study that examined the use of handheld computers by clinical teachers for record keeping and clinical evaluation. Application software programs were designed to facilitate the clinical evaluation of the student nurses in the medical surgical nursing clinical area. The results showed that the clinical teachers embraced the use of the PDA for evaluating and recording student data and saw the electronic method as more efficient and effective than text based. There were some functional issues with the synchronization of the programs to the handheld computer. Synchronization, which involves information exchange between the PDA and a desktop computer, provides a method for educators to monitor the daily journaling of their students, for record keeping, clinical evaluation and other assessments (Cimino & Bakken, 2005).

A wireless PDA based clinical learning tool for professional reflection was designed and evaluated by Garrett and Jackson (2006). Nursing and medical students were able to access clinical expertise and resources remotely, and record their clinical experiences in a variety of media (text, audio and images). The PDA e-portfolio tool was developed to support and enhance clinical learning, promote reflective learning in practice, engage students in the process of knowledge translation, help contextualize and embed clinical knowledge, and to reduce the isolation of students while in supervised clinical practice. The PDA e-portfolio synchronised wirelessly with the user's personal Web based portfolio from any remote location where a cellular telephone signal or wireless connection could be obtained. The evaluation of the tool by nurse practitioner and medical students was positive, yet there were some limits in use due to inherent interface restrictions of the PDA.

In medicine, the educators preload lecture material and display multiple-choice questions as a Webpage while students respond to questions using PDA and wireless Bluetooth cards. This educational modality allows for interactivity and real-time assessment of students' knowledge. The devices were also used for teaching evaluation and student assessment of special activities in the clinical area. Recording such activities in real time avoids much of the recall bias associated with time period evaluations and allows the educators to track a variety of parameters with relative ease (Kho et al.2006).

The descriptive evidence suggests that PDAs are a valuable tool for formal classroom teaching, feedback and evaluation. However there needs to be more rigorous studies undertaken to determine the impact of PDA use on student learning outcomes and patient care, including rates of medication errors. Also there is little evidence from the literature to suggest that the evaluative loop is being closed in practice and that the data is actually being used to provide good feedback or changes in teaching and this appears to be a major obstacle, if the goal is to develop a culture of use by the teachers and the students. Nursing educators can learn from their medical colleagues in this area as they are far more advanced and have implemented quite diverse educational modalities.

Clinical Education

Many nursing academic institutions use PDAs for the clinical education of undergraduate students. The devices are more often used in clinical settings by nursing students and graduates where they use the PDA as a portable resource providing rapid, point of care information to guide patient care and to enhance self directed learning. Wilson, Dignam and Hay (2002) reported on a PDA and personal computer patient care documentation system that was used by undergraduate students in the clinical setting. This initiative contributed to an informatics-integrated curriculum enabling future graduates to better represent practice-based requirements. Miller et al (2005) reported on the use of PDAs by second year undergraduate nursing students. The devices were preloaded with selected software, including drug reference databases, medical laboratory references, and dictionaries. The PDAs were found to be an effective student learning resource. Students made substantial use of their PDAs and the use was linked to access speed and reliability.

Huffstutler, Wyatt, and Wright (2002) explored issues concerning the implementation of handheld technology into their graduate pharmacology course. This study identified challenges associated with changing faculty practice to enable acceptance of PDAs into the program. However, the students primarily perceived the inclusion of handheld technology as a positive feature of the course that enhanced their development of pharmacology knowledge. Greenfield (2007) also focussed on pharmacology knowledge and investigated the use of PDAs to reduce medication error of undergraduate baccalaureate nursing students. The findings showed that the student group using the PDAs were far more accurate in answering drug calculation and drug administration questions than another group using a textbook. Time could also be saved if medication information was in the palm of the nurse's hand rather than in a book.

Farrell and Rose (2008) examined the use of PDAs in improving the pharmacological knowledge of second year undergraduate nursing students in the medical surgical clinical area. Findings showed a slight improvement in the student nurses' pharmacological knowledge however students reported positively on their experience of using handheld mobile technology. The technology improved the efficiency of their nursing practice in real-time with their patients, and improved their overall medical surgical learning experience, although no definitive conclusions can be drawn about any improvement in learning. Students also had little difficulty in using the technology.

Another study undertaken by Farrell (2007) investigated the use of PDAs for improving student nurses' medical surgical knowledge in the clinical area. The findings showed that students were frequent users of the PDAs during patient encounters in medical surgical units, particularly in the area of drug administration. These students medical surgical knowledge showed slight improvement and they all believed the PDAs enhanced their pharmacological knowledge, and to a lesser extent their medical surgical knowledge and saw them as a valuable educational tool to be used in the classroom, clinical area, and at home. Scollin, Patrick, Healey-Walsh, Kafel, Mehta, and Callahan (2007) explored student's attitude toward the use of PDAs - preloaded with medical/nursing databases - during their clinical placements. They found that there were differences in the students' perceptions and acceptance of the PDA as a learning tool.

White et al. (2005) reported on the use of PDAs by student nurses and found that their learning was enhanced in the clinical environment by the rapid and efficient acquisition of relevant information. Furthermore leadership skills and professional confidence were improved by providing students with reinforcement of core knowledge and evidence-based information. In another project PDAs were also provided to student nurses who practiced in medically underserved areas, rural communities and clinics serving migrant/ethnic populations to enhance confidence. The students were able to directly access medical information and databases used in clinical decision making that otherwise would not be available in the rural clinical settings because of a lack of clinical experts and the lack of current technologies (Rice, 2003).

Stolworthy (2003) described an initiative where undergraduate and graduate, students were provided with PDAs, in preparation for their first clinical courses. Graduate students used preloaded reference applications in their precepted clinical courses (six months) and some added additional software applications for their specialty practice setting. Others used the PDAs as reference tools to search for drug information and other clinical information. In addition, 29 percent of the advanced practice nurse preceptors supervising the students owned and used PDAs for their practice, which is slightly higher than the national average of 18 percent of nurses using PDAs. This project is still in progress and all faculties have now been provided with the PDAs to facilitate interaction and support between teachers and students.

MobileNurse, a protype point of care system using a PDA, was developed by Choi, et al.(2004), comprising four modules: patient information management, medical order check, nursing recording and nursing care plan, which was interfaced with the hospital information system. The clinical trial was performed on simulated patients and proved to be helpful and convenient than other non-mobile care systems. To be accepted into real practice the researchers concluded that the system needed an effortless interface and had the ability to replace all paper based nursing records.

In medical education, students and residents use PDAs, like nursing students, as a mobile resource providing rapid, point of care information to direct patient care and to augment self directed learning. Medication reference tools, electronic textbooks and clinical computational programs were the most commonly used applications followed by clinical decision support software, practice guidelines, prediction rules, and physician order sets for common diagnoses. Electronic reference users perceived a time savings of about 1 min/encounter compared with traditional references (Kho et al.2007).

A clinical management approach to evidence based medicine has been applied to PDA use and current studies have been undertaken to determine whether the device could assist this approach at the point of patient care. Medical students were given PDAs preloaded with clinical decision support software (CDSS) or a variety of commercial applications regularly used by physicians. The findings revealed that perceived usefulness of the PDAs with CDSS depended on supportive faculty attitudes, sound knowledge of evidence-based medicine, and enhanced computer literary skills. There was also greater satisfaction with the CDSS than with the commercial applications and this was associated with increased use in a clinical setting and improved success in search rates (Baumgart, 2005; Johnston et al.2004; Sutton, Stockton, McCord, Gilchrist & Fedyna, 2004).

There are numerous clinical decision support systems available for use in clinical practice for all healthcare clinicians, however, there is limited research on how these systems are actually used (Weber, 2007). PDAs uploaded with clinical decision support systems have the potential to facilitate the practice and learning of evidence based medicine and this approach to the clinical education of medical students is an innovation that nursing academics should consider for adoption in nursing programs.

ADVANTAGES OF PDAS

The advantages of PDA use for the clinician and the educator are numerous and many of these have already been discussed. PDAs have become a valuable learning tool and resource for both nursing and medical students and graduates over the past decade. Users of the handhelds appear comfortable and generally satisfied with them. Nursing programs are using PDAs to disseminate references and other course materials, as well as tracking students' clinical exposure (see Table 2). The advantages have been summarised in Table 3 and they reflect only the benefits to the student user but also to the clinician and consumer of health care.

The advantages of PDAs far outweigh the disadvantages (Table 4) yet there are certain aspects that institutions must be aware of when implementing handheld computers. These include security, patient confidentiality and different system interfaces. Other limitations of PDAs include an inability to handle large graphics programs and complete electronic medical records. Acceptance and consistency of use is another potential challenge when utilising PDAs in nursing education (Fischer et al.2003; White et al.2005)

The cost of the devices and initial training are significant disadvantages that may act as barriers to implementation of the devices into new areas. In addition, the relatively small size of handheld computers means they can be easily lost or stolen

Table 2. PDA Applications frequently used by nursing and medical students

Calculators
Evidence based clinical guidelines
Diagnostic tests
Dictionaries
Document readers
Electronic nursing and medical textbooks
Five-minute clinical consults
Nursing and medical literature
Medication references
Physicians' desk reference
Patient-Tracker
Prescription writing
University resources

Table 3. Advantages of PDAs

Portable
Integrated platform for formal education, feedback and evaluation between learner/teacher
Integrated platform for point of care clinical reference, patient management and data communication
Clinical reference programs obtained from Internet and evidence based practice guidelines
Patient management programs allow healthcare professionals to access and store clinical information
Rapid exchange of clinical laboratory results and "efficient patient handovers" through wireless technology
Point-of-care data collection to enhance quality assessment and outcomes in healthcare organisations
Patient education and interaction to prevent and manage diseases such as obesity, diabetes, asthma or urticaria.
Data collection and processing in research

(Lehman, 2003). Another significant disadvantage of PDAs is the short life expectancy due to rapid technological development (Eastes, 2004). Most devices will be obsolete within a two to three year time frame as new technology is released onto the market. PDAs should not be considered as a replacement for the desktop computer; rather they should complement existing hardware and software (Huffstutler, Wyatt, & Wright, 2002).

Barriers to Implementation

The major barriers to PDA adoption in nursing and medical education include small screen size, the

Table 4. Disadvantages of PDAs

Size of screen
Data loss due to battery mishap or failure
Cost and short life of device
Patient confidentiality, security and different system interfaces
Inability to deal with large graphic programs and complete electronic medical records
Acceptance and consistency of use
Small size of device – lost and theft

slow speed of images being obtained, other connectivity problems, lack of available software or programs for specific areas of healthcare, such as critical care, and patient data security concerns.

Other barriers, not related to technical aspects that can cause problems for full adoption of a PDA project is length of time in designing databases and compliance with institutional confidentiality requirements. In regards to users, certain barriers still exist, such as lack of computer experience, a preference for pen and paper, difficulty handling the small device, and concerns about data loss and security. Training and ongoing technical support was identified as a barrier and needs to be increased by nursing education, particularly for clinicians or supervisors in the clinical area, who often lack familiarity with the devices (Farrell & Rose, 2008; Kho et al. 2006). Most nursing programs also lack the full range of technological resources to implement and provide ongoing support for handheld technology use by faculty and students (Koeniger-Donohue, 2008).

In clinical practice the nursing culture does not encourage nurses to use information technology, including PDAs, to manage information. To ensure adoption nurses need to be aware of PDAs, see themselves as users, and understand what PDAs can do. With increased PDA use nurses will shape their own application development by demanding that the technology meets nursing needs. Also educating student and graduate nurses in the use of PDAs contributes to changing the culture in the clinical area.

FUTURE DIRECTIONS

Lindberg and Humphreys (2005) believe the future of information exchange in healthcare education and delivery will be digital and wireless. PDAs will be lighter, have more memory and users will be able to obtain and share opinions on patients with colleagues and international experts with ad-hoc multimedia conferencing. Whatever evolves is uncertain. Baumgart (2005) warns that PDAs are not peripheral brains and are a poor substitute for ad-hoc clinical knowledge and that "no computer system can ever replace dedicated, experienced clinicians and their empathic interaction with patients and families." The fact that healthcare professionals can carry an entire shelf of reference textbooks or a handheld computer's memory card does not automatically mean that clinicians know their contents or can apply their knowledge appropriately in clinical practice. The increasing incidence of this reliance on PDAs is referred to as the residents and medical students' *palmomental reflex* and clinical teachers, and nursing educators need to be aware of this (Crelinsten, 2004). Future research also needs to be conducted that examines the impact of PDA use on patient outcomes including the reduction of nursing and medical errors.

CONCLUSION

This chapter has provided an overview of PDA use in nursing and medical education. These devices are becoming an important and evolving part of the students' resources in nursing and medical education and patient care. Incorporating PDAs in nursing and medical education provides valuable access to point of care information that has the potential to positively impact learning and patient care. The challenge to most educators in nursing education is keeping up with the latest knowledge, including drugs, as most textbooks are outdated even before the student purchases it. Consequently, the question that needs to be asked by nursing academics is: "What resources are best for students to purchase that meets their learning needs yet provides the most current relevant information?" Medicine predicts that the handheld computer will become a necessary part of a physician's equipment like the stethoscope and this trend is likely to extend to nursing and other healthcare professionals. Nursing and medical practice requires instant access to accurate information and because it is possible, through clinical information technologies, it is now becoming necessary. The nursing culture does not encourage the use of information technology so the future lies in the education of our student and graduate nurses, as they will influence the adoption of mobile technologies in the clinical area.

ACKNOWLEDGMENT

I wish to acknowledge the Nurses Board of Victoria and RMIT University for providing funds that have allowed me to conduct research in the use of PDAs in nursing education. Special thanks go to the students who participated in the studies and also to Hewlett Packard and MIMS Australia for providing the handheld computers and the pharmacological databases for the devices.

REFERENCES

Bates, D. W. (2000). Using information technology to reduce rates of medication errors in hospitals. *British Medical Journal*, 320(7237), 788-791.

Baumgart, D. C. (2005). Personal digitial assistants in health care: experienced clinicians in the palm of your hand? *Lancet*, 366(9492), 1210-1222.

Berglund, M., Nilsson, C., Révay, P., Petersson, G., & Nilsson, G. (2007). Nurses' and nurse students' demands of functions and usability in a PDA. *International Journal of Medical Informatics, 76*(7), 530-537.

Blair, R. (2006). Take-along tech and the training of specialty nurses. *Health Management Technology, 27*(3).

Celler, B. G., Lovell, N. H., & Basilakis, J. (2003). Using information technology to improve the management of chronic disease. The *Medical Journal of Australia, 179*(5), 242-246.

Choi, J., Chun, J., Lee, K., Lee, S., Shin, D., Hyun, S., Kim, D., & Kim, D. (2004). MobileNurse: Hand-held information system for point of nursing care. *Computer Methods and Programs in Biomedicine, 74*(3), 245-254.

Cimino, J. J., & Bakken, S. (2005). Personal digital educators. *New England Journal of Medicine, 352*(9), 860-862.

Colevins, H., Bond, D., & Clark, K. (2006). Nurse refresher students get a hand from handhelds. *Computers in Libraries, 26*(4), 6-9.

Courtney, K., Pack, B., & Porter, G. (2004). But will they use it? Nursing utilization of handheld computers. *Journal of Medical Informatics, CD*, 1560.

Crelinsten, G. L. (2004). The intern's palmomental reflex. *New England Journal of Medicine, 350*(10), 1059.

Degroote, S. L., & Doranski, M. (2004). The use of personal digital assistants in the health sciences: results of a survey. *Journal of the Medical Library Association, 92*(3), 341-348.

Eastes, L. (2004). PDAs for the trauma nurse: help or hindrance? *Journal of Emergency Nursing, 30*, 380-3.

Eastes, L. (2001). Use of the personal digitalassistant for point-of-care trauma documentation. *Journal of Emergency Nursing, 27*(5), 516-518.

Farrell, M. J., & Rose, L. (2008). The use of handheld computers in clinical nursing education. *Journal of Nursing Education, 47*(1), 13-19.

Farrell, M. J., Mcgrath, I., D'arcy, M., & Abaloz, E. (2007). Improving Patient Health Outcomes in Acute Care Hospital Units Using Mobile Wireless Technology and Handheld Computers. *Computer Informatics Nursing, 25*(5), 308.

Farrell, M. J. (2007). *Use of handheld computers in medical surgical nursing education.* Final Report. Nurses Board of Victoria, Retrieved

June 10, 2008, from http://www.nbv.org.au/media/67988/m%20farrell%20final%20report%20-%20major%20grant%202006.pdf.

Farrell, M. J. (2006). Nursing and midwifery education using mobile technologies. *Australian Nursing Journal, 14*(1), 25.

Farrell, M. J. (2005). *The evaluation of undergraduate nurses' clinical skills using the latest computer technology*. Final Report, RMIT University.

Fischer, S., Stewart, T. E., Mehta, S., Wax, R., & Lapinsky, S. E. (2003). Handheld computing in medicine. *Journal of the American Medical Informatics Association, 10*(2), 139-149.

Garrett, B.M., & Jackson, C. (2006). A mobile clinical e-portfolio for nursing and medical students, using wireless personal digital assistants (PDAs). *Nurse Education Today, 26*(8), 647-54.

George, L., & Davidson, L. (2005). PDA use in nursing education:Prepared for today, poised for tomorrow. *Online Journal of Nursing Informatics,* 9(2). Retrieved June 10, 2008, from http://eaa-knowledge.com/ojni/ni/9_2/george.htm.

Goss, L., & Carrico, R. (2002). Get a grip on patient safety: outcomes in the palm of your hand. *Journal of Infusion Nurs*ing, *25*(4), 274-279.

Greenfield, S. (2007). Medication error reduction and the use of PDA technology. *The Journal of nursing education, 46*(3), 127-131.

Greenberg, R. (2004). Use of the personal digital assistant (PDA) in medical education. *Medical Education, 38*, 570-571.

Honeybourne, C., Sutton, S., & Ward, L. (2006). Knowledge in the Palm of your hands: PDAs in the clinical setting. *Health Information and Libraries Journal, 23*(1), 51-9.

Huffstutler, S., Wyatt, T. H., & Wright, C. P. (2002). The use of handheld technology in nursing education. *Nurse Educator, 27*(6), 271-275.

Jeffries, P. R. (2005). Technology trends in nursing education: Next steps. *Journal of Nursing Education, 44*(1), 3-4.

Johnston, J.M., Leung, G.M., Tin, K.Y., Ho, L.M. Lam, W., & Fielding, R. (2004). Evaluation of a handheld clinical decision support tools to improve learning of evidence based medicine in medical studies. *British of Medical Journal, 327*, 1090.

Kho, A., Henderson, L. E., Dressler, D. D., & Kripalani, S. (2006). Use of handheld computers in medical education. *Journal of General Internal Medicine, 21*, 531–537.

Koeniger-Donohue, R. (2008). Handheld computers in nursing education: PDA pilot project. *Journal of Nursing Education, 47*(2), 74 -7.

Kuziemsky, C. E., Laul, F., Leung, R. C. (2005). A review on diffusion of personal digital assistants in healthcare. *Journal of Medical Systems, 29*(4), 335 – 342.

Lee, T. T. (2006). Nurses' perceptions of adopting a PDA system--application of Lewin's change theory. *Studies in Health Technology and Informatics, 122*, 958.

Lee, T. T. (2007). Patients' perceptions of nurses' bedside use of PDAs. *Computer Informatics Nursing, 25*(2), 106-11.

Lehman, K. (2003). Clinical nursing instructors' use of handheld computers for student record keeping and evaluation. *Journal of Nursing Education, 42*(1), 41-42.

Lewis, A. (2001). Handheld technology: The newest practice tool for nurses? Online *Journal of Nursing Informatics*. Retrieved February 19, 2007 from http://www.hhdev.psu.edu/nurs/ojni/handheld_technology.htm

Lindberg, D. A. B., & Humphreys, B. L. (2005). 2015 - the future of medical libraries. *New England Journal of Medicine, 352*(11), 1067-1070.

McCord, L. (2003). Using a personal digital assistant to streamline the OR workload. *Association of Perioperative Registerered Nurses Journal,* 78(6):996-1001.

McNeil, B.J., Elfrink, V.L., Bickword,C.J., Peirce, S.T., Beyea, S.C., Averill, C., et al. (20030. Nursing information technology knowledge, skills and, and preparation of student nurses, nursing faculty and clinicians. A U.S. survey. *Journal of Nursing Education, 42,*341-349.

Miller, J., Shaw-Kokot, J. R., Arnold, M. S., Boggin, T., Crowell, K. E., Allegri, F., Blue, J. H., & Berrier, S. B. (2005). A study of personal digital assistants to enhance undergraduate clinical nursing education. *Journal of Nursing Education, 44*(1).

Nursing, PDA, Listserv, & Survey. (2004). Retrieved 15 November, 2007, from http://www.perseus.com/cgi-bin/survsol40.pl.

Rice, M. J. (2003). Bridging the digital divide in medically underserved areas with PDAs [Electronic Version]. Retrieved June 10, 2008, from http://www.pdacortex.com/rural_pdas.htm.

Ruland, C. M. (2002). Handheld technology to improve patient care: Evaluating a support system for preference-based care planning at the bedside. *Journal of the American Medical Informatics Association, 9*(2), 192-201.

Scollin. P., Healey-Walsh. J., Kafel. K., Mehta. A., & Callahan. J. (2007). Evaluating students' attitudes to using PDAs in nursing clinicals at two schools, *Computers, Informatics, Nursing, 25*(4), 228-35.

Shortis, M., McGovern, J., Berry, M., & Farrell, M. J. (2006). Two case studies on the influence of mobile computing on student learning behaviour. *Proceedings of the 17th Annual Conference of the Australasian Association for Engineering Education: Creativity, Challenge, and Change-Partnerships in Engineering Education*, Auckland, New Zealand.

Stolworthy, Y.(2003). *RNs are mobilizing.* Retrieved, June 17, 2004 from www.pdacortex.com/RNs_are_Mobilizing.htm.

Sutton, J., Stockton, L., McCord, G., Gilchrist, V. J., & Fedyna, D. (2004). Hanheld computer use in a family medicine clerkship. *Academic Medicine,* 79, 1114-19.

Tassani, S., Baruffaldi, F., Testi, D., Cacciari, C., Accarisi, S., & Viceconti, M. (2007). Personal digital assistant in an orthopaedic wireless ward: The HandHealth project. *Computer Methods & Programs in Biomedicine, 86*(1), 21-29.

Weber, S. (2007). Clinical decision support systems and how critical care clinicians use them. *Journal of Healthcare Information Management, 21*(2), 41-52.

White, A., Allen, P., Goodwin, L., Breckinridge, D., Dowell, J., & Garvy, R. (2005). Infusing PDA technology into nursing education. *Nurse Educator, 30*(4), 150-154.

Wilson, S., Dignam, D., & Hay, E. (2002). *Addressing the digital divide between nursing practice and education using a personal digital assistant (PDA).* Winds of Changing in the Sea of Learning, Proceedings of the 19th Annual Conference of the Australian Society for Computers in Tertiary Education (ASCILITE), Auckland, New Zealand.

KEY TERMS

Adverse Event: An incident in which unintended harm results to a person receiving health care. The outcome to the person may be a temporary or permanent disability or death. The injury or harm is caused by healthcare management rather than the disease process and includes acts of omission (inaction failure to diagnose or treat) and commission (affirmative actions) from treatment and management. Medication errors, infections, and pressure ulcers are the major areas of harm.

Bluetooth: A telecommunications industry specification describing how mobile computers can be easily interconnected using a short run wireless connection.

Clinical Decision Support Systems: Computer decision support systems are computer software or applications designed to aid health care professionals in making diagnostic and therapeutic decisions in patient care. These systems can simplify access to data needed to make clinical decisions, provide reminders and prompts at the time of a patient encounter, and assist in establishing a diagnosis and in entering appropriate requests. Another advantage is that they can also alert clinicians when new patterns or trends in patient data are recognized. Clinical decision support systems have been shown to be highly effective, sustainable tools for changing clinician behavior.

Functionalities: Practical applications of a PDA - includes basic functions such as an electronic diary, address book, to-do-list, notepad, calculator, expense tracker and alarm clock. Other software and applications used by health care professionals include clinical decision support systems, computerized patient record, patient surveyor tools, clinical data repository, drug reference databases, medical laboratory references, electronic textbooks and clinical practice guidelines.

Mobile Technologies: Mobile technology devices amalgamate hardware, operating systems, networking and software. Personal digital assistants, mobile phones, laptops, notebooks and notepads are all examples of **hardware**. Applications are the **software** programs, **networks** are the infrastructure that supports the transfer of information and the **operating system** manages the tasks and resources on the mobile device.

Personal Digital Assistant (PDAs): A portable computer that is small enough to be held in one's hand. PDAs are small, lightweight, durable, secure, safe, and have low power requirements that do not interfere with medical equipment. There are two types of PDAs, handheld computers and palm sized computers. **Handheld computers** tend to be larger and heavier and use a miniature keyboard, usually in combination with touch-screen technology, for data entry. **Palm sized computers** are smaller and lighter and use stylus/touch-screen technology and handwriting recognition programs for data entry.

Point of Care Technology: Allows clinicians to enter and access data at the point of care. Has the potential to reduce nursing and medical errors and data entry effort, as well as eliminating paperwork. Data is also immediately accessible by administrators, nurses, or other professionals.

Preload, Upload, Download: These terms are used in computing to refer to data transfer. **Preload** is when the handheld device or personal computer is loaded with software programs or applications. **Upload** is the transfer of data from a handheld computer or other mobile devices to a personal computer. **Download** is the transfer of data from a server to a personal computer.

Process Based Education: Focuses on what happens when student learning takes place: the how or why change occurs. Learning "how" or improving ability is not like learning "that" or acquiring information, which is known as content or product based education

Synchronisation: PDAs have the ability to synchronise to personal computers. This is achieved through synchronisation software provided with the handheld. Data synchronization allows users to access the same information on the PDA as the personal computer. Synchronising also prevents the loss of information stored on the device in case it is stolen, lost or destroyed.

Wireless Technology: Wireless refers to telecommunication technology, in which radio waves, instead of cables or wires, are used to carry a signal to connect communication devices. Wireless technology enables users to physically move while using a device, such as a laptop, PDA, paging device, or phone. The Internet, Intranets or Extranets can all be accessed by the PDAs. Healthcare professionals can access and update electronic medical records (EMR) at patients' bedsides, match bar-coded patient wristbands and medication packages to physician orders, and use wireless badges for voice communication. They can also use the Internet and the Intranet to access email, research, patient education, daily schedules, memo writing, voice, dictation, photography, drug calculations, and diagnostic tests and results.

Chapter XVII
Using Information Technology in Nursing Education

Elizabeth Rogerson
University of Dundee, UK

Linda Martindale
University of Dundee, UK

Carolyn Waltz
University of Maryland, USA

ABSTRACT

This chapter addresses issues relating to nursing informatics as used and applied in nursing education. This includes the use of information technology (IT) in delivering nursing education, as well as the teaching of IT and informatics skills to prepare nurses for practice. Drivers associated with the development and use of IT in nursing education are discussed, as well as current use of IT in nursing education and practice, including both mainstream and emerging technologies. Lastly some key issues for the future are identified. Internationalism is regarded as a consistent theme in IT development and occurs as a recurring thread throughout this chapter.

INTRODUCTION

Over the past ten years information technology (IT) has made a substantial impact on the way students learn and how they are taught (Farrell et al, 2007). This evolution has been driven by factors and events internal and external to nursing education, including how nurses practice and how educators and researchers in Higher Education (HE) work together at national and global levels. Evidence also suggests that collaboration and partnership will increasingly play a major part in the use of IT in both education and practice (McCormick et al, 2007).

The nursing profession has long recognised the need for nurses worldwide to possess a basic set of informatics competences if they are to operate effectively in an increasingly technologically driven world (Gassert, 1998; Saranto and Leino- Kilpi, 1997). Over the coming years the use of technology will continue to change the landscape of nursing education, health care delivery and nursing practice (Repique 2007, Brooks and Scott, 2006). It is therefore incumbent on nursing education to ensure that professional registered nurses are prepared for using technology in education and a wide variety of patient care settings, including highly specialised areas of practice. (Bickford et al, 2005). Curriculum design requires to address two distinct but related dimensions of IT use: firstly, how IT can be used to support effective learning; secondly, how students and practising nurses are educationally prepared to apply information and communication technologies (ICTs) in practice.

Increasingly, the education of nurses in IT use goes beyond concerns with the technology to a consideration of pedagogical, professional, social, political and economic consequences and implications of IT integration (Morgan, Rawlinson and Weaver, 2006; Clayton, 2006; and Alexander et al, 2002). This chapter therefore seeks to address three, key, contemporary issues:

- Drivers for the development of IT in nursing education
- Current use of IT in nursing education
- Future focus for IT in nursing education.

DRIVERS FOR IT DEVELOPMENT

Early definitions of nursing informatics described its application to, "... all fields of nursing: nursing services, nurse education, and nursing research." Scholes and Barber 1980, p 73). In 2003 the Canadian Nurses Association issued a more detailed definition of nursing informatics that included the need to manage and deliver educational experiences to support lifelong learning and nursing research (CNA, 2003). Such definitions demonstrate the increasing relevance of nursing informatics in nursing education and evidence-based practice. This is supported by other authoritative voices. According to Smith, Cronenwett and Sherwood (2007), informatics and evidence-based practice need to be intertwining threads in curriculum and programme design, alongside other priority areas such as quality care and patient safety (Cronenwett et al, 2007).

Certain drivers can be identified, which have and will continue to influence use of IT in nursing education:

- Integration of nursing education into HE;
- Increasing use of IT in health care delivery and everyday life;
- Response of the nursing profession to IT;
- Move to standardization (of the basic and specialist skill sets, classification and nursing language);
- Need for lifelong learning.

A final driver for consideration that is intertwined with the above is internationalism. Throughout this chapter internationalism is a recurring theme associated with different aspects of the integration of informatics and IT into nursing education (Killeen and King, 2007).

The collective impact of these drivers on nursing education is complex and will continue to shape the direction and infrastructure of nursing practice, nursing education and health care delivery.

The integration of traditional schools of nursing into Higher Education Institutions (HEIs) over the last four decades has gained global momentum that includes the developing countries. A major advantage of this movement is that nursing education can benefit not only academically (Glen, 1995) but also from the significant funding made available to HEIs to support IT development. In 1993 the UK government supported the creation of the Joint Information Systems Committee (JISC) to oversee networking and specialised information services (JISC, 2007), resulting in a well funded national IT service, that continues to provide core services to HE in the UK, as well as funding for emerging technology solutions, from which nursing education can benefit.

These academic, professional related IT developments are juxtaposed with IT developments in our daily lives from video recording, DVDs and digital television, to mobile phones, email, satellite navigation and virtual reality. This pervasive, societal change naturally extends into work practices and study habits, becoming integral to learning experiences (Bond, 2007). In nursing education the CD-rom led the way in the provision of innovative and interactive content, improving access to literature and bringing technology into the domain of the teacher. For example, the Cumulative Index to Nursing & Allied Health Literature, (Cinahl) introduced a CD-rom in 1989, giving digitised access to its literature database.

By the mid 1990's the internet was beginning to supersede CD-roms as a means of delivering content. Cinahl launched its online database in 1995. In more recent years HE institutions have adopted web-based technologies designed specifically for learning and teaching (McGill and Hobbs, 2007), while concurrently technology has revolutionised communication processes, enabling nurses to communicate more effectively across continents (Killeen and King, 2007). Email became widely used in all levels of education in the 1990s, having originally been designed in its most basic format in the 1960s. In recent years the internet has taken centre stage in global communication and content delivery. These developments inevitably further international goals in nursing education. Academics, professionals and learners can communicate and work together irrespective of geographical location and access to a wide range of information sources is readily and inexpensively available, including search engines for academic publications that provide unprecedented access to peer-reviewed journals and other sources of evidence.

Concurrent with the development of IT in society is the use of IT by the nursing profession to develop health care specific tools. Staggers, Bagley Thompson and Snyder-Halpern (2001) view Computer-based Patient Records (CPR) as central to the contemporary needs of managed care with integrated systems and standardized terminologies for nursing diagnosis and interventions (e.g. the North American Nursing Diagnoses Association (NANDA), the Nursing Outcomes Classification (NOC), and the International Classification for Nursing Practice (ICNP)).

In 2005, the ICNP Version 1 was released, built upon previously published development versions (Hardiker and Coenen, 2007). This development attracted funding from the European Union (EU) for the education and training of nurses in the use of the ICNP and paved the way for subsequent efforts to produce standardised nursing language (SNL). At the present time thirteen SNLs have been approved by the American Nurses Association and are being used worldwide (Lee, Delaney and Moorhead, 2007).

Health care specific tools are also found in areas such as planning and decision-making in nursing care. One example of this is the Creighton Online Multiple Modular Expert System (COMMES). Developed in 1970, this was the predecessor to the Computerised Decision Support Systems (CDSS), which provides a decision-making system that can be used in both education and practice to support nursing diagnosis and development of competence in specific areas, such as managing incontinence in the elderly (Staggers, Bagley Thompson and Snyder-Halpern, 2001).

The Home Health and Ambulatory Care (HHAC) is another example of a health care IT project. Data was collected from 8840 discharged patient records and integrated with the ICNP in Cinahl. This demonstrates the potential for a locally funded initiative for use in both nursing education and practice to be shared and transferred into the international arena using informatics.

This integrated approach to data collection and communication is increasingly in evidence, associated with data integration and managed care across care episodes and over time (Staggers, Bagley Thompson and Snyder-Halpern, 2001).

An example of the increasing sophistication of tools to standardise data is the Master Patient Index (MPI). Computerized prescriber order entry and the creation of medication error databases also serve to improve patient safety (McCartney, 2007).

In nursing education e-learning has been stimulated by other developments such as the growth of distance learning (Rogerson and Harden, 1999) and interest in online learning (Natriello, 2005). Efforts of the international organisations have supported and enhanced these developments. Notable is the EU's Bologna process, which has increased labour mobility, co-operation in development of education standards, competency frameworks and quality assurance across countries. Such approaches serve nursing education well by supporting integrated approaches to education and facilitating efforts to address global health care issues.

Internationalisation predates technological change, dating back to the post-war period, through organisations such as the Council for Trade in Goods, and international agreements such as the General Agreement on Tariffs and Trade (GATT), which became the World Trade Organisation (WTO) in 1993. The concept of the 'global village' is now widely recognised and commonly understood.

Internationalisation impacts on HE and in this context transnationalism is a type of internationalism in which learners are located in a country different from the one where the award-bearing institution is based (Harden, 2006). Transnationalism has many challenges. Koehn and Swick (2006) highlight the multiple and diverse health conditions, policy and social challenges and health disparities. Additionally, in the informatics environment, individual learner differences need to be managed, in terms of IT literacy and availability of technology. From others, such as the International Association of Universities there are concerns about loss of control over standards and quality, as existing national frameworks may be overlooked and local institutions may be driven to lower standards in the interests of global competition.

Transnationalism is also relevant to issues of labour mobility and recruitment and retention, which are now global concerns. While labour mobility policies are beneficial for one community they may have negative effects on others. For example, the EU single market allows EU citizens to work and move freely from one member state to another. In comparison, the impact of migration has been keenly felt in Africa; of 48 African countries 13 have fewer than 5 physicians per 100,000 population (Salafsky, Glasser and Ha, 2005). African countries now need to educate one million nurses and doctors urgently to meet basic health care needs (Joint Learning Initiative, 2004). This comparison exemplifies issues of inequity and poverty identified by the United Nations Millennium Development Goals (Commission for Africa, 2005).

The drivers for IT development identified above can be seen in part to be inter-related, and both affect and are affected by developments in IT. This is particularly so in the case of internationalism, which has been shown to drive IT development in nursing education, but which itself is facilitated by changes in technology.

CURRENT USE OF IT IN NURSING EDUCATION

The rapid pace of change in IT means that the current situation can be viewed as a base from which to plan future changes and these will be discussed in the last section of this chapter. Policies of proactive management in IT are therefore essential, so this section also includes an assessment of emerging technologies in HE. A developing area is closer integration of pedagogy with technology and e-learning. This is manifested in a current focus on end users and is leading to the expectation of benefits to end users (Ehnfors and Grobe, 2004).

A current example of end-user focus is the IMS Global Learning Consortium (IMS GLC). IMS GLC is the leading, global, e-learning standards organisation, which although technologically led employs end user Special Interest Groups (SIGs) to direct development of technology standards. Schools of nursing around the world are active in IMS, discussing needs of end users with other disciplines and with those developing new technologies.

Certain technologies have now become regarded as mainstream in nursing education because of their widespread adoption. Nurse educators therefore have a technology 'tool kit' at their disposal, to suit a variety of learning and teaching situations, including tools such as: virtual learning environments (VLEs), simulation, online assessment tools and electronic portfolios.

In the developed world the VLE is the medium used by most HEIs for technology enhanced learning and teaching. Although VLEs are generally content focused, they are effectively a set of component parts, incorporating opportunities to design interactive learning and assessment experiences and integrate the use of communication and library systems into curriculum delivery. Being web-based VLEs offer flexibility and convenience and provide a secure environment, enabling learners to access information with ease (McGill and Hobbs, 2007).

Anecdotal evidence suggests that early VLE use was limited to posting lecture notes and student hand-outs. This situation is perhaps unsurprising. Teaching staff in HE have typically been subject experts using traditional teaching methods such as lectures, tutorials and seminars. VLEs therefore introduce a radically new vehicle not only for the delivery of programmes but also for the design of creative learning experiences. The effect is to catapult academics into a world of unfamiliar education practices. This process has resulted in a technology – education gap due to variable computer literacy among HE staff, which creates a major barrier to introducing e-learning (Clarke et al 2005).

VLEs have other benefits and in nursing education they can enable teachers to reach students on campus, those studying by distance learning or located across continents and time zones, as well as with local students on clinical placements and/or working unsociable hours. In nursing education the beneficial effects of integrating theory and practice, have been recognised for over a quarter of a century (Bendall, 1975; Alexander, 1982; Alexander, 1983; Derbyshire, 1993; Elkan and Robinson, 1993; Andrews and Jones, 1996 and Williams, 1999). The contemporary debate on integration is extended to include the integration of research into practice (Draper 2000, Glen and Smith 1999, Jarvis 2000, Thomson 2000, Yerrell 2000 and Brennan and Hutt 2001). The flexibility and pedagogical potential of VLEs demonstrates how theory and practice can be taught in an integrated, interactive, flexible and meaningful manner.

VLEs also include tools such as discussion boards and blogs, which enhance communication (Janes, 2006). Discussion boards are a popular means of asynchronous communication and have the advantage of being technically simple, requiring only online access (narrowband or broadband). However an important pedagogical issue is that for meaningful learning to occur the teacher must have skills to set up and facilitate the discussion and be experienced in the design and delivery of structured, interactive learning experiences (Salmon, 2004).

Online communication also offers synchronous communication, as well as asynchronous (Cox, Carr and Hall, 2004; Curran and Fleet,

2005), using technologies such as web conferencing. This allows use of the monitor as a shared workspace so that teachers and learners can view, discuss and work on documents together, regardless of geographic location (Curran and Fleet, 2005). Web conferencing software can also be integrated into the VLE to give seamless use of different technologies.

The use of simulation has gained in popularity in the last decade and in nursing education simulation is used to develop a range of clinical and professional skills (McCallum, 2007). Use of simulation in clinical skills centres supports interprofessional team working (Clemow, 2007) and provides a safe environment for the learner, while protecting the safety of patients (McCallum, 2007). Morgan (2006) studied the perceived benefits to students of clinical skills lab sessions on their first practice placements and found students made a direct link between theory and practice, which improved their confidence in the first placement situation. Similar evidence has been published by Ker (2003).

However there is now an increasingly sophisticated array of technology-enhanced simulation tools available. In the past simulation had one significant drawback; learners needed to be on site to use the simulation models. Simulation now includes web-based solutions, which build virtual patients and practices to provide flexible learning opportunities, often using real data to enhance the experience for learners. The use of virtual tools in education is still in its infancy and their use is generally limited to early adopters and is not yet well understood (JISC, 2007a). Health care education, along with technology partners and other professional disciplines, is leading the way in using and developing standards for virtual patients and virtual communities of practice (JISC, 2007a), in collaboration with organisations such as IMS. Virtual learning will be integrated over time to the mainstream of nursing education using virtual communities such as Second Life, which offer a relatively inexpensive technology for educators to create interactive learning opportunities.

Online assessment can use stand-alone assessment software or can be integrated into VLEs, using either their own tools or embedded proprietary assessment software. Plagiarism can also be monitored for student assignment submissions, using systems such as Turnitin and SafeAssign. Online assessment includes a range of assessment options, from simple multiple choice questions to text-based responses and they can be used to design self, formative and summative assessment.

Electronic portfolios (e-portfolios) increasingly offer the facility of being saved in an electronic format, which allows learners to have access to the e-portfolio beyond the lifespan of a particular course. Portfolios have been used in nursing education to provide a way of collating a range of evidence and can include data on assessment performance, learning behaviour, motivation, persistence and compliance. Mason, Pegler and Weller (2004) argue that e-portfolios are inherently different from their traditional counterparts in that they can be used for different purposes: development of individual learning, presentation to others and assessment in formal learning situations.

With improvements in interoperability it is anticipated that e-portfolios will be able to be built up over time to include all formal learning throughout an individual's career (Beetham, 2005). In terms of nursing education there are key potential benefits of using e-portfolios:

- Promotion of lifelong learning, through building an ongoing comprehensive record of learning and experience
- Ease of access and transfer of information for: the individual; academic institutions (for formal assessment or awarding Accreditation for Prior Learning (APL) and Accreditation for Prior Experiential Learning (APEL); employers (especially with respect

to mandatory update); potential employers; regulatory bodies (such as the Nursing and Midwifery Council (NMC) in the UK, or the National League for Nursing Accrediting Commission (NLNAC) in the US)
- Integration of academic learning and practical experience.

This mainstream of technologies available in nursing education, as described above, have a common advantage in that they provide for more flexible, personalised learning and accommodate the continuum of learning needs from preparation to continuing education. Many, such as e-portfolios, offer opportunities for students, nurses, teachers and employers to work together in planning work experiences around the development of skills, including informatics, and fitness for practice.

A range of emerging technologies is 'waiting in the wings'. The technology for these is already well developed, but adoption into the mainstream of education is just beginning. Some emerging technologies are already well established in everyday life, and have potential application in education settings, whereas others are technologies developed specifically for education. In implementing technologies it is easy to be carried away by the introduction of technology for the sake of technology, rather than appraising and analysing a technology to ascertain what added value it brings. Although there exists already much literature on the use of e-learning in nursing education, there is still a need to build a robust evidence base, to support the pedagogical application of specific technologies. Salmon's work (2004) in use of discussion forums in HE provides a noteworthy example of generating research evidence to support e-learning.

Web 2.0 technologies have been both welcomed and regarded with scepticism in terms of application to education (Skiba, 2006). Web 2.0 has been defined in many different ways, but one generally agreed upon characteristic is that the user is a contributor so the environment is highly collaborative and usually relatively informal. Importantly, these tools can be used to support communication and the building of social structures and networks, including at international level. Examples of Web 2.0 applications include blogs, wikis, and collaborative publishing (Flickr and YouTube being well known examples of these).

Web 2.0 technologies have educational value in sharing and gaining new practice knowledge and learning through the exchange of views and ideas between learners, clinicians and teachers. Thus communities of learners and practitioners can be created, which are not confined to local institutions or national boundaries. In nursing and nursing education such tools may be able to sustain and evolve the internationalisation of nursing and socialization within nursing. Web 2.0 also encourages creativity and can be highly interactive. The caveats are that information and content generated and available through Web 2.0 is of varied reliability and users may not have the skills to be discerning about what is quality, reliable information (Kamel Boulos and Wheeler 2007). These issues relate to nurses as learners and practitioners.

However Web 2.0 technologies are already embedded online, and some tools, such as blogs and wikis, are being adopted into VLEs. The challenge for nursing education seems to be to harness the potential of Web 2.0 while minimising the disadvantages, and at the same time preserving the inherent informality of Web 2.0. To meet this challenge those involved in nursing education will need the skills and knowledge to be able to use Web 2.0 effectively and monitor standards.

Virtual reality tools provide another example of a technology used widely in everyday life, particularly in the gaming industry, which has potential application in education. This is an area which seems to have particular relevance to health care education, where use of simulation is already well established and the potential benefits have been quantified (Morgan, 2006), as discussed above. Virtual reality in health care can comprise virtual patients, virtual practices, virtual hospitals and virtual communities. The application of virtual reality in nursing education has many possibilities, and particularly with respect to problem-based learning (PBL) (Alexander et al, 2002). The potential exists to make problems more life-like, focus learning in and on the elements and challenges of professional practice, allow learners to 'try out' different solutions and evaluate the outcomes, and to reuse scenarios, but with options to customise for a particular clinical situation or culture (Nelson, Sadler and Surtees, 2005). Using PBL in a virtual world also allows groups of learners to work together even if they are geographically dispersed.

The Second Life virtual reality online world allows any individual to adopt an avatar (a virtual persona) and to exist in the virtual world of Second Life. Second Life combines online gaming techniques with communication technologies and although there are already millions of social Second Life users the use of Second Life in education is also being explored and developed (Childress and Braswell, 2006). Second Life is free to users and relatively inexpensive for those who want to develop space within Second Life, thus it can provide a cost effective means for HE to develop virtual learning. The challenges for nursing education appear to be not whether Second Life and other virtual worlds have learning potential, but how nurse educators and students can access, use and develop this technology.

Unlike the other emerging technologies discussed Digital Object Repositories (DORs) have been developed specifically for education. DORs are a specific type of secure content management system and can include Learning Objects (LOs), as well as other content such as research data. They can be thought of as digital libraries that are used to store LOs, which can be anything from a presentation, image or text document to a larger content package, such as a complete module of learning (Liber, 2005). DORs facilitate reuse of digital learning materials and metadata stored with each object provides comprehensive information on objects, from the author to intended level of use to classification information. They can provide a flexible environment for managing learning content and support such functions as multiple classification systems (including standard nursing classification systems or custom designed systems), multiple licence models, integrated image repository, multiple workflows, version control and creation of collections.

The use of DORs is increasing in HE, with many institutions in the developed world now adopting institutional DORs. In some countries the development of DORs is national policy. For example in the UK, JISC has funded ongoing development of JORUM, a free, online repository service for academic staff in Further and Higher Education Institutions. In Ireland the National Digital Learning Repository (NDLR) was set up with nursing as one of the first key areas of development within this repository. Increasing integration of DORs into HE creates potential for reusing and sharing quality resources, especially as issues of intellectual property and digital rights are resolved and internationally agreed models developed.

The potential of DORS also has implications at international level. The collaborative potential of DORs can create a cost-effective approach to technology development and integration, which can be accessed locally and managed at both a national and international level.

There is then already widespread adoption of IT and e-learning solutions into nursing education. These solutions have a common factor of being suitable for use in the range of education activities, from pre-registration and undergraduate curricula to postgraduate and continuing education. Furthermore these technologies can also be used to support students locally, as well as at a distance and have potential to support collaboration at national and international levels.

FUTURE FOCUS FOR IT IN NURSING EDUCATION

As noted in the previous section, it is anticipated that the marriage of technology and pedagogy will develop to benefit end users (Ehnfors and Grobe, 2004) and in this respect nursing education is well positioned because of its history in embracing technology and its deep-rooted commitment to pedagogical strategies (Lavin et al, 2004). This section seeks to identify some key areas which could help nursing education to fully benefit from the use of technology in the HE setting and help to prepare registered nurses to use technology in practice.

Integration with Educational Approaches

A starting point for this final section is that IT has the potential to create learning experiences that have a sound basis in contextual reasoning and professional development as they are based on experience of the real world (Resnick, 1987). This serves to exemplify the need in the future to more clearly align e-learning with educational theory and approaches and in health care education these are also likely to be aligned with practice development.

According to Fetzer (2003), self-actualisation and work experience are key antecedents to the development of professional behaviour, including forming attitudes and values. The relationship between IT and situated learning is therefore worthy of consideration.

Situated learning has its theoretical base in social learning theory and is founded on a belief in the benefits of discovery, exploration in learning, and learning as an active process that empowers (Dewey 1916, Dewey 1925, Dewey 1929, Dewey 1938, Entwistle and Ramsden 1983, Entwistle 1988, Marton and Saljo 1996, and Entwistle and Entwistle 1996). It places learning in the context of authentic practices through the use of learning activities and planned social interaction; thus creating an interactive learning community (Lave and Wenger, 1991; Hay, 1993). Most importantly, it challenges learning that is delivered from a theoretical perspective and lacking a realistic basis (Lave and Wenger, 1991; Hay, 1993; Spouse, 1998(a); Spouse, 1998 (b) and Rogerson, 2003).

Situated learning is founded on a belief that human action is dependent on the context in which it occurs and conceptual knowledge is learned and can be abstracted, from situations in which it is applied (Winn, 1993). Designing learning experiences that place learning in the context of the real world of professional practice are founded in the theory of situated cognition, which views activity, context and culture as intrinsic to the learning experience (Brown 1988, Anderson and Boud 1996). The combination of situated learning and technology enhanced learning in education design and delivery has strong potential for developing meaningful learning experiences. The former acknowledges the importance of the fact that individuals work and learn in communities based on real world situations and that such communities have a definite socio-political and cultural dimension (Lave and Wenger, 1991 and Hay 1993). The contribution of technology is in its potential to 'recreate' the real world, to provide interactive learning and hence to nurture an active learning environment.

Problem-based learning sits in alignment with situated learning but importantly, not if problems are the only focus for learning (Rogerson, 2003). Howard S. Barrows, regarded by many as the father of PBL stressed that while problems are the stimulus for learning, the focus for learning should be practice (Barrows, 1994). Practice-based learning as a species of PBL is particularly suitable for nursing education as it enables holistic assessment of real situations (Rogerson 2003) and provides a valuable strategy for use in virtual learning (Nelson, Sadler and Surtees 2005).

Other learning strategies, which complement situated learning and practice-based learning, are commonplace in nursing education and can be used effectively in e-learning, are outcome-based education (OBE) and competency-based education (CBE). OBE uses clear learning outcomes and can be summarised as "results-orientated thinking" (Harden, et al., 1999). It integrates and makes transparent learning outcomes, including those related to informatics (Reinhard and Moulton 1995). OBE provides a framework to tailor a particular learning situation to meet the individual needs of the student (Anderson and Boud. 1996 and Boak 1998).

Brunt (2007, p6) describes CBE as an approach used " to assess and validate competence." CBE has the structure to build and facilitate education experiences that are learner-centric, real–life orientated, flexible, standards focussed and support structured learning experiences that can be measured. Such learning approaches provide a scaffold for teachers to move away from traditional, narrow, didactic, and content focussed teaching styles and for learners to have the opportunity to personalise their learning experience (Rogerson 2003, Nelson, Sadler and Surtees 2005). The new technologies are reported to have the same effect (Ehnfors and Grobe, 2004). These educational approaches also fit well with the post-modern paradigm of nursing education, which seeks to liberate the nurse from the confines of the classroom (Lister 1997, Lister 1999, Marks-Maran and Rose 1997, Marks-Maran and Rose 1999 and Rolfe 1999).

A variety of learning strategies therefore exist that have the potential to stand in a complementary and aligned relationship with technology tools. Integration of such educational approaches with e-learning provides an opportunity to create meaningful and timely learning experiences, provide students with learning signposts, retain alignment of assessment, facilitate knowledge acquisition and transfer and address the requirements for diagnostic appraisal and remediation.

Self-directed learning is also an area attracting increasing attention, particularly with respect to online learning. In this respect, lessons can be learned from the design of traditional paper-based study guides, which were traditionally used to facilitate self-directed learning (Laidlaw and Harden 1990, Harden and Smythe 1994, Rowntree 1996 and Harden et al, 1999).

Principles of study guide design include the three components: content delivery, management of the learning experience and provision of interactive learning (Harden and Smythe, 1994, Harden et al, 1999 and Rogerson and Harden, 1999). These three components together with considerations of time, resources, skills and expertise, are highly relevant to effective and creative e-learning design (Speziale and Jacobson, 2005 and Koehler, Mishra and Yahya 2007). This demonstrates the potential to build on the existing evidence-base in nursing education to inform future development of e-learning resources.

In the previous section a technology – education gap was identified. Future focus on embedding well-established and research educational strategies into e-learning frameworks will help to close this gap, benefiting students and educators alike.

Informatics Education

A gap also appears to exist between theory learning and practice learning in terms of informatics education (Greiner and Knebel, 2003) and there is a need in the future to address in a better way this area of nursing education. This gap can be bridged in the design of technology enhanced learning by applying the principles of situated learning and practice-based learning when designing learning and teaching resources. Of relevance to this goal is that nurses are apparently more prepared to use and develop technologies for managing information if the outcomes relate directly to patient benefits (Gassert, 1998). Recognising this challenge, the Division of Nursing in the Health Resources and Services Administration of the Department of Health and Human Services in the USA, set out to develop information technologies in a manner that will match the supply and distribution of qualified nurses with the needs of patients (Gassert, 1998). Linked also to these approaches are developments in internet, satellite and portable computing devices, which will be increasingly pivotal in matching technology use to the growing accessibility for providers and users to health care information services (Jadad, 1999).

In 2001 the Institute of Medicine (IOM) also reported a major gap between, *"...what we know is good quality care and what the norm is in practice"*. (Stead, Kelly and Kolodner 2005, p113) The IOM in the same report recommended a systematic approach through the better management of clinical data to reduce spiralling costs of health care and the increasing number of people without access. (Stead Kelly and Kolodner, 2005). The IOM identified as a core competency the understanding of the value and use of informatics to all areas of health care, to reduce errors, manage knowledge and information, and make decisions and communicate (Staggers, Bagley Thompson and Snyder-Halpern,2001).

Stead, Kelly and Kolodner (2005) propose a Three Dimensions model of health care data gathering, which supports these goals. This three dimensional model consists of the health care provider dimension, the population health dimension and the personal health dimension. With due consideration to confidentiality, intellectual property and digital rights management such data systems can be used to enhance nursing practice and patient care services and for the purposes of education to consider the use of outcome-based education and the use of 'real' scenarios in virtual learning. The IOM report and the subsequent analysis by Greiner and Knebel (2003) and Stead, Kelly and Kolodner (2005) however highlight the complexities of designing learning experiences that match the needs of professional practice.

This evidence supports the view that there is a need to provide quality education in informatics and health care related IT systems in the HE system, to ensure a workforce competent in the necessary informatics skills and to benefit patient care and safety.

International Perspectives

The international dimension is an important future consideration. Its relevance for the informatics movement and the nursing profession relate to the general move to globalisation in which a number of factors play a central role in decision making, including: spiralling costs of education and health care; health disparities; social deprivation; labour mobility; and recruitment and retention.

International partnerships in nursing education offer the possibility of creating a relatively cost-effective and safe infrastructure, for developing technology enhanced learning that provides local value and relevance. O'Neil and Krauel (2004) outline the benefits and demands of entering into a range of dynamic, partnership arrangements to match different strategic and operational goals. This complements the belief that success in an organisation is dependent on: learning and adapting quickly; creating new knowledge consistently; disseminating knowledge swiftly; and embodying learning in all new technologies and products.

The growth of informatics and internationalism are also both linked to the growing awareness of the needs of the developing world and the need to adapt to ongoing technological change. Governments world-wide have made a commitment to the Millennium Development Goals, which outline clearly the social, political and economic objectives for the developing world (Commission for Africa, 2005). International partnerships in nursing education support these goals as do many charitable organisations. Indeed many grants awarding bodies in the area of technology enhanced learning actively encourage applications which are built on partnership between educational institutions at international level or which will make digital content openly accessible. The British Council, EU and the Hewlett Foundation provide examples of this approach.

Harden (2006, p522), considering the growth of internationalism, puts forward a three dimensional model for the future based on the components of the student, the teacher and the curriculum, "...*in which internationalism is integrated and embedded within a curriculum and involves collaboration between a number of schools in different countries*".

While the arguments surrounding internationalism and transnationism continue the position of nursing education is that a 'both and' approach rather than 'either or' is required. In this respect, it is important to be cognizant of the potential for IT to ensure that education reaches all nurses irrespective of where they are located geographically, as well as reducing the migration of nurses from countries where their skills are desperately needed. Conversely, it is important to recognise that many countries wish to offer opportunities for nurses to gain international experiences by spending time outside their own culture. For example, the Australian government encourages student and academic mobility and transferability of qualifications.

A review of ninety-seven articles on the issue of informatics literacy concluded that international cooperation and a wide range of efforts was needed to ensure effective educational programmes in health informatics and enhance the knowledge and skills in computer use among health care professionals (Saranto and Hovenga, 2004). Working together to develop and share resources and professional expertise can provide global partners access to a community of practice that is worldwide and supports international social awareness and networking.

CONCLUSION

Nursing education has to respond to the two perspectives of information use in practice and in education. In terms of practice, nursing education has a duty to prepare students and nurses for using IT in the practice situation, whereas in education the use of IT comprises principally use of a range of IT tools as a vehicle for learning. In this chapter a range of issues, historic, current and future have been discussed, relating to these two perspectives. The overlap between these two areas suggests that the education experience can help students to develop generic IT skills, while learning technology skills that could be transferred to professional and clinical practice.

It is therefore incumbent on nursing education to understand the needs of informatics education and to realise the potential of technology in the education setting. Nurses require quality education and training in the use of technology that benefits professional practice (Lofstrom and Nevgi, 2007), including support to engage in higher order thinking using problem-solving and critical thinking. With such skills nurses will be able to fully exploit technology in practice and in learning situations and will be able to fully participate in helping to address the global health challenges of the present and the future.

REFERENCES

Alexander, J. G., McDaniel, G. S., Baldwin, M. S., & Money, B. J. (2002). Promoting, applying and evaluating problem-based learning in the undergraduate nursing curriculum. *Nursing Education Perspectives, 23*(5), 248-253.

Alexander, M. (1983). *Learning to Nurse: Integrating Theory and Practice.* Edinburgh: Churchill Livingston.

Alexander, M. (1982). Integrating theory and practice - 2. *Nursing Times, 23*, 69 - 71.

Anderson, G., & Boud, D. (1996). Introducing learning contracts: a flexible way to learn. *Innovations in Education and Training, 33*, 221 - 227.

Andrews, M., & Jones, P.R. (1996). Problem-based learning in an undergraduate nursing programme: A case study. *Journal of Advanced Nursing, 23*, 357 - 365.

Barrows H. S. (1994). *Practice-based learning: Problem-based learning applied to medical education.* Springfield, Illinois: Southern Illinois University School of Medicine.

Beetham, H. (2005). *E-portfolios in post-16 learning in the UK: developments, issues and opportunities.* JISC. Retrieved November 13, 2007, from http://www.jisc.ac.uk/media/documents/themes/elearning/eportfolioped.pdf

Bendall, E. (1975). *So You Passed Nurse*. London: Royal College of Nursing.

Bickford, C. J., Smith, K., Ball, M. J., Frantz, G., Panniers, T. L., Newbold, S. K., Knecht, K. L., Farish-Hunt, H., & Cortes-Comerer, N. (2005). Evaluation of a nursing informatics training program shows significant changes in nurses' perception of their knowledge of information technology. *Health Informatics Journal, 11*(3), 255-235.

Boak, G. (1998). *A complete Guide to Learning Contracts.* Hampshire: Gower Publishing.

Bond, C. S. (2007). Nurses' requirements for information technology: a challenge for educators. *International Journal of Nursing Studies, 44*, 1075-1078.

Brennan, A-M., & Hutt, R. (2001). The challenges and conflicts of facilitating learning in practice: the experience of two clinical nurse educators. *Nurse Education Today, 21*, 181 - 188.

Brown, L. A. (1988). Maintaining professional practice - is continuing education a cure or merely a tonic? *Nurse Education Today, 8*, 251 - 257.

Brooks, F., & Scott, P. (2006). Knowledge work in nursing and midwifery: an evaluation through computer-mediated communication. *International Journal of Nursing Studies, 43*, 83-97.

Brunt, B. (2007). *Competencies for staff educators*. Marblehead, MA: HCPro Inc.

Childress, M. D., & Braswell, R. (2006). Using Massively Multiplayer Online Role-Playing Games for Online Learning. *Distance Education, 27*(2), 187-196

Clarke, A., Lewis, D., Cole, I., & Ringrose, L. (2005). A strategic approach to developing e-learning capability for healthcare. *Health Information and Libraries Journal, 22*, 33–41.

Clayton, L. H. (2006). Concept mapping: an effective, active teaching-learning method. *Nursing Education Perspectives, 27*(4), 197-203.

Clemow, R. (2007). An illuminative evaluation of skills rehearsal in a mentorship course. *Nurse Education Today, 27*, 80-87.

CNA. (2003). Retrieved November 13, 2007, from http://dlthede.net/Informatics/Chap01/NIDefinitions.htm#CNA2

Commission for Africa. (2005). *Our common interest. Report of the commission for Africa.* Commission for Africa.

Cox, G., Carr, T., & Hall, M. (2004). Evaluating the use of synchronous communication in two blended courses. *Journal of Computer Assisted Learning, 20*, 183-193.

Cronenwett, L., Sherwood, G., Barnsteiner, J., Disch, J., Johnson, J., Mitchell, P., Sullivan, D.T., & Warren, J. (2007). Quality and Safety Education for Nurses. *Nursing Outlook, 55*(3), 122-31.

Curran, V. R., & Fleet, L. (2005). A review of evaluation outcomes of web-based continuing medical education. *Medical Education, 39*(6), 561-567

Darbyshire, P. (1993). In defense of pedagogy: A critique of the notion of andragogy. *Nurse Education Today, 13*, 310 - 314.

Dewey, J. (1916). *Education and democracy.* New York: The Free Press.

Dewey, J. (1925). *Experience and nature.* In: Boyston, J. A.. (1981). *John Dewey the later works, 1925-1953, 1: 1925.* Carbondale, Southern Illinois: University Press.

Dewey, J. (1929). *The quest for certainty.* New York: Minton.

Dewey J. (1938). *Experience and education.* New York: Macmillan.

Draper, P. (2000). The practitioner-researcher in nursing. *Nurse Education Today, 20,* 43 - 44.

Ehnfors, M., & Grobe, S. (2004). Nursing curriculum and continuing education:future directions. *International Journal of Medical Informatics, 73,* 591—598.

Elkan, R., & Robinson, J. (1993). Project 2000: the gap between theory and practice. *Nurse Education Today, 13,* 295-298.

Entwistle, N. J. (1988). *Styles of learning and teaching.* Chichester, England: Wiley.

Entwistle, N. J., & Entwistle, A. C. (1996). *Revision and the experience of understanding.* In: Marton, F., Hounsell, D. J., & Entwistle, N. J. (eds). *The experience of learning.* (Second edition). Edinburgh: Scottish Academic Press.

Entwistle, N. J., & Ramsden, P. (1983). *Understanding students learning.* London: Croom Helm.

Farrell, G. A., Cubit, K. A., Bobrowski, C. L., & Salmon P. (2007). Using the WWW to teach undergraduate nurses clinical communication. *Nurse Education Today, 27,* 427-435.

Fetzer, S. J. (2003). Professionalism of associate degree nurses: the role of self-actualization. *Nursing Education Perspectives, 24*(3), 139-143.

Gassert, C. (1998). The challenge of meeting patients' needs with a national nursing informatics agenda. *The Journal of the American Medical Informatics Association, 5*(3), 263-268.

Glen, S. (1995). Towards a New Model of Nursing Education. *Nurse Education Today,* 15, 90-95.

Glen, S., & Smith, K. (1999). Towards new models of teaching and researching nursing: the research practitioner. *Nurse Education Today, 19,* 628 - 632.

Greiner, A., & Knebel, E. (Eds.). (2003). *Health Professionals Education: Bridge to Quality, IOM.* Retrieved on November 13, 2007, at http://www.nap.edu/catalog/10681.html .

Harden, R.M. (2006). International medical education and future directions: a global perspective. *Academic Medicine,* 81(12), S22-S28.

Harden, R. M. & Smythe, J. J. (1994). Computer - based study guides II: educational components and advantages. *Medical Teacher, 16,* 315 - 321.

Harden, R. M., Laidlaw, J. M., & Hesketh, A. (1999). *Study Guides: Their use and preparation.* AMEE Education Guide No.16. Dundee, UK: Association for Medical Education in Europe.

Hardiker, N. R., & Coenen, A. (2007) Interpretation of an international terminology standard in the development of a logic-based compositional terminology. *International Journal of Medical Informatics, 76,* S274–S280.

Hay, K. E. (1993). Legitimate peripheral participation, instructionism and constructionism: whose situation is it anyway? *Educational Technology* (March) 33 - 38.

Jadad, A. (1999). Promoting partnerships: challenges for the internet age. *British Medical Journal, 319,* 761 - 764

Janes, G. (2006). Addressing the learning needs of multidisciplinary students at a distance using a virtual learning environment (VLE): A novice teacher reflects. *Nurse Education in Practice, 6,* 87-97.

Jarvis, P. (2000). The practitioner - researcher in nursing. *Nurse Education Today, 20*, 30 - 35.

Jarvis, P. (2002). *The theory and practice of teaching.* Eds. London: Kogan Page Limited.

JISC. (2007). About us. Retrieved November 13, 2007, from http://www.jisc.ac.uk/aboutus/about_jisc/history.aspx .

JISC. (2007a). Briefing paper: game-based learning. Retrieved November 13, 2007, from http://www.jisc.ac.uk/publications/publications/pub_gamebasedlearningBP/pub_gamebasedlearningBP_content.aspx .

Joint Learning Initiative. (2004). *Human resources for health: overcoming the crisis Sustainability, mobilisation and increased knowledge key to strengthened health work force.* Global Health Trust.

Kamel Boulos, M.N. & Wheeler, S. (2007). The emerging Web 2.0 social software: an enabling suite of sociable technologies in health and health care Education. *Health Information and Libraries Journal, 24*, 2-23.

Ker, J.S. (2003). Developing professional clinical skills for practice - the results of a feasibility study using a reflective approach to intimate examination. *Medical Education*, 37*(Suppl 1)*, 34-41.

Killeen, M. B., & King, M. M. (2007). Viewpoint: Use of King's conceptual system, nursing informatics, and nursing classification systems for global communication. *International Journal of Nursing Terminologies and Classifications, 18*(2), 51-57.

Koehler, M. J. Mishra, P., & Yahya, K. (2007). Tracing the development of teacher knowledge in a design seminar: Integrating content, pedagogy and technology. *Computers & Education, 49*, 740–762.

Koehn, P. H., & Swick, H. M. (2006). Medical education for a changing world: moving beyond cultural competence into transnational competence. *Academic Medicine, 81*(6), 548-556.

Laidlaw, J. M., & Harden, R. M. (1990). What is ...a study guide? *Medical Teacher, 12* (1), 7-12.

Lave, J., & Wenger, E. (1991). *Situated learning: Legitimate peripheral participation.* Cambridge, M.A: Cambridge University Press.

Lavin, M. A., Avant, K., Craft-Rosenberg, M., Herdman, T. H., & Gebbie, K. (2004). Contexts for the study of economic influence of nursing diagnoses on patient outcomes. *International Journal of Nursing Terminologies and Classifications, 15*(2), 39-47.

Lee, M., Delaney, C., & Moorhead, S. (2007). Building a personal health record from a nursing perspective. *International Journal of Medical Informatics, 76*, S308-S316.

Liber, O. (2005). Learning objects: Conditions for viability. *Journal of Computer Assisted Learning, 21*, 366-373.

Lister, P. (1997). The art of nursing in a 'post-modern' context. *Journal of Advanced Nursing, 25*, 38 - 44.

Lister, P. (1999). A taxonomy for developing cultural competence. *Nurse Education Today, 19*, 313 - 318.

Lofstrom, E, & Nevgi, A. (2007). From strategic planning to meaningful learning: diverse perspectives on the development of web-based teaching and learning in higher education. *British Journal of Educational Technology, 38*(2), 312-324.

Marks-Maran, D., & Rose P. (1997). *Reconstructing nursing: beyond art and science.* London: Bailliere Tindall and RCN.

Marks-Maran & Rose, D. (1999). Reconstructing nursing: evidence, artistry and the curriculum. *Nurse Education Today, 19*, 668 - 672.

Marton, F., & Saljo, R. (1996). *Approaches to learning.* In: Marton, F.D., Hounsell, J. & Entwistle, N. J. (Eds), *The experience of learning.* (Second edition). Edinburgh: Scottish Academic Press.

Mason, R., Pegler, C., & Weller, M. (2004). E-portfolios: an assessment tool for online courses. *British Journal of Educational Technology, 35*(6), 717–727.

McCallum, J. (2007). The debate in favour of using simulation education in pre-registration adult nursing. *Nurse Education Today, 27,* 825-831.

McCartney, P. R. (2007). Nursing informatics then and now. Keeping readers "Plugged in". *The Association of Women's Health, Obstetric and Neonatal Nurses, 11*(1), 80-82.

McCormick, K., Delaney, C., Brennan, P., Effken, J., Kendrick, K., Murphy, J., Skiba, D., Warren, J., Weaver, C., Weiner, B., & Westra, B. (2007) Guideposts to the Future—An Agenda for Nursing Informatics. *Journal of the American Medical Informatics Association, 14*(1), 19-24.

McGill, T. J., & Hobbs, V. J. (2007). (In press). How students and instructors using a virtual learning environment perceive the fit between technology and task. *Journal of Computer Assisted Learning.*

Morgan, J., Rawlinson, M., & Weaver, M. (2006). Facilitating online reflective learning for health and social care professionals. *Open Learning, 21*(2), 167-176.

Morgan, R. (2006). Using clinical skills laboratories to promote theory–practice integration during first practice placement: an Irish perspective. *Journal of Clinical Nursing, 15,* 155-161.

Natriello, G. (2005) Modest Changes, Revolutionary Possibilities: Distance Learning and the Future of Education. *Teachers College Record, 107*(8), 1885-1904.

Nelson, L. Sadler, L., & Surtees, G. (2005). Bringing problem based learning to life using virtual reality. *Nurse Education in Practice, 5,* 103-108.

O'Neil, E., & Krauel, P. (2004). Building transformational partnerships in nursing *Journal of Professional Nursing, 20*(5), 295-299.

Reinhard, S.C., & Moulton, P.J. (1995). Integrating informatics into the graduate community health nursing curriculum. *Public Health Nursing, 12*(3), 151-158.

Repique, R. J. R. (2007). Computers and information technologies in psychiatric nursing. *Perspectives in Psychiatric Care, 43*(2), 77-83.

Resnick, L. B. (1987). Learning in school and out. The 1987 AERA Presidential address. *Educational Researcher, 16,* 13 - 20.

Rogerson, E. (2003). *The role and facilitation of problem-based learning in a distance learning programme leading to the award of Bachelor of Nursing.* Thesis presented for the degree of Doctor of Philosophy, University of Dundee Scotland.

Rogerson, E., & Harden, R. M. (1999). Seven Years On: Distance learning courses for first level nurses and midwives. *Nurse Education Today, 19,* 286 - 294.

Rolfe, G. (1999). The pleasure of the bottomless: postmodernism, chaos and paradigm shifts. *Nurse Education Today, 19,* 668 - 672.

Rowntree, D. (1996). *Exploring open and distance learning.* The Open University. London: Kogan Page.

Salafsky, B., Glasser, M., & Ha, J. (2005). Addressing issues of maldistribution of health care workers. *Annals of the Academy of Medicine, 34*(8), 520-525.

Salmon G. (2004). *E-moderating: the key to teaching and learning online* (2nd edition) London: RoutledgeFalmer.

Saranto, K., & Hovenga, E.J. (2004). Information literacy-what it is about?; Literature review of the concept and the context. *International Journal of Medical Informatics, 73*(6), 503-13.

Saranto, K., & Leino-Kilpi, H. (1997). Computer literacy in nursing: developing the information technology syllabus in nursing education. *Journal of Advanced Nursing, 25*, 377-385.

Scholes, M., & Barber, B. (1980). *Towards nursing informatics*. In Lindberg, D.A.D., & Kaihara, S. (Eds.) *MEDINFO: 1980*. Amsterdam, Netherlands: North-Holland, 7-73.

Skiba, D. J. (2006). Web 2.0: Next Great Thing or Just Marketing Hype. *Nursing Education Perspectives, 27*(4), 212-214.

Smith, E. L., Cronenwett, L., & Sherwood, G. (2007). Current assessments of quality and safety education in nursing. *Nursing Outlook, 55*(3), 132-7.

Speziale, H. J., & Jacobson, L. (2005). Trends in registered nurse education programs 1998-2008. *Nursing Education Perspectives, 26*(4) 230-235.

Spouse, J. (1998). Learning to nurse through legitimate peripheral participation. *Nurse Education Today, 18*, 35 - 39.

Spouse, J. (1998a). Scaffolding student learning in clinical practice. In Entwistle, N. J. (1995). Frameworks for understanding as experienced in essay writing and in preparing for examinations. *Educational Psychologist, 30*, 47 - 54.

Staggers, N., Bagley Thompson, C., & Snyder-Halpern, R. (2001). History and trends in clinical information systems in the United States. *Journal of Nursing Scholarship, 33*(1), 75-81.

Stead, W. W., Kelly, B. J., & Kolodner, R. M. (2005). Achievable Steps Toward Building a National Health Information Infrastructure in the United States *Journal of the American Medical Informatics Association, 12*(2), 113-120.

Thomson, P. (2000). Implementing evidence-based healthcare: the nurse teachers' role in supporting the dissemination and implementation of SIGN clinical guidelines. *Nurse Education Today, 20*, 39 - 40.

Williams, A. F. (1999). An antipodean evaluation of problem-based learning by clinical educators. *Nurse Education Today, 19*, 659 - 667.

Winn, W. (1993). Instructional design and situated learning: paradox or partnership. *Educational Technology*, March, 16 - 21.

Yerrell, P. (2000). The practitioner-researcher in nursing: there won't be too many. Kilgore Trouts. *Nurse Education Today, 20*, 36 - 38.

KEY TERMS

E-Learning: Learning and teaching which is delivered using information technology.

Educational Approach: A theoretically-based strategy to use as a framework for delivering learning.

Emerging Technologies: Technologies which are beginning to be use by early adopters in education to support teaching and learning.

Information Technology: Computer-based systems which deliver content and information to others and which can be used for communication purposes

Internationalism: Activities in nursing education and health service delivery conducted in countries other than that in which the institution is located, including collaborative work with other education partners, non-governmental organisations and health service providers.

Nursing Education: The continuum of formal learning available to nurses, from pre-registration and undergraduate programmes to postgraduate and continuing education courses.

Virtual Learning Environment: A web-based software application, used in educational settings to deliver learning and teaching resources to student.

Compilation of References

Aarts, J., & Gorman, P. (2007). IT in Healthcare: Sociotechnical Approaches "To Err is System"; Editorial. *International Journal of Medical Informatics*, 76(Supp lement 1)S1-S3.

Aarts, J., Doorewaard, H., & Berg, M. (2004). Understanding implementation: The case of a computerized physician order system in a large Dutch university. *Journal of the American Informatics Association, 11*, 207-216.

Active Voice (2003). *The New Americans*. {Information posted on the website}. Retrieved November 18, 2007 from the web: http://www.activevoice.net.

Adams, T. (1987, February). Dementia is a Family Affair. *Community Outlook*, 7-8.

Agency for Healthcare Research and Quality. (2007). Retrieved May 25, 2008, from http://www.ahrq.gov/clinic/epcix.htm

Agrawal, K., Kapur, D., & McHale, J. (2004). *Defying Distance: Examining the Influence of the Diaspora on Scientific Knowledge Flows*. Queen's School of Business, Queen's University, ON. Presented at the Fourth Annual Roundtable for Engineering Entrepreneurship Research, Georgia Institute of Technology, College of Management, December 4, 2004.

Ahrens, J., Feldman, P. H., & Frey, D. (2002). Preventing medication errors in home care. *Centre for Home Care policy & Research Policy Brief, 12*, 1-6.

AIHW. (2007). *Australia's Health 2006*. Camberra: Australian Institute of Health and Welfare.

Alexander, J. G., McDaniel, G. S., Baldwin, M. S., & Money, B. J. (2002). Promoting, applying and evaluating problem-based learning in the undergraduate nursing curriculum. *Nursing Education Perspectives, 23*(5), 248-253.

Alexander, M. (1982). Integrating theory and practice - 2. *Nursing Times, 23*, 69 - 71.

Alexander, M. (1983). *Learning to Nurse: Integrating Theory and Practice.* Edinburgh: Churchill Livingston.

Ali, N. S., Hodson-Carlton, K., & Ryan, M. (2004). Students' perceptions of online learning: Implications for teaching. *Nurse Educator, 29*, 111-115.

Ali, N. S., Hodson-Carlton, K., Ryan, M., Flowers, J., Rose, M. A., & Wayda, V. (2005). Online education: Needs assessment for faculty development. *The Journal of Continuing Education in Nursing, 36*(1), 32-38.

Allan, J., & Englebright, J. (2000). Patient-centered documentation: An effective and efficient use of clinical information systems. *J Nurs Adm, 30*(2), 90-95.

Allen, I. E., & Seaman, J. (2007). Online *nation: Five years of growth in online learning.* Needham, MA: Sloan Consortium.

Altman, G. (2004). *Delmar's fundamental and advanced nursing skills* (2nd ed.). Toronto: Thompson Delmar Learning.

AMA. (2007). *Rural doctors have their say on key solutions to improve rural health care delivery*: Australian Medical Association.

American Association of Colleges of Nursing (1997). *Joint position statement on nursing administration education.* Retrieved December 11, 2007 from http://www.aacn.nche.edu/Publications/positions/nae.htm.

American Association of Colleges of Nursing (1996). *Essentials of master's education.*

American Hospital Association (2007). The *2007 state of America's Hospitals: Taking the pulse.* Retrieved November 24, 2007 from http://www.aha.org/aha/research-and-trends/index.html

American Medical Informatics Association. (2007). Retrieved October 26, 2007, from http://www.amia.org/

American Medical Student Association. (2007). Health Care Delivery: Rural vs. Urban Communities. Retrieved April 9, 2007, from http://www.amsa.org/programs/gpit/ruralurban.cfm

American Nurses Association (ANA) Recognized terminologies and data elements set (2006, May 11). *ANA nursing practice information infrastructure.* Retrieved May, 25, 2008, from http://www.nursingworld.org/npii/terminologies.htm

American Organization of Nurse Executives, (2005). AONE nurse executive competencies. *Nurse Leader.* February 2005, 15-21.

Ammenwerth, E., Eichstädter, R., Happek, T., Hoppe, B., Iller, C,, Kandert, M., Kutscha, A., Kutscha, U., Mansmann, U., Luther, G., & Mahler, C. (2002). Auswirkungen EDV-gestützter Pflegedokumentation – Ergebnisse von Studien am Universitätsklinikum Heidelberg. PrInternet, 11/02, 85-92.

Ammenwerth, E., Eichstädter, R., Haux, R., Pohl, U., Rebel, S., & Ziegler, S. (2001). A Randomized Evaluation of a Computer-based Nursing Documentation System. Method Inform Med. *40*, 61-68.

Ammenwerth, E., Mansmann, U., Iller, C., & Eichstädter, R. (2003). Factors Affecting and Affected by User Acceptance of Computer-based Nursing Documentation: Results of a Two-year Study. *Journal of the American Medical Informatics Association, 10*(1), 69-84.

Anderson, G., & Boud, D. (1996). Introducing learning contracts: a flexible way to learn. *Innovations in Education and Training, 33*, 221 - 227.

Anderson, J. G., & Aydin, C. E. (2005). *Evaluating the organizational impact of healthcare information systems* (2nd ed.). New York: Springer.

Andersson, G., Stromgren, T., Strom, L., & Lyttkens, L. (2002). Randomized controlled trial of internet-based cognitive behavior therapy for distress associated with tinnitus. *Psychosom Med.,* 64(5), 810-816.

Andrews, M., & Jones, P.R. (1996). Problem-based learning in an undergraduate nursing programme: A case study. *Journal of Advanced Nursing, 23*, 357 - 365.

Angell Y. S, & Cetron, M. S (2005). Health Disparities among Travelers Visiting Friends and Relatives Abroad. *Ann Intern Med. January 4, 2005; 142*(1) 67-72.

ANU. (2006). *Responding to the primary healthcare workforce shortage*: Australian National University.

Arbaugh, J. (2001). How instructor immediacy behaviours affect student satisfaction and learning in web-based courses. *Business Communication Quarterly, 64*(4), 42-54.

Arlington, K. (2004). Health Minister gets stony awakening to nursing care. *Nursing Review.* Canberra: 3.

Ash, J. S., Berg, M., & Coiera, E. (2004). Some Unintended Consequences of Information Technology in Health Care: The Nature of Patient Care Information System-related Errors. *J Am Med Inform Assoc, 11*, 104-112.

Ash, J. S., Sittig, D. F., Dykstra, R. H., Guappone, K., Carpenter, J. D., & Seshadri, V. (2007). Categorizing the unintended sociotechnical consequences of computerized provider order entry. *International Journal of Medical Informatics, 76*(1), 21-7.

Ashby, W. R. (1967). Self Regulation and Requisite Variety. In F. E. Emery (Ed.), *System Thinking.* Penguin: Harmondsworth.

ATA's Federal Policy Recommendations for Home Telehealth and Remote Monitoring. (n/d). Retrieved

October 20, 2007, from http://www.americantelemed.org/news/policy_issues/FINA_%20DRAFTHome_Telehealth_Policy_ver3.5.pdf

Atack, L. (2003). Becoming a Web-based learner: Registered nurses' experience. *Journal of Advanced Nursing, 44*, 289-297.

Atack, L., & Rankin, J. (2002). A descriptive study of registered nurses' experiences with Web-based learning. *Journal of Advanced Nursing, 40*, 457-465.

Atkinson, C. (2000). The Soft Information Systems and Technologies Methodology (SISTeM): A Contingency Approach to Integrated Decision Making and Development, In (Eds.) Altmann, G., Lamp, J., Love, P., et al. *Proceedings of ICSTM2000: International Conference on Systems Thinking in Management*, Geelong, November 8-10, 2000.

Australian Council of Deans of Education (ACDE). (1998). *Preparing a profession: Report of the national standards and guidelines for initial teacher education project*. Canberra: ACDE.

Avison, D., & Wood-Harper, T. (1990). Multiview methodology. Oxford: Blackwell Scientific Publishers.

Bailey, R. (2002). *Demographics of Immigrants in Guilford County, NC*. {Report posted on the Web}.Retrieved December, 2007 from the CNNC web.

Balas, E. A., & Boren, S. A. (2000). Managing clinical knowledge for health care improvement. In *Yearbook of Medical Informatics 2000: Patient-Centered Systems* (pp. 65-70). Stuttgart, Germany: Schattauer.

Baldwin, K. M., & Burns, P. G. (2004). Development and implementation of an online CNS program. *Clinical Nurse Specialist, 18*(5), 248-254.

Barber, J. W., King, W. D., Monroe, K. W., & Nichols, M. H. (2000). Evaluation of emergency department referrals by telephone triage. *Pediatrics, 105*(4 Pt 1), 819–21.

Barr, A. (1984, January). Hospital nursing establishments and costs. *Hospital and Health Services Review*, 31-37.

Barriteau, E. (2003). *Confronting power, theorizing gender: Interdisciplinary perspectives in the Caribbean*. University of West Indies Press.

Barrows H. S. (1994). *Practice-based learning: Problem-based learning applied to medical education*. Springfield, Illinois: Southern Illinois University School of Medicine.

Bartholomeyczik, S. (2004). Operationalisierung von Pflegebedürftigkeit – Assessments und ihre Möglichkeiten. In: Bartholomeyczik, S., Halek, S. (Hrsg.) (2004). *Assessmentinstrumente in der Pflege*. Hannover: Schlütersche, 11-20.

Bartholomeyczik, S. (2006). *Pflegediagnostik, Assessment und Klassifikationen: Funktionen und Grenzen. PrInternet*, 9/06, 453-458.

Basler, B. (2007, April). *Care in the express lane*. AARP (American Association of Retired Persons Publications) Bulletin, 48(4), 12-14. New York: American Association of Retired Persons Publications.

Bates, D. W. (2000). Using information technology to reduce rates of medication errors in hospitals. *British Medical Journal*, 320(7237), 788-791.

Baumgart, D. C. (2005). Personal digital assistants in health care: Experienced clinicians in the palm of your hand? *Lancet, 366(9492)*, 1210-1222.

Baumgart, D. C. (2005). Personal digitial assistants in health care: experienced clinicians in the palm of your hand? *Lancet*, 366(9492), 1210-1222.

Baumlein, G. (2003). *Teaching strategies and student outcomes in Web-based instruction in nursing: A case study of expert nurse educators*. Unpublished doctoral dissertation. The University of Akron, Ohio.

Beat, J. W. S. (1970). Ward analysis. *Nursing Times* 66(29), Supp 101-104.

Beetham, H. (2005). *E-portfolios in post-16 learning in the UK: developments, issues and opportunities*. JISC. Retrieved November 13, 2007, from http://www.jisc.ac.uk/media/documents/themes/elearning/eportfolioped.pdf

Behrman, J. R., Foster, A. D., Rosenzweig, M. R., & Vashishtha, P. (1999). Women's schooling, home teaching, and economic growth. *Journal of Political Economy, 107(4)*, 632–714.

Beitz, J. M., & Snarponis, J. A. (2006). Strategies for online teaching and learning: Lessons learned. *Nurse Educator, 31*(6), 20-25.

Belfield, G., & Colin-Thome, D. (2004). *Improving chronic disease management.* Department of Health, UK National Health Service. Retrieved October 20, 2007, from http://www.dh.gov.uk/en/Publicationsandstatistics/Publications/PublicationsPolicyAndGuidance/DH_4075214.

Bell, C., Devarajan, S., & Gersbach, H. (2004). Thinking about the long-run economic costs of AIDS. In *The Macroeconomics of HIV/AIDS*, M. Haacker, (Ed.). (pp. 96–133). Washington, DC: International Monetary Fund.

Benatar, D., Bondmass, M., Ghitelman, J., & Avitall, B. (2003). Outcomes of chronic heart failure. *Arch Intern Med., 163*(3), 347-52.

Bendall, E. (1975). *So You Passed Nurse*. London: Royal College of Nursing.

Bennett, M. (1990). Nursing research in Australia: development of patient dependency scales. *Nursing Research for Nursing Practice*. Melbourne, Australia, Chapman and Hall: 145-161.

Bensink, M. E., Armfield, N., Russell, T. G., Irving, H., & Wootton, R. (2004). Paediatric palliative home care with Internet-based video-phones: lessons learnt. *Journal of Telemedicine and Telecare, 10*(Suppl. 1), 10-13.

Bensink, M., Hailey, D., & Wootton, R. (2006). A systematic review of successes and failures in home telehealth: preliminary results. *Journal of Telemedicine and Telecare, 12*(Suppl. 3), 8-16.

Bensink, M., Hailey, D., & Wootton, R. (in press). A systematic review of successes and failures in home telehealth. Part 2: final quality rating results. *Journal of Telemedicine and Telecare* 2006 (Accepted for publication August 2007).

Bensink, M., Shergold, J., Lockwood, L., Little, M., Irving, H., Russell, T., et al. (2006). Video-phone support for an 8-year-old boy undergoing paediatric bone marrow transplantation. *Journal of Telemedicine and Telecare, 12*(5), 266-268.

Bensink, M., Wootton, R., Irving, H., Hallahan, A., Theodoros, D., Russell, T., et al. (2007). Investigating the cost-effectiveness of video-telephone based support for newly diagnosed paediatric oncology patients and their families: design of a randomised controlled trial. *BMC Health Services Research, 7*(38):doi:10.1186/1472-6963-7-38.

Beolchi, L. (Ed.) (2003). *Telemedicine Glossary (5th ed.).* Brussels: The European Commission, Information Society Directorate-Generale.

Berg, A., Fleischer, S., & Behrens, J. (2005). Development of two search strategies for literature in MEDLINE-PubMed: Nursing diagnoses in the context of evidence-based nursing. *International Journal of Nursing Terminologies and Classifications, 16(2)*, 26-32.

Berg, M. (1999a). Patient care information systems and health care work: A sociotechnical approach. *International Journal of Medical Informatics, 55*(2), 87-101.

Berg, M. (1999b). Accumulating and according: Occasions for information technology in medical work. *Computer Supported Cooperative Work, 8*, 373-401.

Berg, M. (2002). Patients and professionals in the information society: what might keep us awake in 2013. *Int J Med Inform, 66*(1-3), 31-37.

Berg, M., & Goorman, E. (1999). The contextual nature of medical information. *International Journal Medical Informatics, 56*, (1-3), 51-60.

Berg, M., Langenberg, C., Berg, I., & Kwakkernaat, J. (1998). Considerations for sociotechnical design: Experiences with an electronic patient record in a clinical context. *International Journal of Medical Informatics, 52*(1), 243-251.

Berglund, M., Nilsson, C., Révay, P., Petersson, G., & Nilsson, G. (2007). Nurses' and nurse students' demands of functions and usability in a PDA. *International Journal of Medical Informatics, 76*(7), 530-537.

Berlin, E., & Fowkes, W. (1983). Teaching Framework for Cross Cultural Care. An Application in Family Practice. *West J.Med., 139*(6), 934-938.

Bhasale, A. L., Miller, G. C., Reid, S. E., & Britt, H. C. (1998). Analysing potential harm in Australian general practice: an incident-monitoring study. *Med J Aust, 169*(2), 73-76.

Bickford, C. J., Smith, K., Ball, M. J., Frantz, G., Panniers, T. L., Newbold, S. K., Knecht, K. L., Farish-Hunt, H., & Cortes-Comerer, N. (2005). Evaluation of a nursing informatics training program shows significant changes in nurses' perception of their knowledge of information technology. *Health Informatics Journal, 11*(3), 255-235.

Bijker, W. E., Hughes, T. P., & Pinch, T. J. (Eds.) (1987). *The Social Construction of Technological Systems: New Directions in the Sociology and History of Technology.* Cambridge, MA: MIT Press.

Billings, D. M., (2007). Optimizing distance education in nursing. *Journal of Nursing Education, 46*(6), 247-248.

Bjorneby, S. (2000). Smart houses: can they really benefit older people? *Signpost.* 5, 36-38.

Blackboard Academic Suite hardware sizing guide (2004). Retrieved November 7, 2007 from http://library.blackboard.com/docs/r6/6_1/admin/bbls_rel61_hardware_sizing_guide.pdf

Blair, R. (2006). Take-along tech and the training of specialty nurses. *Health Management Technology, 27*(3).

Blair, W. (2000). Australian Industrial Relations Commission – Record of Proceedings. Cited on ANF Victoria website Retrieved April 6 2004 from www.anfvic.asn.au/news_briefs/news_ratios.htm

Boak, G. (1998). *A complete Guide to Learning Contracts.* Hampshire: Gower Publishing.

Bond, C. S. (2007). Nurses' requirements for information technology: a challenge for educators. *International Journal of Nursing Studies, 44,* 1075-1078.

Boned-Ombuena, A. (2007). *Development Assistance to Health Information Systems Strengthening.* Washington, DC: Health, Nutrition and Population Unit in Human Development Network, World Bank.

Borsook, T. K., & Higginbotham-Wheat, N. (1991). Interactivity: What is it and what can it do for computer-based instruction? *Educational Technology, 37*(5), 11-17.

Bortoft, H. (1996). *The Wholeness of Nature: Goethe's Way of Science.* Floris Books.

Borycki, E. M., & Kushniruk, A. W. (2006). Identifying and preventing technology-induced error using simulations: Application of usability engineering techniques. *Healthcare Quarterly, 8,* 99-105.

Borycki, E. M., & Lemieux-Charles, L. (2008). *Does a hybrid electronic-paper record environment impact upon health professional information seeking?* Conference Proceedings for Medical Informatics Europe, Goteborg, Sweden., May 26-28.

Borycki, E. M., Kushniruk, A. W., Kuwata, S., & Kannry, J. (2006). Use of simulation in the study of clinician workflow. *AMIA Annual Symposium,* 61-65.

Brain Injury Resource Foundation (2008). *Functional Independence Measure™ and Functional Assessment Measure Brain Injury.* Retrieved from http://www.birf.info/pdf/tools/-famform.pdf (18.03.2008)

Brandenburg, H., (2004). Das Resident Assessment Instrument (RAI) Eine Chance für die Pflege in Deutschland. In: Bartholomeyczik S., Halek S. (2004), *Assessmentinstrumente in der Pflege. Hannover: Schlütersche,* 69-89

Brennan, A-M., & Hutt, R. (2001). The challenges and conflicts of facilitating learning in practice: the experience of two clinical nurse educators. *Nurse Education Today, 21,* 181 - 188.

Bricon-Souf, N., & Newman, C. R. (2007). Context awareness in healthcare: A review. *International Journal of Medical Informatics, 76*(1), 2 – 12.

bridges.org. (2003). *The Satellife PDA project*. Retrieved March 12, 2007 from http://www.bridges.org/case_studies/351

Brinkerhoff, J. M. (2006). Diasporas, mobilization factors, and policy options. In *Converting Migration Drains into Gains: Harnessing the Resources of Overseas Professionals*, C. Wescott and J. Brinkerhoff (Eds.). (pp. 127–53). Manila: Asian Development Bank.

Britt, R. (2006). Online education: A survey of faculty and students. *Radiologic Technology, 77*(3), 183-190.

Brobst, R., Clarke Coughlin, A. M., Cunningham, D., Feldman J. M. Hess, R. G., Mason J. E., Fenner McBride, L. A., Romano C. A., Warren, J. J., & Wright, W. (2007). *Der Pflegeprozess in der Praxis, 2.* aktualisierte Auflagc. Bern: Verlag Hans Huber.

Brooks, F., & Scott, P. (2006). Knowledge work in nursing and midwifery: an evaluation through computer-mediated communication. *International Journal of Nursing Studies, 43*, 83-97.

Brown, L. A. (1988). Maintaining professional practice - is continuing education a cure or merely a tonic? *Nurse Education Today, 8*, 251 - 257.

Bruffee, K. (1984). *Collaborative learning: Higher education, interdependence, and the authority of knowledge.* Baltimore, MD: The Johns Hopkins University.

Brunt, B. (2007). *Competencies for staff educators.* Marblehead, MA: HCPro Inc.

Bryant, M. (2002). *The expanding role of ICTs in HIV/AIDS program design and implementation.* Retrieved November 13, 2005 from http://topics.developmentgateway.org/hiv/sdm/previewDocument.do~activeDocumentID

Bryant-Lukosius, D., DiCenso, A., Browne, G., & Pinelli, J. (2004). Advanced practice nursing roles: development, implementation and evaluation. *J Adv Nurs, 48*(5), 519-529.

Bryson, C., & Hand, L. (2007). The role of engagement in inspiring teaching and learning. *Innovations in Education and Teaching International, 44*(4), 349-363.

Bu, D., Pan, E., Johnston, D., Walker, J., Adler-Milstein, J., Kendrick, D., et.al. (2007). *The value of information technology-Enabled diabetes management.* Charlestown, MA: Healthcare Information and Management System Society.

Buchan, J. (2004). A certain ratio? Royal College of Nursing: 3. United Kingdom.

Buchan, J. (2004). What Difference Does ("Good") HRM make? *Human Resources for Health*, 2:6 (7 June 2004), World Health Organization, Geneva, Switzerland.

Burke, L., & Weill, B. (2005). *Information Technology for the Health Professions. 2nd Ed.* Chicago, IL: Prentice Hall.

Cam, K. M., Efthimiadis, E. N., & Hammond, K. W. (2008, January 7-10, 2008). An Investigation on the Use of Computerized Patient Care Documentation: Preliminary Results. *Paper presented at the 41st Annual Hawaii International Conference on System Sciences,* Waikoloa, Big Island, Hawaii.

Campion, T. R., Weinberg, S. T., Lorenzi, N. M., & Waitman, L. R. (2007). Analysis of a computerized sign-out tool: Identification of Unanticipated Uses. *Paper presented at the 2007 National Library of Medicine Fellowship Conference.*

Canadian Nurses Association. (2006). *E-Nursing Strategy for Canada.* Ottawa: Author.

Carbone, D., Sharkey, L., & Scully, A. (2007). Building research capacity in a small rural hospital: Benchmarking computer literacy levels. *Paper presented at the Sydney GP & PHC Research Conference: Working Together,* Sydney.

Caselli, F., & Coleman, W. J. (2001).Cross-country technology diffusion: The case of computers. *American Economic Review Papers and Proceedings, 91(2)*, 328–35.

CCSAA (2001). *Clinical Costing Standards Version 5.* Frankston, Vic, Australia, Clinical Costing Standards Association of Australia.

Celler, B. G., Lovell, N. H., & Basilakis, J. (2003). Using information technology to improve the management of chronic disease. The *Medical Journal of Australia, 179*(5), 242-246.

Center for Rural Health Practice. (2004). *Bridging the Health Divide: The Rural Public Health Research Agenda*: University of Pittsburgh.

Chakravorty, R. (2006, March). MobiCare: A Programmable Service Architecture for Mobile Medical Care. *Proceedings of UbiCare 2006: The First Workshop on Ubiquitous and Pervasive Healthcare.*

Chaudhry, B., Wang, J., Wu, S., Maglione, M., Mojica, W., Roth, E., et al. (2006). Systematic review: impact of health information technology on quality, efficiency, and costs of medical care. *Ann Intern Med, 144*(10), 742-752.

Checkland P. (1981). *Systems Thinking, Systems Practice.* Wiley, Chichester.

Checkland, P. B. (1981). *Systems thinking, systems practice.* Chinchester: John Wiley.

Checkland, P. B., & Scholes, J. (1990). *Soft systems methodology in action.* Chinchester: John Wiley and Sons.

Chen, M. (1995). A methodology for characterizing computer-based learning environments. *Instructional Science, 23*(1), 183-220.

Chevalier (2003). *Tips for Working Effectively with Interpreters.* Center for New North Carolinians.

Chickering, A., & Ehrmann, S. (1996). Implementing the seven principles: technology as lever. *AAHE Bulletin*, 3-6.

Child, J. (1972). Organization Structure and Strategies of Control: A Replication of the Aston Study. *Administrative Science Quarterly, 17*, 163 – 77.

Child, J., & Faulkner, D. (1998). *Strategies of Cooperation: Managing Alliances, Networks and Joint Ventures.* Oxford: Oxford University Press.

Childress, M. D., & Braswell, R. (2006). Using Massively Multiplayer Online Role-Playing Games for Online Learning. *Distance Education, 27*(2), 187-196

Choi, J., Chun, J., Lee, K., Lee, S., Shin, D., Hyun, S., Kim, D., & Kim, D. (2004). MobileNurse: Hand-held information system for point of nursing care. *Computer Methods and Programs in Biomedicine, 74*(3), 245-254.

Chumbler, N. R., Vogel, W. B., Garel, M., Qin, H., Kobb, R., & Ryan, P. (2005). Health Services Utilization of a Care Coordination/Home-Telehealth Program for Veterans With Diabetes: A Matched-cohort Study. *J Ambul Care Manage, 28*(3), 230-240.

Cimino, J. (2001). Delivery of just in time information. *American Medical Informatics Association, 2001 Spring Congress Final Program, Developing a National Agenda for Public Health Informatics.* (p.13). Bethesda, Maryland: American Medical Informatics Association.

Cimino, J. J., & Bakken, S. (2005). Personal digital educators. *New England Journal of Medicine, 352*(9), 860-862.

Clark, R. A., Inglis, S., C., McAlister, F. A., Cleland, J. G. F., & Stewart, S. (2007). Telemonitoring or structured telephone support programmes for patients with chronic heart failure: systematic review and meta-analysis. *BMJ* (Clinical research ed.) *334*(7600), 910-911.

Clarke, A., Lewis, D., Cole, I., & Ringrose, L. (2005). A strategic approach to developing e-learning capability for healthcare. *Health Information and Libraries Journal, 22*, 33–41.

Clarke, M. (2004). Systematic reviews and the Cochrane Collaboration. Retrieved November 12, 2007, from http://www.cochrane.org/docs/whycc.htm.

Clayton, L. H. (2006). Concept mapping: an effective, active teaching-learning method. *Nursing Education Perspectives, 27*(4), 197-203.

Clemensen, J., Larsen, B., Kirkevold, M., & Ejskjær, N. (2007). Telemedical teamwork between home and hospital: A synergetic triangle emerges. In Westbrook J.I., Coiera E.W., Callen J.L., & Aarts J. (Eds.) *Information Technology in Health Care 2007 - Proceedings of the 3rd International Conference on Information Technology in Health Care: Socio-technical Approaches. Studies in Health Technology and Informatics, 130*, 81-89.

Clemow, R. (2007). An illuminative evaluation of skills rehearsal in a mentorship course. *Nurse Education Today, 27*, 80-87.

CNA. (2003). Retrieved November 13, 2007, from http://dlthede.net/Informatics/Chap01/NIDefinitions.htm#CNA2

Coakes, E., Willis, D., & Lloyd-Jones R. E. (Eds.) (2000). *The New Sociotech: Graffiti on the Long Wall*: London: Springer-Verlag.

Cochrane, T. (2005). *Podcasting: Do It Yourself Guide*. Indianapolis, IND: Wiley Publishing Inc.

Cockerill, R., O'Brien-Pallas, L., Bolley, H., & Pink, G. (1993). Measuring nursing workload for case costing. *Nursing Economic$* 11(6), 342-349.

Coiera E. (1997). *Guide to medical informatics, the Internet and telemedicine*. Chapman and Hall Medical.

Coiera, E. (2000). When conversation is better than computation. *J Am Med Inform Assoc, 7*(3), 277-286.

Coiera, E., Westbrook, J. I., & Wyatt, J. (2006). The Safety and Quality of Decision Support Systems. *Methods Inf Med, 45*(Suppl 1), S20-25.

Colevins, H., Bond, D., & Clark, K. (2006). Nurse refresher students get a hand from handhelds. *Computers in Libraries, 26(4)*, 6-8; 46-48.

Colevins, H., Bond, D., & Clark, K. (2006). Nurse refresher students get a hand from handhelds. *Computers in Libraries, 26*(4), 6-9.

Commission for Africa. (2005). *Our common interest. Report of the commission for Africa.* Commission for Africa.

Commonwealth, Department of Health and Aging (2003). Trends in hospital activity Australia, 1991-2 to 2000-2001. *Occasional papers.* Canberra.

Conrad, D. (2002). Deep in the hearts of learners: Insights into the nature of online community. *Journal of Distance Education, 17*(1).

Conrick, M. (2006) Health informatics, transforming healthcare with technology, Thomson, South Melbourne, Victoria..

Cook, K. (1977). Exchange and Power in Networks of Interorganizational Relations. *Sociological Quarterly, 18*, 62 – 82.

Cooley, M. (1987). *Architect or Bee? The Human Price of Technology*. The Hogarth Press, p.117.

Coppel, J., Dumont, J., & Visco, I. (2001). Trends in Immigration and Economic Consequences. *OECD Economics Department Working Papers*, No. 284, OECD Publishing. Doi: 10.1787/553515678780.

Corrigan, J., Kohn, L., & Donaldson, M. (Eds.) (2000). *To err is human: Building a safer health system.* National Academies Press: Washington, D.C.

Courtney, K., Pack, B., & Porter, G. (2004). But will they use it? Nursing utilization of handheld computers. *Journal of Medical Informatics, CD*, 1560.

Cox, G., Carr, T., & Hall, M. (2004). Evaluating the use of synchronous communication in two blended courses. *Journal of Computer Assisted Learning, 20*, 183-193.

Cox, W. (2005). Commonwealth Secretariat: Towards a trade and development approach in the Caribbean region. Retrieved March 12, 2007 from http://www.thecommonwealth.org/speech/34293/35178/152062/152049/143178/towards_a_trade_address_to_the_symposium.htm

Crelinsten, G. L. (2004). The intern's palmomental reflex. *New England Journal of Medicine, 350*(10), 1059.

Cronenwett, L., Sherwood, G., Barnsteiner, J., Disch, J., Johnson, J., Mitchell, P., Sullivan, D.T., & Warren, J. (2007). Quality and Safety Education for Nurses. *Nursing Outlook, 55*(3), 122-31.

Cubbon, J. (2007). Personal communication November, 12, 2007.

Cuellar, N. (2002). The transition from classroom to online teaching. *Nursing Forum, 37*(3), 5-13.

Cultural Competency for Health Care Providers (2007). Champlain Valley Area Health Education Center, 2007.

Curran, V. R., & Fleet, L. (2005). A review of evaluation outcomes of web-based continuing medical education. *Medical Education, 39*(6), 561-567

Currell, R., & Urquhart, C. (2003). Nursing record systems: effects on nursing practice and health care outcomes. *Cochrane Database Syst Rev,* (3), CD002099.

Dabbagh, N. (2004). Distance learning: Emerging pedagogical issues and learning designs. *The Quarterly Review of Distance Education, 5*(1), 37-49.

Darbyshire, P. (1993). In defense of pedagogy: A critique of the notion of andragogy. *Nurse Education Today, 13,* 310 - 314.

Darkins, A., Dearde, C. H., Rocke, L. G., Martin, J. B., Sibson, L., & Wootton, R. (1996). An evaluation of telemedical support for a minor treatment centre. *Journal of Telemedicine and Telecare, 2*(2), 92-99.

Davenport, C.B. (2004). *What Nurses Need to Know about Personal Digital Assistants (PDAs).* Retrieved March 20, 2007 from http://eaa-knowledge.com/ojni/ni/8_3/davenport.htm

Davenport, T. H., & Prusak, L. (1997). Working Knowledge: How Organizations Manage What They Know, *Harvard Business School.* Boston: HBS Press.

Davenport, T. H., Long, D. W. D., & Beers, M. C. (1998). Successful Knowledge Management Projects. *Sloan Management Review, 39*(2).

Dee, C. R., Teolis, M., & Todd, A. (n.d.). Multi-state study of health professionals' use of the personal digital assistant (PDA). Retrieved on October 22, 2005 from http://www.mc.vanderbuilt.edu/biblio/scmla/pres/dee.pdf

Degroote, S. L., & Doranski, M. (2004). The use of personal digital assistants in the health sciences: results of a survey. *Journal of the Medical Library Association, 92*(3), 341-348.

Demakis, J. G., Beauchamp, C., Cull, W. L., Denwood, R., Eisen, S. A., Lofgren, R., et al. (2000). Improving Residents' Compliance With Standards of Ambulatory Care: Results From the VA Cooperative Study on Computerized Reminders. *JAMA: the journal of the American Medical Association, 284*(11), 1411-1416.

Department of Health. (2000). *The NHS Plan: A plan for investment, a plan for reform.* London: The Stationary Office.

Devineni, T., & Blanchard, E. B. (2005). A randomized controlled trial of an internet-based treatment for chronic headache. *Behav Res Ther, 43*(3), 277-92.

Dewey J. (1938). *Experience and education.* New York: Macmillan.

Dewey the later works, 1925-1953, 1: 1925. Carbondale, Southern Illinois: University Press.

Dewey, J. (1916). *Education and democracy.* New York: The Free Press.

Dewey, J. (1925). *Experience and nature.* In: Boyston, J. A.. (1981). *John*

Dewey, J. (1929). *The quest for certainty.* New York: Minton.

Dickinson, J. (2002). General Practice. *MJA, 176*(1), 17.

Diekelmann, N., & Mendias, E. P. (2005). Being a supportive presence in online courses: Knowing and connecting with students through writing. *Journal of Nursing Education, 44*(8), 344-346

Diers, D. (1992). Diagnosis-Related Groups and the measurement of nursing. charting nursing's future, Agenda for the 1990's. L. Aiken and C. Fagin. Philadelphia, J. B. Lippincott: 139-156.

Diers, D. (2003). Personal communications.

Diers, D. (2004). Speaking of Nursing. Sudbury, MA: Jones and Bartlett.

Dipietro, L., & Caspersen, C. (1991). National Estimates of Physical Activity among White and Black Americans. *Journal of Med Science Sports Exercise*, (23).

Dixon, J., & Welch, N. (2000). Researching the Rural-Metropolitan Health Differential Using the 'Social Determinants of Health'. *Australian Journal of Rural Health, 8*(5).

Doarn, C. R., Lavrentyev, V. A., Orlov, O. I., Nicogossian, A. E., Grigoriev A. I., Ferguson E. W., & Merrell R. C. (2003). Evolution of telemedicine in Russia: The influence of the space program on modern telemedicine programs. *Telemed J E Health, 9*(1), 103-9.

Doncliff, B. (2001). Making nursing visable and valueable. *KAI TIAKI nursing New Zealand* December/January.

Doolan, D. F., & Bates, D. W. (2002). Computerized physician order entry system in hospitals: mandates and incentives. *Health Affairs, 21*(4), 180-188.

Dørup, J. (2004). Experience and Attitudes towards Information Technology among First-Year Medical Students in Denmark: Longitudinal Questionnaire Survey. *Journal Medical Internet Research, 6*(1), 10.

Dossia gains momentum toward providing employees with personal, private, portable and secure health records (2007, October 3). [Press release] Retrieved May 25, 2008, from http://www.dossia.org/home/Dossia_Gains_Momentum_Sept_07.pdf

Dowding, D. (2007). Computerized decision support systems in nursing. In N. Cullum, D. Ciliska, B. Haynes & S. Marks (Eds.), *Evidence-based nursing: an introduction*. Oxford: Blackwell.

Dowding, D., Lattimer, V., Randell, R., Mitchell, N., Foster, B., Thompson, C., et al. (2007). How do nurses use new technologies to inform their decision making? Final Report, University of York, York.

Draper, P. (2000). The practitioner-researcher in nursing. *Nurse Education Today, 20*, 43 - 44.

Drummond M. F., & Jefferson T. O. (1996). Guidelines for authors and peer reviewers of economic submissions to the BMJ. *British Medical Journal,* 313, 275–83.

Duffy, J. (2007). Dimensions of caring: Psychometric evaluation of the caring assessment tool. *Advances in Nursing Science, 30*(3), 235-245.

Earl, M. J., & Skyrme, D. J. (1990, May). Hybrid Managers: What should you do? *Computer Bulletin*, 19-21.

Eason, K. D. (1988). *Information technology and organizational change.* London: Taylor & Francis.

Eason, K.D., & Harker, S. (1989). *An open systems approach to task analysis*. Internal Report, HUSAT Research Centre, Loughborough University of Technology.

Eastes, L. (2001). Use of the personal digitalassistant for point-of-care trauma documentation. *Journal of Emergency Nursing, 27*(5), 516-518.

Eccles, M., Hawthorne, G., Whitty, P., Steen, N., Vanoli, A., Grimshaw, J., et al. (2002). A randomised controlled trial of a patient based Diabetes Recall and Management system: The DREAM trial: a study protocol. *BMC Health Services Research, 2*(1), 5.

Eccles, M., McColl, E., Steen, N., Rousseau, N., Grimshaw, J., Parkin, D., et al. (2002). Effect of computerized evidence based guidelines on management of asthma and angina in adults in primary care: cluster randomised controlled trial. *British Medical Journal, 325*, 941.

Edirippulige, S., Smith, A. C., Young, J., & Wootton, R. (2006). Knowledge, perceptions and expectations of nurses in e-health: results of a survey in a children's hospital, *Journal of Telemedicine and Telecare, 12*(Suppl. 3), S3, 35-38.

Edirippulige, S., Smith, A., Beattie, H., Davies, E., & R., W. (2007). Pre-registration nurses: An investigation of knowledge, experience, and comprehension of E-Health. *Australian Journal of Advanced Nursing, 25*(2), 78-83.

Edirippulige, S., Smith, A., Beattie, H., Davies, E., & Wootton, R. (2007). Preregistration nurses: an investigation of knowledge, experience and comprehension of e-health. *Australian Journal of Advanced Nursing,* 25(2), 78-83.

Education. *Health Information and Libraries Journal, 24*, 2-23.

Eedy, D. J., & Wootton, R. (2001). Teledermatology: A review. *Br J Dermatol., 144*(4), 696-707.

Effken, J. A. (2002). Different lenses, improved outcomes: a new approach to the analysis and design of healthcare information systems. *International journal of medical informatics, 65*(1), 59-74.

Effken, J., Loeb, R., Johnson, K., Johnson, S., & Reyna, V. (2001). Using cognitive work analysis to design clinical displays. *Medinfo. MEDINFO, 10*(Pt), 127-131.

Egger, M., Smith, G., & Altman, D. G. (2001). *Systematic Reviews in Health Care: Meta-analysis in Context.* 2 ed. London: BMJ Publishing Group.

Ehnfors, M., & Grobe, S. (2004). Nursing curriculum and continuing education:future directions. *International Journal of Medical Informatics, 73*, 591—598.

Ehrlich, A. I., Kobrinsky, B. A., Petlakh, V. I., Rozinov, V. M., & Shabanov, V. E. (2007). Telemedicine for a Children's Field Hospital in Chechnya, *J Telemed Telecare, 13*(1), 4-6.

Elbaz, F. (1991). Research on teacher's knowledge: The evolution of a discourse. *Journal of Curriculum Studies, 23*, 1-19.

Electronic Research Service/ United States Department of Agriculture (ERS/USDA) Research Emphasis (2007). *An enhanced quality of life for rural Americans.* Retrieved October 21, 2007, from http//www.ers.usda.gov/emphases/rural/

Elfrink, V. L., Davis, L. S., Fitzwater, E., Castleman, J., Burley, J., Gorney-Moreno, M. J., et al. (2000). A comparison of teaching strategies for integrating information technology into clinical nursing education. *Nurse Educator, 25*(3), 136-144.

El-Hassen, O., & Fiadeiro, J. L. (2007). Role-based Architectural Modelling of Socio-Technical Systems. *Electronic Notes in Theoretical Computer Science,181*, 5–17.

Elkan, R., & Robinson, J. (1993). Project 2000. the gap between theory and practice. *Nurse Education Today, 13*, 295-298.

Emery, F. E., & Trist, E. L. (1960). Socio-technical Systems. *Management Sciences Models and Techniques, 2.*

Entwistle, N. (1991) Approaches to learning and perceptions of the learning environment-introduction to the special issue, *Higher Education, 22*, 201-204.

Entwistle, N. J. (1988). *Styles of learning and teaching.* Chichester, England: Wiley.

Entwistle, N. J., & Entwistle, A. C. (1996). *Revision and the experience of understanding.* In: Marton, F., Hounsell, D. J., & Entwistle, N. J. (eds). *The experience of learning.* (Second edition). Edinburgh: Scottish Academic Press.

Entwistle, N. J., & Ramsden, P. (1983). *Understanding students learning.* London: Croom Helm.

Escarce, J., & Kapur, K. (2006). Access to and quality of healthcare. In M. Tienda & F. Mitchell (Eds.), *Hispanics & the American Future (pp. 410-446).* Washington, D.C.: National Academies Press.

Evidence-based Practice Centers Overview (2007, July). *Agency for Healthcare Research and Quality*, Rockville, MD. Retrieved August 19, 2007 from, http://www.ahrq.gov/clinic/epc/

Fang, D., & Wisniewski, S. W. (2007). American Association of Colleges of Nursing: Special survey of AACN membership on vacant faculty positions for academic year 2007-2008. Retrieved November 25, 2007 from http://www.aacn.nche.edu/IDS/pdf/vacancy07.pdf.

Farrell, G. A., Cubit, K. A., Bobrowski, C. L., & Salmon P. (2007). Using the WWW to teach undergraduate nurses clinical communication. *Nurse Education Today, 27*, 427-435.

Farrell, M. J. (2005). *The evaluation of undergraduate nurses' clinical skills using the latest computer technology.* Final Report, RMIT University.

Farrell, M. J. (2006). Nursing and midwifery education using mobile technologies. *Australian Nursing Journal, 14*(1), 25.

Farrell, M. J. (2007). *Use of handheld computers in medical surgical nursing education.* Final Report. Nurses Board of Victoria, Retrieved June 10, 2008, from http://

www.nbv.org.au/media/67988/m%20farrell%20final%20report%20-%20major%20grant%202006.pdf.

Farrell, M. J., & Rose, L. (2008). The use of handheld computers in clinical nursing education. *Journal of Nursing Education, 47*(1), 13-19.

Farrell, M. J., Mcgrath, I., D'arcy, M., & Abaloz, E. (2007). Improving Patient Health Outcomes in Acute Care Hospital Units Using Mobile Wireless Technology and Handheld Computers. *Computer Informatics Nursing, 25*(5), 308.

Fetzer, S. J. (2003). Professionalism of associate degree nurses: the role of self-actualization. *Nursing Education Perspectives, 24*(3), 139-143.

Feuerstein, I., & Fritz, E. (2007). *Die Anwendung des RAI-HC 2.0 in der Steiermark – Ergebnisse einer Befragung von diplomierten Pflegepersonen.* Vortrag am 24.10.2007 beim Amt der Steiermärkischen Landesregierung FA 8 B - Gesundheitswesen (Sanitätsdirektion) Graz.

Finnigan, S., Abel, M., Dobler, T., Hudson, L., & Terry, B. (1993). Automated patient acuity. linking nursing systems and quality measurement with patient outcomes. *Journal of Nursing Administration, 23*(5), 62-71.

Fischer, S., Stewart, T. E., Mehta, S., Wax, R., & Lapinsky, S. E. (2003). Handheld computing in medicine. *Journal of the American Medical Informatics Association, 10*(2), 139-149.

Fitzmaurice, D., Hobbs, R., Murray, E., Holder, R., Allan, T., & Rose, P. (2000). Oral anticoagulation management in primary care with the use of computerized decision support and near-patient testing. *Archives of Internal Medicine, 160*, 2343-2348.

Flesner, M. K. (2004). Care of the elderly as a global nursing issue, *Nursing Administration Quarterly*, 28(1), 67-72.

Foresto C. (2004). *La comunicazione organizzativa: spunti di riflessione, appunti di lavoro, resoconto di un'esperienza alla Michelin Italia.* Milano: Centro Studi Logos.

Fowler (1998). Providing Primary to Health Care Immigrants and Refugees: The North Hamilton Experience. *Canadian Medical Association, 159*(4), 388-391.

Frey, H. (2006). *Charticle: The Milken Institute Review.*

Friedman, C. P., & Wyatt, J. C. (1997). *Evaluation methods in medical informatics.* New York: Springer.

Fritz, E., Müller, G., & Them, C. (2007). Assessment für die Pflege? *Österreichische Pflegezeitschrift, 5*(7), 8-12.

Fulton, J., & Kellinger, K. (2004). An ethics framework for nursing education on the Internet. *Nursing Education Perspectives, 25*(2), 62-66.

Fung, C. H., Woods, J. N., Asch, S. M., Glassman, P., & Doebbeling, B. N. (2004). Variation in Implementation and Use of Computerized Clinical Reminders in an Integrated Healthcare System. *American Journal of Managed Care, 10*(2), 878-885.

Furlong, E., & Smith, R. (2005). Advanced nursing practice: Policy, education and role development. *J Clin Nurs, 14*, 1059-1066.

Gaba, D. M. (2000). Structural and organizational issues in patient safety: A comparison of health care to other high-hazard industries. *California Management Review, 43*(1), 83-102.

Galbraith, J. R. (1973). *Designing Complex Organizations.* Reading, MA: Addison-Wesley.

Gärdenfors, P. (2000). *Conceptual Spaces: The Geometry of Thought.* MIT Press.

Garg, A. X., Adhikari, N. K. J., McDonald, H., Rosas-Arellano, M. P., Devereaux, P. J., Beyene, J., et al. (2005). Effects of computerized clinical decision support systems on practitioner performance and patient outcomes: A systematic review. *JAMA: The journal of the American Medical Association, 293*(10), 1223-1238.

Garms-Homolovà (2005). *RAI-System als Voraussetzung der Erfüllung zeitgemäßer Qualitäts und Planungserfordernisse.* Retrieved from http://www.

igk-forschung.de/RAI-GERMANY/ rai-germany.html (15/12/2005).

Garms-Homolovà, V., & Gilgen, R. (Hrsg.) (2000). RAI 2.0 Resident Assessment Instrument. Bern, Verlag Hans Huber

Garrett, B.M., & Jackson, C. (2006). A mobile clinical e-portfolio for nursing and medical students, using wireless personal digital assistants (PDAs). *Nurse Education Today, 26*(8), 647-54.

Garrison, D. R. (2006). *Online community of inquiry review: Social, cognitive, and teaching presence issues.* Unpublished manuscript, University of Calgary. Retrieved November 20, 2007 from http://www.communitiesofinquiry.com/documents/Community%20of%20Inquiry%20Issues.pdf

Gassert, C. (1998). The challenge of meeting patients' needs with a national nursing informatics agenda. *The Journal of the American Medical Informatics Association, 5*(3), 263-268.

Gavagan, T., & Brodyaga, J. (1998). Medical Care for Immigrants and Refugee. *American Family Physicians, 57*(5).

Gelhaus, I. (2002). High-tech homes mean a brighter future for seniors. *Provider*, 28, 40-42.

Gellert, G. A. (1993). International migration and control of communicable diseases. Soc Sci Med 1993, 37(12), 1489-99.

George, L., & Davidson, L. (2005). PDA use in nursing education:Prepared for today, poised for tomorrow. *Online Journal of Nursing Informatics,* 9(2). Retrieved June 10, 2008, from http://eaa-knowledge.com/ojni/ni/9_2/george.htm.

Gerber, S., & Scott, L. (2007). Designing a learning curriculum and technology's role **in it.** *Educational Technology, Research and Development, 55*(5), 461-479.

Gerrish, K., Chau, R., Sobowale, A., & Birks, E. (2004). Bridging the language barrier: the use of interpreters in primary care nursing. *Health & Social Care in the Community* 12 (5), 407–413.

Gibson, F. (2003). Seven Oakes: friendly design and sensitive technology. *Journal of Dementia Care, 11*, 27-30.

Giddens, A. (1984). *The Constitution of Society: Outline of the Theory of Structuration.* Berkeley, University of California Press.

Gideon, J. (2006). Integrated gender interests into health policy. *Development and Change, 37(2)*, 329-352.

Gillett, S. (2001). *Nursing intensity in Victorian public hospitals.* Unpublished.

Glen, S. (1995). Towards a New Model of Nursing Education. *Nurse Education Today*, 15, 90-95.

Glen, S., & Smith, K. (1999). Towards new models of teaching and researching nursing: the research practitioner. *Nurse Education Today, 19*, 628 - 632.

Goffman, E. (1974). *Frame analysis: An essay on the organization of experience.* London: Harper and Row.

Goldberg, S. I., Mahanek, A. O., & Novikov, I. D. Dispatcher-consultative systems. Main characteristics and an example of realization. (1991). *Vest. Vsesoyuzn. Obsh. Informat. I Vych. Tech,. 1*, 46-52 [in Russian].

Goldstein, M. K., Coleman, R. W., Tu, S. W., Shankar, R D., O'Connor, M. J., Musen, M. A., et al. (2004). Translating research into practice: Organizational issues in implementing automated decision support for hypertension in three medical centers. *Journal of the American Medical Informatics Association, 11*(5), 368-376.

Goodhue, D. L., & Thompson, R. L. (1995). "Task-Technology Fit and Individual Performance". *MIS quarterly: management information systems., 19*(2), 213.

Goossen, W. T. F. (2000). *Towards strategic use of nursing information in The Netherlands.* The Haag, Gegevens Koninklijke.

Goossen, W. T., Epping, P. J., Dassen, T. W., Hasman, A., & van den Heuvel, W. J. (1997). Can we solve current problems with nursing information systems? *Comput Methods Programs Biomed, 54*(1-2), 85-91.

Goss, L., & Carrico, R. (2002). Get a grip on patient safety: outcomes in the palm of your hand. *Journal of Infusion Nursing*, *25*(4), 274-279.

Gottschalck, T. (2003). Assessmentinstrumente zur pflegerischen Beurteilung des Mundes. *Pflege, 16*, 273–282.

Granger, C. V., Hamilton, B. B., Linacre, J. M., Heinemann, A. W., & Wright, B. D. (1993). Performance profiles of the functional independence measure. *Am.J Phys Med Rehabil, 72*(2), 84-89.

Greatbatch, D., Hanlon, G., Goode, J., O'Cathain, A., Strangleman, T., & Luff, D. (2005). Telephone triage, expert systems and clinical expertise. *Sociology of Health & Illness, 27*(6), 802-830.

Green, D., & Kenyon, B. (1991). Rigidity and fragility of large socio-technical systems: Advanced information technology, the dominant coalition, and paradigm shift at the end of the 20th century. *Behavioral Science, 36*(1), 64-79.

Greenberg, R. (2004). Use of the personal digital assistant (PDA) in medical education. *Medical Education, 38*, 570-571.

Greenfield, S. (2007). Medication error reduction and the use of PDA technology. *The Journal of nursing education, 46*(3), 127-131.

Greiner, A., & Knebel, E. (Eds.). (2003). *Health Professionals Education: Bridge to Quality, IOM*. Retrieved on November 13, 2007, at http://www.nap.edu/catalog/10681.html .

Griffin, R. (1980). Relationships among individual, task design, and leader behavior variables. *Academy of Management Journal, 23*, 665-683.

Gubler, E. V. (1990). *Informatics in pathology, clinical medicine, and paediatrics.* Leningrad: Meditsina. [in Russian]

Guigoz, Y., Vellas B. J., & Garry, P. J. (1994). Mini Nutrional Assessment: A practical assessment tool for grading the nutritional state of elderly patients. *Facts and research in gerontology, Supplement on Nutrition an Aging, 2*, 15-59. New York: Springer Publishing Co.

Gutkin, C. (2008). Family physician shortages Are nurses the answer? *Can Fam Physician, 54*(3), 480

Haas, U., Mayer, H., & Evers, G. C. M. (2002). Die Interrater Reliabiliät des. Functional Independence Measure. (FIM) bei Patienten mit Schädel-Hirn-Verletzungen. In: *Pflege 2002, 15*, 191-197.

Hager, M. H. (2006). Centers for MediCare & MedicAid Services Telehealth Coverage of MNT—What ADA Members Need to Know. *J Am Diet Assoc., 4*(106), 513-6.

Hajioff, S. (1998). Computerized decision support systems: an overview. *Health Informatics Journal, 4*, 23-28.

Halek, M. (2003). *Wie misst man Pflegebedürftigkeit?* Hannover: Schlütersche.

Hall, M. J., Owings, M. F., & Shinogle, J. A. (2006). Inpatient Care in Rural Hospitals at the Beginning of the 21st Century. *The Journal of Rural Health, 22*(4), 331–338.

Halter, M. J., Kleiner, C., & Hess, R.F. (2006). The experience of nursing students in an online doctoral program in nursing: A phenomenological study. *International Journal of Nursing Studies, 43*, 99-105.

Hammer, M., & Champy, J. (1993). *Reengineering the corporation.* New York: HarperBusiness.

Hanlon, G., Strangleman, T., Goode, J., Luff, D., O'Cathain, A., & Greatbatch, D. (2005). Knowledge, technology and nursing: The case of NHS Direct. *Human Relations, 58*(2), 147-171.

Hansebo, G., Kihlgren, M., Ljunggren, G., & Winblad, B. (1998). Staff views on the Resident Assessment Instrument, RAI/MDS, in nursing homes, and the use of the Cognitive Performance Scale, CPS, in different levels of care in Stockholm, Sweden. *Journal of Advanced Nursing, 28*(3), 642-653.

Harden, R. M. & Smythe, J. J. (1994). Computer - based study guides II: educational components and advantages. *Medical Teacher, 16*, 315 - 321.

Harden, R. M., Laidlaw, J. M., & Hesketh, A. (1999). *Study Guides: Their use and preparation.* AMEE Education Guide No.16. Dundee, UK: Association for Medical Education in Europe.

Harden, R.M. (2006). International medical education and future directions: a global perspective. *Academic Medicine*, 81(12), S22-S28.

Hardiker, N. R., & Coenen, A. (2007) Interpretation of an international terminology standard in the development of a logic-based compositional terminology. *International Journal of Medical Informatics*, *76*, S274–S280.

Harris, B. L. (1990). Becoming deprofessionalized: one aspect of the staff nurse's perspective on computer-mediated nursing care plans. *ANS Adv Nurs Sci, 13*(2), 63-74.

Harris, K., Fleming, M., Hunter, R., Rosser, B., & Cushman, A. (1998). *The Knowledge Management Scenario: Trends and Directions for 1998-2003*. Technical report, Gartner Group.

Harris, k., Huber, D., Jones, R., Manojlovich, M., Reineck, C. (2006). Future nursing administration graduate curricula, part 1: Call to action. *Journal of Nursing Administration, 36*(10), 435-440.

Hawes, C., Mor, V., Phillips, C. D., Fries, B. E., Morris, J. N., Steele-Friedlob, E., Greene, A. M., & Nennstiel, N. (1997). The OBRA-87 Nursing Home Regulations and Implementation of the Resident Assessment Instrument: Effects on Process Quality. *JAGS, 45*, 977-985.

Hay, K. E. (1993). Legitimate peripheral participation, instructionism and constructionism: whose situation is it anyway? *Educational Technology* (March) 33 - 38.

Hayes, G., & Barnett, D. (Eds.) (2008). *UK Health Computing: Recollections and Reflections*, BCS.

Healthcare Terminologies and Classification: An action agenda for the United States (2006). *American Medical Informatics Association and American Health Information Management Association*. Retrieved May, 2008 from, http://www.amia.org/inside/initatives/docs/terminologiesandclassifications.pdf

Hebda, T., Szar, P., & Mascara, C. (2005). Handbook of informatics for nurse and health care professionals 3rd Ed, Pearson Prentice Hall, New Jersey.

Hebert, M. (n.d.) National nursing informatics project discussion paper [Electronic version]. Retrieved on December 8, 2003 from http://www.cna-nurses.ca/pages/resources/nni/nni_discussion_paper.doc

Hegney, D., Buikstra, E., Eley, R., Fallon, T., Gilmore, V., & Soar, J. (2007). *Nurses and information technology: Final Report*: Australian Nursing Federation and Australian Government Department of Health and Ageing.

Henderson, K. (2006). TelEmergency: Distance emergency care in rural emergency departments using nurse practitioners. *J Emerg Nurs. 32*(5), 388-93.

Henderson, L. E., Dressler, D. D., & Kripalani, S. (2006). Use of handheld computers in medical education. *Journal of General Internal Medicine*, *21*, 531–537.

Hersh, W. (2006). Who are the Informaticians? What We Know and Should Know. *Journal of the American Medical Informatics Association, 13*, 166-170.

Heuschmann, P.U., Kolominsky-Rabas, P.L., Nolte, C.H., Hünermund, G., Ruf, H.U., Laumeir, I., Meyrer, R., Alberti, T., Rahmann, A., Kurth, T., & Berger, K. (2005). Untersuchung der Reliabilität der deutschen Version des Barthel-Index sowie der Entwicklung einer postalischen und telefonischen Fassung für den Einsatz bei Schlaganfall-Patienten. *Fortschr Neurol Psychiat, 73*, 74-82.

Hinchcliffe, S. M. (Ed.) (1989). *Nursing Practice and Health Care*, [1st Edition only], London, Edward Arnold.

Hinshaw, A. S. (2008). Navigating the perfect storm: balancing a culture of safety with workforce challenges. *Nurs Res, 57*(1 Suppl), S4-10.

Hobbs, S. D. (2002). Measuring Nurses' Computer Competency: An Analysis of Published Instruments. *Computer Informatics Nursing, 20*(2), 63-73.

Hodge, E., Bosse, M.J., Faulconer, J., & Fewell, M. (2006). Mimicking proximity: The role of distance education in forming communities of learning. *International Journal of Instructional Technology and Distance Learning.* Retrieved November 19, 2007 from http://www.itdl.org/Journal/Dec_06/article01.htm

Hogenbirk, J. C., Pong, R. W., & Lemieux, S. K. (2005). Impact of telephone triage on medical service use: implications for rural and remote areas. *J Agric Saf Health, 11*(2), 229-37.

Holmström, I. (2007). Decision aid software programs in telenursing: not used as intended? Experiences of Swedish telenurses. *Nursing and Health Sciences, 9*(1), 23–28.

Honeybourne, C., Sutton, S., & Ward, L. (2006). Knowledge in the Palm of your hands: PDAs in the clinical setting. *Health Information and Libraries Journal, 23*(1), 51-9.

Horrocks, S., Anderson, E., & Salisbury, C. (2002). Systematic review of whether nurse practitioners working in primary care can provide equivalent care to doctors. *BMJ, 324*, 819-823.

Houck, J. B. (2001). PDAs-Stat-for busy nurses. Retrieved October 22, 2005 from http://www.wirelessnewsfactor.com

Hovenga, E. J. S. (1994). *Casemix, hospital nursing resource usage and costs: The basis for a nurse staffing and costing system*. Sydney, The University of New South Wales: 269.

Hovenga, E. J. S. (1983). *Patient dependency and nurse staffing for Victorian hospitals*. Victoria, Health Department.

Huffstutler, S., Wyatt, T. H., & Wright, C. P. (2002). The use of handheld technology in nursing education. *Nurse Educator, 27*(6), 271-275.

Hung, D. (2001). Theories of learning and computer-mediated instructional technologies. *Education Media International, 38*(4), 281-287.

Hunt, E.C. (2002). The value of a PDA to a nurse. Retrieved October 22, 2005 from http://www.unc.edu5/~dbailey1/CON1/nsgpdavalue.doc

Hutchins, H. (2003). Instructional immediacy and the seven principles: Strategies for facilitating online course. *Online Journal of Distance Learning Administration*, 4(3), 1-11.

Hyde, A., & Murray, (2005). Nurses' experiences of distance education programmes. *Journal of Advanced Nursing, 49*, 87-95.

Iams, J., Johnson, F., & O'Shaughnessy, R. (1988). A prospective random trial of home uterine activity monitoring in pregnancies at increased risk of preterm labor Part II. *Am J Obstet Gynecol., 159*, 595-603.

Information Technology Association of America E-Health Committee (2004). *Chronic care improvement: How Medicare transformation can save lives, save money and stimulate an emerging technology industry*, ITAA May 2004. Retrieved October 20, 2007 from http://www.itaa.org/isec/docs/choniccare.pdf

Institute of Medicine (1999). *To err is human: Building a Safer Health System.* Washington, DC: National Academies Press.

Institute of Medicine (2001). *Crossing the Quality Chasm: A New Health System for the 21st century.* Washington, D C: National Academies Press.

Institute of Medicine (2003). *The future of the public's health in the 21st Century.* Washington, D.C.: National Academies Press. Institute of Medicine, Committee on the Future of Rural Healthcare. (2005). *Quality through collaboration: The future of rural health.* Washington, D.C.: National Academies Press.

Institute of Medicine (2003). *Health Professions Education: A Bridge to Quality,* Washington, D C: National Academies Press.

Institute of Medicine (IOM) (2007). *Nutrigenomics and beyond: Informing the future.* Washington, DC: The National Academies Press.

Institute of Medicine, Committee on Quality of Health Care in America (2001). *Crossing the quality chasm: A new health system for the 21st Century.* Washington, D.C.: National Academies Press.

The International Council of Nurses. The ICN Definition of Nursing. Retrieved June 16, 2008, from http://www.icn.ch/definition.htm

International Council of Nurses (2005). *International Classification for Nursing Practice, Version 1*. Geneva, Switzerland: Author.

International Development Research Centre. (2004). *Uganda Health Information Network*. Technical report – IDRC Grant No. 102136-001. Ottawa, ON: IDRC.

International Medical Informatics Association – Nursing Informatics. (2008). The Nursing Special Interest Group. Retrieved March 20, 2008 from http://www.imiani.org/

The International Council of Nurses. The ICN Definition of Nursing. Retrieved June 16, 2008, from http://www.icn.ch/definition.htm Isfort, M., & Weidner, F. (2001). Pflegequalität und Pflegeleistungen I. Zwischenbericht zur ersten Phase des Projektes. *Entwicklung und Erprobung eines Modells zur Planung und Darstellung von Pflegequalität und Pflegeleistungen. Deutsches Institut für angewandte Pflegeforschung* (dip), Köln. http://www.dip-home.de/material /downloads/bericht-pflegeleistung1.pdf (18.003.2008).

Isfort, M., Klug, E., & Weidner, F. (2002). Pflegequalität und Pflegeleistungen II Zwischenbericht zur zweiten Phase des Projektes. *Entwicklung und Erprobung eines Modells zur Planung und Darstellung von Pflegequalität und Pflegeleistungen*. Deutsches Institut für angewandte Pflegeforschung (dip), Köln. http://www.dip-home.de/material /downloads/bericht-pflegeleistung2.pdf (18.003.2008).

Issenberg, S. B., McGaghie, W. C., Petrusa, E. R., Gordon, D. L., & Scalese, R. J. (2005). Features and uses of high-fidelity medical simulations that lead to effective learning: A BEME systematic review. *Medical Teacher, 27*(1), 10-28.

Ivanitskaya, L., O'Boyle, I., & Casey, A. (2006). Health Information Literacy and Competencies of Information Age Students: Results From the Interactive Online Research Readiness Self-Assessment (RRSA). *J Med Internet Res, 8*(2), e6.

Jacobs, S. K., Rosenfeld, P., & Haber, J. (2003). Information literacy as the foundation for evidence-based practice in graduate nursing education: a curriculum-integrated approach. *Journal of Professional Nursing, 19*(5), 320-328.

Jadad, A. (1999). Promoting partnerships: challenges for the internet age. *British Medical Journal, 319*, 761 - 764

Jairath, N., & Stair, N. (2004). A development and implementation framework for Web-based nursing courses. *Nursing Education Perspectives, 25*(2), 67-72.

Janes, G. (2006). Addressing the learning needs of multidisciplinary students at a distance using a virtual learning environment (VLE): A novice teacher reflects. *Nurse Education in Practice, 6*, 87-97.

Janes, R., Arroll, B., Buetow, S., Coster, G., McCormick, R., & I., H. (2005). Few rural general practitioners use the Internet frequently in regard to patient care. *N Z Med J*(118), 1212.

Jarvis, P. (2000). The practitioner - researcher in nursing. *Nurse Education Today, 20*, 30 - 35.

Jarvis, P. (2002). *The theory and practice of teaching*. Eds. London: Kogan Page Limited.

Jayasuriya, R., & Caputi, P. (1996). Computer attitude and computer anxiety in nursing. Validation of an instrument using an Australian sample. *Computer Informatics Nursing, 14*(6), 340-345.

Jeffries, P. R. (2005). Technology trends in nursing education: Next steps. *Journal of Nursing Education, 44*(1), 3-4.

Jenkins, R. L., & White, P. (2001). Telehealth advancing nursing practice. *Nursing Outlook, 49*(2), 100-105.

Jesuit Distance Education Network. (n.d.). *Competency Assessment in Distributed Education*. Retrieved November 10, 2007 from http://www.ajcunet.edu/index.aspx?sid=21.

JISC. (2007). About us. Retrieved November 13, 2007, from http://www.jisc.ac.uk/aboutus/about_jisc/history.aspx .

JISC. (2007a). Briefing paper: game-based learning. Retrieved November 13, 2007, from http://www.jisc.ac.uk/publications/publications/pub_gamebasedlearningBP/pub_gamebasedlearningBP_content.aspx .

Joanna Briggs Institute. (2006). strategies to reduce medication errors with reference to older adults. *Aust Nurs J, 14*(4), 26-9.

Johnson Pettinari, C., & Jessopp, L. (2001). Your ears become your eyes: Managing the absence of visibility in NHS Direct. *Journal of Advanced Nursing, 36*(5), 668-675.

Johnson, M. E., Brems, C., Warner, T. D., & Roberts, L. W. (2005). Rural–Urban Healthcare Provider Disparities in Alaska and New Mexico. *Administration and Policy in Mental Health and Mental Health Services Research, 33*(4), 504-507.

Johnston, J.M., Leung, G.M., Tin, K.Y., Ho, L.M. Lam, W., & Fielding, R. (2004). Evaluation of a handheld clinical decision support tools to improve learning of evidence based medicine in medical studies. *British of Medical Journal, 327*, 1090.

Joint Learning Initiative. (2004). *Human resources for health: overcoming the crisis Sustainability, mobilisation and increased knowledge key to strengthened health work force*. Global Health Trust.

Jones, M. (Ed.). (1999). *Nurse Prescribing: Politics to Practice*. London: Harcourt Publishers.

Jones, P. (1996). Humans, Information, and Science. *Journal of Advanced Nursing, 24*(3), 591-598.

Jones, P. (1998). *Hodges' Health Career Care Domains Model*. Retrieved June 8, 2008, from http://www.p-jones.demon.co.uk

Jones, P. (2000a). *Hodges' Health Career Care Domains Model, Structural Assumptions*. Retrieved June 8, 2008, from http://www.p-jones.demon.co.uk/theory.html

Jones, P. (2000b). *Hodges' Health Career Care Domains Model, Theoretical Assumptions*. Retrieved June 8, 2008, from http://www.p-jones.demon.co.uk/struct.html

Jones, P. (2004). Viewpoint: Can Informatics And Holistic Multidisciplinary Care Be Harmonised? *British Journal of Healthcare Computing & Information Management, 21*, 6, 17-18.

Jones, P. (2008). Exploring Serres' Atlas, Hodges' Knowledge Domains and the Fusion of Informatics and Cultural Horizons, In Kidd, T., Chen, I. (Eds.) *Social Information Technology Connecting Society and Cultural Issues*. IGI Global.

Jordan, H., Roderick, P., Martin, D., & Barnett, S. (2004). Distance, rurality and the need for care: Access to health services in South West England. *International Journal of Health Geographics, 3*, 21.

Kadel, R. (2006). Coursecasting: The wave of the future? ... Bit by bit: Podcasting with purpose. Retrieved May 20, 2008 from InfoTrac OneFile database.

Kaiser Daily. (2006). Short of health care workers in developing countries undermines essential services. Retrieved May 20, 2008 from http://www.kaisernetwork.org/daily_reports/rep_index.cfm?DR_ID=44073

Kaleidoscope (2003). Cultural Diversity in Guilford County. *A training handbook for Health and human service providers.*

Kamel Boulos, M.N. & Wheeler, S. (2007). The emerging Web 2.0 social software: an enabling suite of sociable technologies in health and health care

Kaner, C., Falk, J., & Nguyen, H. Q. (1999). *Testing computer software* (2nd ed.). New York: Wiley.

Kankaanranta M (2005). International perspectives on the pedagogically innovative uses of technology. *Human Technology, 1(2),* 111–116.

Kaplan, B., Brennan, P. F., Dowling, A. F., Friedman, C. P., & Peel, V. (2001). Toward an Informatics Research Agenda: Key People and Organizational Issues. *Journal of the American Medical Informatics Association, 8*, 235-241.

Kaplan, S., Rosenfeld, P., & Haber, J. (2003). Information literacy as the foundation for evidence-based practice in graduate nursing education: a curriculum-integrated approach. *Journal of Professional Nursing 19*(5), 320-328.

Kaplan-Leiserson, E. (2005). Trend: Podcasting in Academic and Corporate Learning. Retrieved May 20, 2007 from http://www.learningcircuits.org/2005/jun2005/0506_trends

Karliner, L. S., Jacobs, E. A., Chen, A. H., & Mutha, S. (2007). Do Professional Interpreters Improve Clinical Care for Patients with Limited English Proficiency. *A Systematic Review of the Literature Health Services Research, 42*(2), 727–754.

Katz, S., Ford, A.B., Moskowitz, R. W., Jackson, B.A., & Jaffe, M. W. (1963, September). Studies of Ilness in the Aged. The Index of ADL: Standardized Measure of Biological and Psychosocial Function. *JAMA, 21*, 185, 914-9.

Kaul, I. (2002). Kaul Report. Retrieved May 20, 2008 from www.undp.org/globalpublicgoods/globalization/pdfs/Kaul%20162-180.pdf

Kawamoto, K., Houlihan, C. A., Balas, E. A., & Lobach, D. F. (2005). Improving clinical practice using clinical decision suppoıt systems: A systematic review of trials to identify features critical to success. *BMJ, 330*(7494), 765-772.

Kenner, C., Androwich, I. M, & Edwards, P. A. (2003). Innovative educational strategies to prepare nurse executives for new leadership roles. *Nursing Administration Quarterly, 27*(2), 172-179.

Kenny, A. (2002). Online learning: Enhancing nursing education? *Journal of Advanced Nursing, 38*(2), 127-135.

Ker, J.S. (2003). Developing professional clinical skills for practice - the results of a feasibility study using a reflective approach to intimate examination. *Medical Education*, 37*(Suppl 1)*, 34-41.

Khoury, M., & Mensah, G. (2005, April). Genomics and the prevention and control of common chronic diseases: Emerging priorities for public health action. *Preventing Chronic Disease: Publ'c Health Research, Practice and Policy, 2(2)1- 11.* Retrieved June 8, 2005, from, http://www.cdc.gov/pcd/ issues/2005/apr/05_0011.htm

Killeen, M. B., & King, M. M. (2007). Viewpoint: Use of King's conceptual system, nursing informatics, and nursing classification systems for global communication. *International Journal of Nursing Terminologies and Classifications, 18*(2), 51-57.

Kimball, B., & O'Neil, E. (2003). *Healthcare's human crisis: The American nursing shortage.* Robert Woods Johnson Foundation. Retrieved May 25, 2008, from, http://www.rwjf.org/files/publications/other/NursingReport.pdf

Kingma, M. (2004). *Nurses on the move, Migration and the global health care economy*, Cornell University Press, Ithaca.

Klein G. B. (1998). Osservare e valutare la comunicazione nelle organizzazioni. *Rassegna Italiana di Valutazione*. 10.

Kobb, R., Hilsen, P., & Ryan, P. (2003). Assessing technology needs for the elderly: finding the perfect match for home. *Home Healthc Nurs, 1*, 666-73.

Kobrinskiy, B.A., & Matveev, N.V. (2006). Teleconsultations at the Moscow Research Institute for Paediatrics and Children's Surgery. In *The 6th International Conference on Successes and Failures in Telehealth* (pp.193-194). Brisbane, Australia.

Koeckeritz, J., Malkiewicz, J., & Henderson, A. (2002). The seven principles of good practice: Applications for online education in nursing. *Nurse Educator, 27*(6), 283-287.

Koehler, M. J. Mishra, P., & Yahya, K. (2007). Tracing the development of teacher knowledge in a design seminar: Integrating content, pedagogy and technology. *Computers & Education, 49*, 740–762.

Koehn, P. H., & Swick, H. M. (2006). Medical education for a changing world: moving beyond cultural competence into transnational competence. *Academic Medicine, 81*(6), 548-556.

Koeniger-Donohue, R. (2008). Handheld computers in nursing education: PDA pilot project. *Journal of Nursing Education, 47*(2), 74 -7.

Kolodner, R. M., & Douglas, J. V. (1997). *Computerizing large integrated health networks the VA success*. New York: Springer.

Koppel, R., Metlay, J. P., Cohen, A., Abaluck, B., Localio, A. R., Kimmel, S. E., & Strom, B. L. (2005). Role of computerized physician order entry systems in facilitating medication errors. *JAMA, 293*(10), 1197-1203.

Kreijns, K., Kirschner, P., & Jochems, W. (2002). The sociability of computer-supported collaborative learning environments. *Educational Technology and Society, 5*(1), 8-22.

Kuperman, G. L., & Gibson, R. F. (2003). Computer physician order entry: Benefits, costs and issues. *Ann Intern Med. 139*(16), 31-39.

Kurtz, C. F., & Snowden, D. J. (2003) The new dynamics of strategy: Sense-making in a complex and complicated world. *IBM Systems Journal, 42,* 3.

Kushniruk, A. (2002). Evaluation in the design of health information systems: Application of approaches emerging from usability engineering. *Computers in Biology and Medicine, 32*(3), 141-149.

Kushniruk, A. W., & Patel, V. L. (2004). Cognitive and usability engineering methods for the evalution of clinical information systems. *Journal of Biomedical Informatics, 37*, 56-76.

Kushniruk, A. W., Borycki, E., Kuwata, S., & Kannry, J. (2006). Predicting changes in workflow resulting from healthcare information systems: Ensuring the safety of healthcare. *Healthcare Quarterly, 9*, 114-118.

Kushniruk, A. W., Patel, V. L., & Cimino, J. J. (1997). Usability testing in medical informatics: Cognitive approaches to evaluation of information systems and user interfaces. In *Proceedings of the 1997 AMIA Annual Fall Symposium: The Emergence of 'Internetable' Health Care, Systems that Really Work, 21,* 218-222). Philadelphia: Hanley and Belfus.

Kushniruk, A., Triola, M., Stein, B., Borycki, E., & Kannry, J. (2004). The relationship of usability to medical error: An evaluation of errors associated with usability problems in the use of a handheld application for prescribing medications. In M. A. Musen, C. P. Friedman & J. M. Teich (Eds.), *AMIA/MedInfo 2004 Symposium: Building High Performance Health Care Organizations, 28*, 1073-1076. San Francisco: American Medical Informatics Association.

Kuwata, S., Kushniruk, A., Borycki, E., & Watanabe, H. (2006). Using simulation methods to analyze and predict changes in workflow and potential problems in the use of a bar coding medication order entry system. *AMIA Annual Symposium*, 994.

Kuziemsky, C. E., Laul, F., Leung, R. C. (2005). A review on diffusion of personal digital assistants in healthcare. *Journal of Medical Systems, 29*(4), 335 – 342.

Lacere, F., Jensen, L., & Biddlecom, A. (1994). Healthcare Utilization, Family Context, and Adaptation among Immigrants to the United States. *Journal of Health & Social Behavior, 35*(4), 370-384.

LaDuke, S. (2001). Online nursing documentation: finding a middle ground. *J Nurs Adm, 31*(6), 283-286.

Laidlaw, J. M., & Harden, R. M. (1990). What is ...a study guide? *Medical Teacher, 12* (1), 7-12.

Lane, D. C., & Oliva, R. (1998). The greater whole: Towards a synthesis of system dynamics and soft systems methodology. *European Journal of Operational Research, 107*, 214-235.

Lange, A., Rietdijk, D., Hudcovicova, M., van de Ven J-P., Schrieken, B., & Emmelkamp, P. M. G. (2003). Interapy: A controlled randomized trial of the standardized treatment of posttraumatic stress through the internet. *Journal of Consulting and Clinical Psychology, 71*(5), 901-999.

Lapointe, L., & Rivard, S. (2006). Getting physicians to accept new information technology: Insights from case studies. *CMAJ, 174*(11), 1573-1578.

Laschinger, H. K. S. (2008). Effect of empowerment on professional practice environments, work satisfaction, and patient care quality: Further testing the nursing worklife model. *Journal of Nursing Care Quality, 20.*

Lattimer, V., George, S., Thompson, F., Thomas, E., Mullee, M., Turnbull, J., et al. (1998). Safety and effectiveness of nurse telephone consultation in out of hours primary care: randomised controlled trial. *British Medical Journal, 317*, 1054-1059.

Lauesen, S. (2007). *Guide to requirements SL-07.* Lauesen Publishing.

Laurant, M. (2000). Evidence based substitution of doctors by nurses in primary care? *British Medical Journal, 320*(7241), 1078.

Laurant, M., Reeves, D., Hermens, R., Braspenning, J., Grol, R., & Sibbald, B. (2007). Substitution of doctors by nurses in primary care. *The Cochrane Database of Systematic Reviews*(1).

Lave, J., & Wenger, E. (1991). *Situated learning: Legitimate peripheral participation.* Cambridge, M.A: Cambridge University Press.

Lavin, M. A., Avant, K., Craft-Rosenberg, M., Herdman, T. H., & Gebbie, K. (2004). Contexts for the study of economic influence of nursing diagnoses on patient outcomes. *International Journal of Nursing Terminologies and Classifications, 15*(2), 39-47.

Lawrence, P., & Lorsch, J. W. (1967). *Organizations and environment.* Boston: Division of Research, Graduate School of Business Administration, Harvard University.

Lawton, M. P., & Brody, E. M. (1969). Assessment of older people: self-maintaining and instrumental activities of daily living. *Gerontologist, 9*(3), 179-86.

Lee, J., Carter-Wells, J., Glaeser, B., Ivers, K., & Street, C. (2006). Facilitating the development of a learning community in an online graduate program. *The Quarterly Review of Distance Education, 7*(1), 13-33.

Lee, M., Delaney, C., & Moorhead, S. (2007). Building a personal health record from a nursing perspective. *International Journal of Medical Informatics, 76*, S308-S316.

Lee, T. T. (2006). Nurses' perceptions of adopting a PDA system--application of Lewin's change theory. *Studies in Health Technology and Informatics, 122*, 958.

Lee, T. T. (2007). Patients' perceptions of nurses' bedside use of PDAs. *Computer Informatics Nursing, 25*(2), 106-11.

Lee, Y., & Nguyen, H. (2007). Get your degree from an educational ATM: An empirical study in online education. *International Journal on E-Learning, 6*(1), 31-40.

Lehman, K. (2003). Clinical nursing instructors' use of handheld computers for student record keeping and evaluation. *Journal of Nursing Education, 42*(1), 41-42.

Leininger, M., & McFarland, M. M. (2006). Culture Care Diversity and Universality: A Worldwide Nursing Theory. Sudbury: Jones and Barlett publishers.

Lemieux-Charles, L., & McGuire, W. L. (2006). What do we know about health care team effectiveness? A review of the literature. *Medical Care Research and Review, 63*(3), 263-300.

Levitt, P., & Nyberg-Sorenson, N. (2004). *The transnational turn in migration studies.* Global Commission on International Migration: Global Migration Perspectives, No. 6.

Lewis, A. (2001). Handheld technology: The newest practice tool for nurses? Online *Journal of Nursing Informatics.* Retrieved February 19, 2007 from http://www.hhdev.psu.edu/nurs/ojni/handheld_technology.htm

Lewis, A. (2001). Handheld technology: The newest practice tool for nurses? Online *Journal of Nursing Informatics.* Retrieved February 19, 2007 from http://www.hhdev.psu.edu/nurs/ojni/handheld_technology.htm

Liber, O. (2005). Learning objects: Conditions for viability. *Journal of Computer Assisted Learning, 21*, 366-373.

Lindberg, D. A. B., & Humphreys, B. L. (2005). 2015 - the future of medical libraries. *New England Journal of Medicine, 352*(11), 1067-1070.

Lindsay, C. (2001). PDAs give nurses more time. *Nurse Week*, August 8, 2001.

Lister, P. (1997). The art of nursing in a 'postmodern' context. *Journal of Advanced Nursing, 25*, 38 - 44.

Lister, P. (1999). A taxonomy for developing cultural competence. *Nurse Education Today, 19*, 313 - 318.

Littlejohns, P., Wyatt, J. C., & Garvican, L. (2003). Evaluating computerised health information systems: Hard lessons still to be learnt. *BMJ: British Medical Journa,* (326), 860-863.

Liu, J., Wyatt, J., & Altman, D. G. (2006). Decision tools in health care: Focus on the problem, not the solution. *BMC Medical Informatics and Decision Making, 6*(4).

Liu, X., Magjuka, R. J., Bonk, C. J., & Lee, S. (2007). Does sense of community matter? An examination of participants' perception of building learning communities in online courses. *The Quarterly Review of Distance Education, 8*(1), 9-24.

Lofstrom, E, & Nevgi, A. (2007). From strategic planning to meaningful learning: diverse perspectives on the development of web-based teaching and learning in higher education. *British Journal of Education Technology, 38*(2), 312-324.

Lohrmann, C. (2004). Die Pflegeabhängigkeitsskala. In: Bartholomeyczik S., Halek S. (2004): Assessmentinstrumente in der Pflege. *Hannover, Schlütersche*, 55-60.

Lohrmann, C., & Dijkstra, D. T. (2003). The Care Dependency Scale An Assessment Instrument for Elderly Patients in German Hospitals. *Geriatr Nurs, 24*, 40-3.

Lorenzi, N. M. (2004). Beyond the gadgets: Non-technological barriers to information systems need to be overcome too. *BMJ, 328*, 1146-1147.

Lowndes, V., & Skelcher, C. (1998). The Dynamics of Multi-Organizational Partnerships: An Analysis of Changing Modes of Governance. *Public Administration, 76*, 313 – 33.

Lynch, K. (2006). Readiness to Communicate in a Digital World. *Issues in Informing Science and Information Technology, 3*.

Maag, M. (2006). Nursing students' attitudes toward technology: A national study. *Nurse Educator, 31*(3), 112-118.

Maat, M. B. (1997). A group Art Therapy Experience for Immigrant Adolescents. *American Journal of Arts Therapy, 36*, 11-19.

Macdonald, I. J. (2003). Immigrant and Refugee Community Organization: Project interwoven tapestry. *Paper presented at the Annual meeting of the Society for Applied Anthropology*, Portland Oregon.

Macpherson, D. W. (1993). Immigrant health issues: assessment guidelines for the Physician. *Can J Contin Med Education,* (5) 59-66.

Magruder,C., Burke, C., Hann, N., and Ludovic, J., (2005) Using information technology to improve the public health system. *Journal of Public Health Management Practice, 11*(2), 123-130.

Mahoney, F. I., & Barthel, D. W. (1965). Functional Evaluation. The Barthel Index. *MD State Med J, 14*, 61-65.

Malizia, P. (1993). *Parola e sistema: saggio su comunicazione ed organizzazione.* Roma: Bulzoni Editore.

Mancuso-Murphy, J. (2007). Distance education in nursing: An integrated review of online nursing students' experiences with technology-delivered instruction. *Journal of Nursing Education, 46*(6), 252-261.

Manfredi, M. (1993). The development of nursing in Latin America: A strategic view. *Review Latin American Enfermagem, 1(1)*, 23-35.

March, J. G., & Simon, H. A. (1958). *Organizations.* New York: John Wiley & Son.

Marklund, B., Ström, M., Månsson, J., Borgquist, L., Baigi, A., & Fridlund, B. (2007). Computersupported telephone nurse triage: An evaluation of medical quality and costs. *J Nurs Manag., 15*(2),180–7.

Marks-Maran & Rose, D. (1999). Reconstructing nursing: evidence, artistry and the curriculum. *Nurse Education Today, 19*, 668 - 672.

Marks-Maran, D., & Rose P. (1997). *Reconstructing nursing: beyond art and science.* London: Bailliere Tindall and RCN.

Marmot, M., & Wilkinson, R. (Eds.). (1999). *Social determinants of health.* Oxford OX2: Oxford University Press.

Martin, K., & Scheet, N. (1992). *The Omaha System: Applications for community health nursing and The Omaha System: A pocket guide for community health nursing.* Philadelphia: Saunders.

Martin, S. (2003). News: Pulse. *Canadian Medical Association Journal, 169 (9).* Retrieved February 5, 2004 from http://www.cmaj.ca/cgi/content/full/169/9/952a

Marton, F., & Saljo, R. (1996). *Approaches to learning.* In: Marton, F.D., Hounsell, J. & Entwistle, N. J. (Eds), *The experience of learning.* (Second edition). Edinburgh: Scottish Academic Press.

Mason, R., Pegler, C., & Weller, M. (2004). E-portfolios: an assessment tool for online courses. *British Journal of Educational Technology, 35*(6), 717–727.

Massaro, T. A. (1993). Introducing physician order entry at a major academic medical centre: Impact on organizational culture and behaviour. *Academic Medicine, 68*(1), 20-30.

Masys, D. R., Brennan, P. F., Ozbolt, J. G., Corn, M., & Shortliffe, E. H. (2000). Are Medical Informatics and Nursing Informatics Distinct Disciplines? The 1999 ACMI Debate. *Journal American Medical Informatics Association,* (7), 304-312.

Matveev, N. V. Automatic color correction of digital skin images in teledermatology. (2006). *J Telemed and Telecare, 12*(Suppl. 3), 62-63.

Mayer H., Nonn C., Osterbrink J., & Evers G. (2004). Qualitätskriterien von Assessmentinstrumenten – Cohen's Kappa als Maß der Interrater – Reliabilität (Teil 1). *Pflege, 17,* 36-46.

McCallum, J. (2007). The debate in favour of using simulation education in pre-registration adult nursing. *Nurse Education Today, 27,* 825-831.

McCartney, P. R. (2007). Nursing informatics then and now. Keeping readers "Plugged in". *The Association of Women's Health, Obstetric and Neonatal Nurses, 11*(1), 80-82.

McCord, L. (2003). Using a personal digital assistant to streamline the OR workload. *Association of Perioperative Registerered Nurses Journal,* 78(6):996-1001.

McCormick, K. A., Delaney, C. J., Brennan, P. F., Effken, J. A., Kendrick, K., Murphy, J., et al. (2007). Guideposts to the Future-An Agenda for Nursing Informatics. *Journal of the American Medical Informatics Association, 14,* 19-24.

McCormick, K., Delaney, C., Brennan, P., Effken, J., Kendrick, K., Murphy, J., Skiba, D., Warren, J., Weaver, C., Weiner, B., & Westra, B. (2007) Guideposts to the Future—An Agenda for Nursing Informatics. *Journal of the American Medical Informatics Association, 14*(1), 19-24.

McGee, M. (2007, May 28). Urgent care. *Information Week, 140*(1), 40-50.

McGill, T. J., & Hobbs, V. J. (2007). (In press). How students and instructors using a virtual learning environment perceive the fit between technology and task. *Journal of Computer Assisted Learning.*

McKesson Corporate: Healthcare Providers (2008). Retrieved May 25, 2008, from http://www.mckesson.com/en_us/McKesson.com/For+Healthcare+Providers/Home+Care/Telehealth+Solutions/McKesson+Telehealth+Advisor+Components/Health+Buddy+Appliance.html

McLaughlin, C. P., & Kaluzny, A. D. (2006). *Continuous quality improvement in health care: Theory, implementations and applications* (3rd ed.). Toronto: Jones and Bartlett.

McMurray, A., Gilbert, C., Reis, B., Chueh, H., Kohane, I., & Mandl, K. (2007). A self-scaling, distributed information architecture for public health, research and clinical care. *Journal of the American Informatics Association, 14*(4), 527-533.

McNeil, B. J., Elfrink V., Beyea S. C., Pierce S. T., & Bickford C. J. (2006). Computer Literacy Study: Report of Qualitative Findings. *J Prof Nurs. 22*(1), 52–9.

McNeil, B., Elfrink, V., Beyea, S., Pierce, S., & Bickford, C. (2006). Computer literacy study: report of qualitative findings. *Journal of Professional Nursing, 22*(1), 52-59.

McNeil, B.J., Elfrink, V.L., Bickword,C.J., Peirce, S.T., Beyea, S.C., Averill, C., et al. (20030. Nursing information technology knowledge, skills and, and preparation of student nurses, nursing faculty and clinicians. A U.S. survey. *Journal of Nursing Education, 42*,341-349.

Melton, G. B., Parsons, S., Morrison, F. P., Rothschild, A. S., Markatou, M., & Hripcsak, G. (2006). Inter-patient distance metrics using SNOMED CT defining relationships. *Journal of Biomedical Informatics, 39*, 6, 697-705.

Mendes, I. A. C., & Marziale, M. H. (2008). Shortage of qualified health workers: a call to action for nurses. *Rev Latino-Am Enfermagem., 2*(16), 173-4.

Merriam-Webster online dictionary. (2007). Retrieved November 18, 2007 from http://dictionary.reference.com/browse/relationship

Miller, A. (2004). A work domain analysis framework for modelling intensive care unit patients. *Cognition, Technology, and Work, 6*, 207-222.

Miller, G. A. (1956). The magic number seven plus or minus two: Some limits of our capacity for information processing. *Psychological Review, 63*(2), 87-87.

Miller, J. (2003). *Doctors say PDAs improves [sic] medical care*. Retrieved on October 22, 2005 from Rim Road: News at http://www.rimroad.com

Miller, J., Shaw-Kokot, J. R., Arnold, M. S., Boggin, T., Crowell, K. E., Allegri, F., Blue, J. H., & Berrier, S. B. (2005). A study of personal digital assistants to enhance undergraduate clinical nursing education. *Journal of Nursing Education, 44*(1).

Miller, J., Shaw-Kokot, J. R., Crowell, K. E., Allegri, F., Arnold, M. S., Blue, J. H., Boggin, T., Koyanagi, M., Berrier, S. B., & Sommers, H. (2005). A study of personal digital assistants to enhance undergraduate clinical nursing education. *Journal of Nursing Education, 44(1)*, 19-26.

Mintzberg, H. (1983). An emerging strategy of 'direct' research. In Van Maanen J. (Ed.), *Qualitative methodology.* Beverly Hills, CA: Sage.

Moher, D., Schulz, K., & Altman, D. (2001). Revised recommendations for improving the quality of reports of parallel group randmoized trials. *Annals of Internal Medicine, 134*(8), 657-662.

Mold, J. W., & Peterson, K. A. (2005). Primary care practice-based research networks: Working at the interface between research and quality improvement. *Annals of Family Medicine, 3*(1), 12-20.

Moo, S., & Fletcher, J. (2007). Northern Territory HealthConnect: Shared electronic health record service implementation experiences and benefits realised in indigenous health. *Medinfo, 12*(1), 297-301.

Moore, P., & Hart, L. (2004). Strategies for teaching nursing research online. *International Nursing Review, 51,* 123-128.

Moore, R. S., Britton, B. & Chetney, R. (2005). Wound care using interactive telehealth. *Home Health Care Manage Pract, 17*(3), 203-12.

Morgan, J., Rawlinson, M., & Weaver, M. (2006). Facilitating online reflective learning for health and social care professionals. *Open Learning, 21*(2), 167-176.

Morgan, R. (2006). Using clinical skills laboratories to promote theory–practice integration during first practice placement: an Irish perspective. *Journal of Clinical Nursing, 15*, 155-161.

Morgans, A., Archer, F., Walker, T., & Thuma, E. (2005). Barriers to accessing ambulance services in rural Victoria for acute asthma: Patients' and medical professionals' perspectives. *Australian Journal of Rural Health, 13*(2), 116-120.

Morieson, B. (2003). *Secretary of the Victorian Branch of the Australian Nursing Federation.* Personal Interview. South Melbourne.

Morrison, J. C., & Chauhan, S. P. (2003). Current status of home uterine activity monitoring. Clinics in Perinatology, *30*, 751-80.

Mueller, C. (2001). Masters in nursing students' experiences as a member of a virtual classroom on the Internet. *Dissertation Abstracts International, 62*(08), 3557B.

Mullan, B., Snyder, M., Lindgren, B., Finkelstein, S. M., & Hertz, M. I. (2003). Home monitoring for lung transplant candidates. *Prog Transplant, 13*(3), 176-82.

Mullen, P. (2007, June). A conservation with Jonathan Weiner, DrPH: Mixing population-based care with market controls. *Managed Care*, *16*(6), 1-7. Retrieved August 8, 2007, from http://www.managedcaremag.comarchives/0706/0706.qna_weiner.html

Müller-Staub, M., Needham, I., Odenbreit, M., Lavin, M.A., & van Achterberg, T. (2007). Improved Quality of Nursing Documentation: Results of a Nursing Diagnosis, Interventions, an Outcomes Implementation Study. International *Journal of Nursing Technologies and Classifications, 18*, 1, 5-17.

Mumford, E. (1983). *Designing Human Systems for New Technology - The ETHICS Method,*

Mumford, E. (1996). *Systems Design Ethical Tools for Ethical Change*, Macmillan.

Murray, V. (1997). Interorganizational Collaboration in the Non-Profit Sector. In Shafritz J. M. (Ed.), *International Encyclopaedia of Public Policy and Administration*, 2. Boulder, CO: Westview Press, 192 – 6.

Nagarajan, K. V. (2004). Rural and remote community health care in Canada: beyond the Kirby Panel Report, the Romanow Report and the federal budget of 2003. *Canadian Journal of Rural Medicine, 9*(4), 245-251.

Nagykaldi, Z., & Mold, J. W. (2007). The Role of Health Information Technology in the Translation of Research into Practice: An Oklahoma Physicians Resource/Research Network (OKPRN) Study. *The Journal of the American Board of Family Medicine, 20*(2), 188-195.

Narciss, S., Proske, A., & Körndle, H. (2007). Interactivity and learners' achievement in Web-based learning. *Journal of Interactive Learning Research, 18(*4), 511-532.

National Advisory Council on Nurse Education and Practice. (1997). *A National Informatics Agenda for Nursing Education and Practice: Report to the Secretary of Health and Human Services.* Rockville, MD: U.S. Department of Health and Human Services, Health Resources and Services Administration, Bureau of Health Professions, Division of Nursing.

National Health Expenditures Aggregate Amounts and Average Annual Percent. Retrieved October 15, 2007 from http://www.cms.hhs.gov/NationalHealthExpendData/downloads/tables.pdf

National nursing and nursing education taskforce. (2005). Maximising education pathways: Our Duty of Care - Recommendation 12. Retrieved January 5, 2008, from http://www.nnnet.gov.au/work/rec12.htm

National Office of Public Health Genomics [CDC] (2007). Retrieved August 10, 2007, from http://www.cdc.gov/genomics/activities.htm

Natriello, G. (2005) Modest Changes, Revolutionary Possibilities: Distance Learning and the Future of Education. *Teachers College Record, 107*(8), 1885-1904.

Nelson, L. Sadler, L., & Surtees, G. (2005). Bringing problem based learning to life using virtual reality. *Nurse Education in Practice*, *5*, 103-108.

Nemeth, C., Nunnally, M., Connor, M. O., Klock, P. A., & Cook, R. (2005). Getting to the point: developing IT for the sharp end of healthcare. *J. of Biomedical Informatics, 38*(1), 18-25.

Netting the Evidence (2007). Retrieved August 19, 2007, from http://www.shef.ac.uk/=scharr/ir/netting/

Nevárez, J. (2008). *The Reversal of Technology.* In Kidd, T., Chen, I. (Eds.) *Social Information Technology Connecting Society and Cultural Issues.* IGI Global.

Nightingale, F. (1992). *Notes on nursing: What it is, and what it is not.* London: Harris. (original work published in 1959)

Niland, J. C., Rouse, L., & Stahl, D. C., (2006). An Informatics Blueprint for Healthcare Quality Information Systems. *Journal of the American Medical Informatics Association, 13*(4), 402–417.

Norredam, M., Mygind, A., Nielsen, S. N, Bagger, J., & Krasnik, A. (2007). Motivation and relevance of emergency room visits among immigrants and patients of Danish origin. *The European Journal of Public Health* 2007, *17*(5), 497-502.

North America Nursing Diagnosis Association-International (NANDA-I) (2007-2008). *Nursing diagnosis: Definitions and classifications.* Philadelphia: NANDA.

North American Nursing Diagnosis Association (NANDA) (1990). *Definition of Nursing Diagnosis.* http://www.enotes.com/nursing-encyclopedia/nursing-diagnosis (28.05.2008).

Numerof, R., Abrams, M., & Ott, B., (2004). Building a nursing leadership infrastructure. *Nurse Leader, 2*(1), 33-37.

Nursing, PDA, Listserv, & Survey. (2004). Retrieved 15 November, 2007, from http://www.perseus.com/cgi-bin/survsol40.pl.

O'Cathain, A., Sampson, F. C., Munro, J. F., Thomas, K. J., & Nicholl, J. P. (2004). Nurses' views of using computerized decision support software in NHS Direct. *Journal of Advanced Nursing, 45*(3), 280-286.

O'Neil, E., & Krauel, P. (2004). Building transformational partnerships in nursing *Journal of Professional Nursing, 20*(5), 295-299.

OECD (1999). *Trends in International Migration*, Australian Department of Immigration and Multicultural Affairs (DIMA), Citizenship and Immigration Canada, New Zealand Immigration Service, U.S. Immigration and Naturalization Service, European Migration Centre (EMZ).

Olade, R. (2004). Evidence-based practice and research utilization activities among rural nurses. *J Nurs Scholarsh, 36*(3), 220-225.

Olsen, R. (2007). *Design Patterns in Ruby*, Addison-Wesley, Chapter 16.

Orleans, C., Schoenbach, V., Wagner, E., Quade, D., Salmon, M., Pearson, D., et al. (1991). Self-help quit smoking interventions: effects of self-help materials, social support instructions, and telephone counselling. *J Consult Clin Psychol, 59*(3), 439-448.

Orlikowski W. J. (1991). Integrated information environment or matrix of control? The contradictory implications of information technology. *Accounting, Management, and Information Technology, 1*(1), 9 – 42.

Orlikowski, W. J. (1992). The duality of technology: Rethinking the concept of technology in organizations. *Organizational Science, 3*(3), 398-427.

Orlikowski, W. J., & Gash, D. C. (1994). Technological Frames: Making Sense of Information Technology in Organization. *ACM Transactions on Information Systems, 12*(2), 174-207.

Orlikowski, W. J., & Robey, D. (1991). Information Technology and the Structuring of Organizations. *Information Systems Research, 2*(2).

Ornes, L., & Gassert, C. (2007). Computer competencies in a BSN program. *J Nurs Educ, 46*(2), 75-78.

Orr, L. V. (n.d.) *Computer anxiety: University of Southern Main, Communication 499.* Retrieved on January 26, 2004 from http://www.usm.maine.edu/~com/lindap~1.htm

Otieno, O.G., Toyama, H., Asonuma, M., Kanai-Pak, M., & Naitoh, K. (2007). Nurses' views on the use, quality and user satisfaction with electronic medical records: questionnaire development. *Journal of Advanced Nursing, 60*(2), 209-219.

Ouchi, W. G. (1980) Markets, Bureaucracies, and Clans. *Administrative Science Quarterly, 25*(1), 129 – 141.

Ouzts, K. (2006). Sense of community in online courses. *The Quarterly Review of Distance Education, 7*(3), 285-296. Retrieved November 2, 2007 from http://0-web.ebscohost.com.aupac.lib.athabascau.ca/ehost/pdf?vid=3&hid=104&sid=b8254076-4ede-4f7c-9949-46a8720b2147%40sessionmgr107

Pan American Health Organization. (1999). *Setting up healthcare services information systems: A guide for requirement analysis, application specification, and procurement.* Washington, DC: Essential Drugs and Technology Program, Division of Health systems and Services Development. PAHA/WHO.

Pan American Health Organization. (2004). *Nursing and Midwifery Services Contributing to Equity, Access, Coverage, Quality, and Sustainability in the Health Services.* Washington, DC: Health Services Organization (OS) - Technology and Health Services Delivery (THS).

Parker, E. B., & Howland, L. C. (2006). Strategies to manage the time demands of online teaching. *Nurse Educator, 31*(6), 270-274.

Parrish, M. (1997). Medical advice is available for ships at sea. *BMJ. 315*(7114), 1020.

Parsons T. (1951). *The Social System.* Glencoe, IL: Free Press.

Patel, V. L., Kushniruk, A. W., Yang, S., & Yale, J-F. (2001). Impact of a computer-based patient record system on data collection, knowledge organization, and reasoning. *JAMIA, 7*(6), 569-585.

Patterson, E. S., Nguyen, A. D., Halloran, J. P., & Asch, S. M. (2004). Human Factors Barriers to the Effective Use of Ten HIV Clinical Reminders. *J Am Med Inform Assoc, 11*, 50-59.

Patterson, E. S., Rogers, M. L., Chapman, R. J., & Render, M. L. (2002). Improving patient safety by identifying side effects from introducing bar coding in medication administration. *JAMIA, 9*, 540-553.

Patton, R. (2001). *Software testing.* SAMS: Indianapolis, Indiana.

PDA Cortex. (2004). *Analysis of PDAs in nursing: benefits and barriers.* Available at: http://pdacortex.com/Analysis_PDAs_Nursing.htm

PDA Cortex.com (2002). First hand intelligence. *Journal of Mobile Informatics.* Retrieved November 13, 2005 from http://www.pdacortex.com

PDA Cortex.com (2003). *Adopting mobile technology to enhance patient care.* Retrieved on October 22, 2005 from http://www.pdacortex.com/issues_and_attitudes.htm

Pearsall, J., et al. (Eds.) (1998). The New Oxford Dictionary of English, OUP. p. 468.

Peltu, M., Eason, K., & Clegg, C. (2008). How a Socio-technical approach can help NPfIT deliver better NHS patient care, Report produced following BCS Workshop 7 February 2008. Retrieved 8 June 2008, from http://www.bcs.org/server.php?show=nav.9932

Pelz, B. (2004). Three principles of effective online pedagogy. *Journal of Asynchronous Learning Networks, 8*(3), 33-46.

Penley, L. E. (1982). An investigation of the information processing framework of organizational communication. *Human Communication Research, 8*(4), 348-365.

Perlin, J. B., Kolodner, R. M., & Roswell, R. H. (2004). The Veterans Health Administration: quality, value, accountability, and information as transforming strategies for patient-centered care. *The American journal of managed care, 10*(11), 828-836.

Perry, B., & Edwards, M. (2005). Exemplary online educators: Creating a community of inquiry. *Turkish Online Journal of Distance Education, 6(2),* Retrieved October 6, 2007 from http://tojde.anadolu.edu.tr/tojde18/articles/article6.htm.

Peterson, M. (2004). PDA and its future in nursing. *Kansas Nurse*, October.

Petraglia, J. (1998). The real world on a short leash: The (mis)application of constructivism to the design of educational technology. *Educational Technology Research and Development, 46*(3), 53-65.

Petrucka, P., Bassendowski, S., & James, T. (2007). The role of ICTs in enhancing diasporic citizenry and connectedness: A Caribbean exemplar. *The International Journal of Technology, Knowledge and Society, 2(7)*, 43-48.

Piaget, J. (1967). *Logique et Connaissance scientifique.* Paris: Gallimard.

Picone, D., Phillips, K., Hathaway, V., & Parkes, R. (1993). *National nursing service weight study.* Canberra, Commonwealth Department of Human Services and Health, Casemix Development Program.

Pinsonneault, A., & Kraemer, K. L. (1997). Information Technology and Middle Management Downsizing: A Tale of Two Cities, CRITO Working Paper URB-115, 4/16/97. Retrieved June 8, 2008 from http://repositories.cdlib.org/cgi/viewcontent.cgi?article=1090&context=crito

Plummer, V. (2005). *An analysis of patient dependency data utilizing the TrendCare system.* Monash university, Melbourne, Australia

Ponce, N. A., Hays, R. D., & Cunningham, E. W. (2006). Linguistic Disparities in Health Care Access and Health Status among Older Adults. *Journal of General Internal Medicine, 21*(7), 786–791.

Population Estimates Program, Bureau of the Census, Department of Commerce, Washington, DC, May 2006

Portes, A., & Rumbaut, R. G. (1996). Immigrant America, Berkeley, CA: University of California –Press.

Prado, M., J. Reina-Tosina, and L. Roa (2002). Distributed intelligent architecture for falling detection and physical activity analysis in the elderly. In: *Proceeding of the Second Joint EMBS/BMES Conference, 3*, 1910–1911.

Prandelli, E., & Verona, G. (2006). *Marketing in rete 2/ed - Oltre Internet verso il nuovo Marketing.* Milano: McGraw-Hill.

Preece, J., Sharp, H., Benyon, D., Holland, S., & Carey, T. (1994). *Human-computer interaction.* Toronto: Addison-Wesley.

Priest, H., Roberts, P., & Woods, L. (2003). An overview of three different approaches to the interpretation of qualitative data. Part 1: Theoretical issues. *Nurse Researcher, 10*(1), 30-43. Retrieved November 3, 2007 from http://www.nursing-standard.co.uk/nurseresearcher-archive/nr_archive/nrv10n1-2002/nrv10n1p4351.pdf

Primo Braga, C. A., Daly, J., and Sareen, B. (2003). The Future of Information and Communication Technologies for Development. *Paper presented at the Information and Communications Technology Development Forum*, Petersburg, Germany, May 21.

Public Health Informatics Institute (2006). *Common ground: Transforming public health information systems* (2006, August 1). Retrieved September 10, 2007, from http://commongroundprogram.org/

Public Health Informatics Institute (2006). *Taking care of business: A collaboration to define local health department business processes.* Decatur: GA: Public Health Institute.

Putnam, L. L., Phillips, N., & Chapman, P. (1996). Metaphors of Communication and Organization. In Clegg, S. R., Hardy, C. & Nord W. (Eds.), *Handbook of Organizational Studies.* London: Sage.

Rafnsson, S. B., & Bhopal, R. J. (2008, May). *Public Health, 122(5), 532-534.*

Ragin, C. C. (1994). *Constructing Social Research: The Unity and Diversity of Method*, Pine Forge Press.

Raider-Roth, M. (2004). Taking the time to think: A portrait of reflection. *Teaching and Learning, 18*(5), 79-97.

Raider-Roth, M. (2005). *Trusting what you know: The high stakes of classroom relationships.* San Francisco: Jossey-Bass.

Randell, R., Mitchell, N., Dowding, D., Cullum, N., & Thompson, C. (2007). Effects of computerized decision support systems on nursing performance and patient outcomes. *Journal of Health Services Research and Policy, 12*(4), 242-249.

Randell, R., Mitchell, N., Thompson, C., McCaughan, D., & Dowding, D. (In press-a). From pull to push: Understanding nurses' information needs *Health Informatics Journal.*

Randell, R., Mitchell, N., Thompson, C., McCaughan, D., & Dowding, D. (In press-b). Supporting nurse decision making in primary care: exploring use of and attitude to decision tools *Health Informatics Journal.*

Raskin J. D. (2002). Constructivism in psychology: Personal construct psychology, radical constructivism, and social constructionism. In Raskin J. D. and Bridges S. K. (Eds.), *Studies in meaning: Exploring constructivist psychology.* New York: Pace University Press, 1 – 25.

Rasmussen, J., Pejtersen, A. M., & Goodstein, L. P (1994). *Cognitive Systems Engineering.* New York: Wiley.

Reed K. Telemedicine: Benefits to Advanced Practice Nursing and the Communities They Serve. *J Am Acad Nurse Pract., 17*(5), 176-80.

Reed, K. (2005). Telemedicine: Benefits to advanced practice nursing and the communities they serve. *Clinical Practice.* 17(5), 176-180.

Refugee and Immigrant Service Center (1995). *Working Effectively with Interpreters: A Guide for Service Providers.* Olympia, W.A.

Reinhard, S.C., & Moulton, P.J. (1995). Integrating informatics into the graduate community health nursing curriculum. *Public Health Nursing, 12*(3), 151-158.

Repique, R. J. R. (2007). Computers and information technologies in psychiatric nursing. *Perspectives in Psychiatric Care, 43*(2), 77-83.

Resnick, L. B. (1987). Learning in school and out. The 1987 AERA Presidential address. *Educational Researcher, 16*, 13 - 20.

Rialle, V. Rumeau, P, Ollivet, C. & Hervé, C. (2006). Smart homes. In Wootton R, Kvedar J & Dimmick SL. *Home Telehealth: Connecting care within community,* 65-75. RSM, London,

Rice, M. J. (2003). *Bridging the Digital Divide in Medically Underserved Areas with PDAs.* Retrieved May 3, 2005, from www.pdacortex.com/rural_pdas.htm

Rice, M. J. (2003). Bridging the digital divide in medically underserved areas with PDAs [Electronic Version]. Retrieved June 10, 2008, from http://www.pdacortex.com/rural_pdas.htm.

Richards, D., Godfrey, L., Tawfik, J., Ryan, M., Meakins, J., Dutton, E., et al. (2004). Direct versus general practice based triage for same day appointments in primary care: Cluster randomised controlled trial. *British Medical Journal, 329*, 774.

Richardson, G., & Maynard, A. (1995). Fewer doctors? More nurses? A review of the knowledge base of doctor-nurse substitution. 135. from http://ideas.repec.org/p/chy/respap/dp135.html

Richardson, J., & Swan, K. (2003). Examining social presence in online courses in relation to students' perceived learning and satisfaction. *Journal of Asynchronous Learning Networks,*7(1), 68-88. Retrieved October 5, 2007 from http://www.sloan-c.org/publications/jaln/v7n1/pdf/v7n1_richardson.pdf

Ricketts, S., Gesler, W. & Osborne, D. (Eds.). (1994). *Geographic methods for health services research. A focus on the rural-urban continuum.* Maryland: United Press of *America, Inc.*

Rinehart, J. (1999). Turning theory into theorizing: Collaborative learning in a sociological theory course. *Teaching Sociology, 27*(3), 216-233.

Robbins, D. & Brill, J. (2005, May-June). *Blending ethics and empowerment with consumer-driven healthcare.* Patient Safety & Quality Healthcare. Retrieved August 4, 2007, from http://www.psqh.com/mayjun05/ethics.html

Robert Wood Johnson Foundation. (2007). *Improving the health & healthcare of all Americans Project.* Retreived from http://www.rwjf.org/programareas//resources/product.jsp?id=21131&pid=1140&gsa=pa1140

Robley, L., Farnsworth, B., Flynn, J., & Horne, C. (2004). This new house: Building knowledge through online learning. *Journal of Professional Nursing, 20*, 333-343.

Rogers, C. (2002). Seeing student learning: Teach change and the role of reflection. *Harvard Educational Review, 72*(2), 230-255.

Rogerson, E. (2003). *The role and facilitation of problem-based learning in a distance learning programme leading to the award of Bachelor of Nursing.* Thesis presented for the degree of Doctor of Philosophy, University of Dundee Scotland.

Rogerson, E., & Harden, R. M. (1999). Seven Years On: Distance learning courses for first level nurses and midwives. *Nurse Education Today, 19*, 286 - 294.

Rolfe, G. (1999). The pleasure of the bottomless: post-modernism, chaos and paradigm shifts. *Nurse Education Today, 19*, 668 - 672.

Romano C. (2006). Informatics is on the national agenda and nurses need to be informed and involved. *Nurs Outlook., 54*(5), 303-5.

Ronaldson, S. (2004). Untangling critical thinking in educational cyberspace. Unpublished doctoral dissertation. The University of British Columbia, Canada.

Rood, E., Bosnan, R., van der Spoel, J., Taylor, P., & Zandstra, D. (2005). Use of a computerized guideline for glucose regulation in the intensive care unit improved both guideline adherence and glucose regulation. *Journal of the American Informatics Association, 12*(2), 172-180.

Rorty R. (1980). *Philosophy and the Mirror of Nature.* Princeton: Princeton UniversityPress.

Rosen, R., & Mountford, L. (2002). Developing and supporting extended nursing roles: the challenges of NHS walk-in centres. *Journal of Advanced Nursing, 39*(3), 241-248.

Rosenzweig, M. R., & Wolpin, K. I. (1994). Are there increasing returns to the intergenerational production of human capital? Maternal schooling and child intellectual achievement. *Journal of Human Resources 29 (2),* 670–93.

Rourke, G, Garrison, D., Anderson, T., & Archer, W. (2001). Critical thinking, cognitive presence, and computer conferencing in distance education. *American Journal of Distance Education, 15*(1).

Rourke, G., Garrison, D., Anderson, T., & Archer, W. (2000). Critical inquiry in a text-based environment: Computer conferencing in higher education. *The Internet and Higher Education, 2*(2-3), 87-105.

Rovai, A. (2002). Building sense of community at a distance. *International Review of Research in Open and Distance Learning, 3*(1). Retrieved October 4, 2007 from http://www.irrodl.org/index.php/irrodl/article/viewFile/79/153

Rowntree, D. (1996). *Exploring open and distance learning.* The Open University. London: Kogan Page.

Ruland, C. M. (2002). Handheld technology to improve patient care: Evaluating a support system for preference-based care planning at the bedside. *Journal of the American Medical Informatics Association, 9(2)*, 192-201.

Ruland, C. M. (2002). Handheld technology to improve patient care: Evaluating a support system for preference-based care planning at the bedside. *Journal of the American Medical Informatics Association, 9*(2), 192-201.

Ryan, M., Carlton, K. H., & Ali, N. S. (2004). Reflections on the role of faculty in distance learning and changing pedagogies. *Nursing Education Perspectives, 25*(2), 73-80.

Ryan, M., Hodson-Carlton, K., & Ali, A. S. (2005). A model for faculty teaching online: Confirmation of a dimensional matrix. *Journal of Nursing Education, 44*(8), 357-365.

Ryan, P., Kobb, R., & Hilsen, P. (2003). Making the right connection: matching patients to technology. *Telemed J E Health, 9*, 81-8.

Saba, V. (2006). *Clinical care classification (CCC) system manual. A guide to nursing documentation.* New York: Springer Publishing.

Saba. V. (1991). *Home health care classification project.* Washington, D.C.: Georgetown University (NTIS Pub. #PB92-177013/AS).

Sackett D.L. et al. (1996). Evidence based medicine: what it is and what it isn't. *BMJ, 312*(7023), 71-72.

Salafsky, B., Glasser, M., & Ha, J. (2005). Addressing issues of maldistribution of health care workers. *Annals of the Academy of Medicine, 34*(8), 520-525.

Saleem, J. J., Patterson, E. S., Militello, L., Render, M. L., Orshansky, G., & Asch, S. M. (2005). Exploring Barriers and Facilitators to the Use of Computerized Clinical Reminders. *JAMIA, 12*, 438-447.

Salisbury, C., Chalder, M., Scott, T. M., Pope, C., & Moore, L. (2002). What is the role of walk-in centres in the NHS? *BMJ, 324*, 399-402.

Salmon G. (2004). *E-moderating: the key to teaching and learning online* (2nd edition) London: Routledge-Falmer.

Salmon, G. (2005). Flying not flapping: a strategic framework for e-learning and pedagogical innovation in higher education institutions. *ALT-J, Research in Learning Technology, 13*(3), 201-218.

Sapolsky, R. (2005). Sick of poverty. *Scientific American, 293(6)92-99.* NewYork: Scientific American, Inc.

Saranto, K., & H., L.-K. (1997). Computer literacy in nursing: developing the information technology syllabus in nursing education. *Journal of Advanced Nursing, 25*(2), 377-385.

Saranto, K., & Hovenga, E.J. (2004). Information literacy-what it is about?; Literature review of the concept and the context. *International Journal of Medical Informatics, 73*(6), 503-13.

Saranto, K., & Leino-Kilpi, H. (1997). Computer literacy in nursing: developing the information technology syllabus in nursing education. *Journal of Advanced Nursing, 25*, 377-385.

Sarbaugh-Thompson M., & Feldman, M. S. (1998). Electronic Mail and Organizational Communication. *Organization Science*, *9*(6), 685 – 698.

Sastry, C.L.R. (2003). *India Health Care Project: An application of IT in rural health care at grass root level.* Retrieved March 12, 2007 from www.iimahd.ernet.in/egov/ifip/jun2003/article4.htm

Satellife. (2005). *Handhelds for health: Satellife's experience in Africa and Asia.* Ottawa, ON: IDRC.

Satzinger, J. W., & Orvik, T. U. (2001). *The object-oriented approach.* Thompson Learning: Canada.

Sauter, D., Abderhalden, C., Needham, I., & Wolff, S. (2006). *Lehrbuch psychiatrische Pflege*. Bern: Verlag Hans Huber.

Scalvini, S., Capomolla, S., Zanelli, E., Benigno, M., Domenighini, D., Paletta, L., et al. (2005). Effect of home-based telecardiology on chronic heart failure: costs and outcomes. *J Telemed Telecare, 11*(Suppl 1), 16-8.

Scardamalia, M. (2002). Collective cognitive responsibility for the advancement of knowledge. In B. Smith (Ed.), *Liberal education in a knowledge society* (pp. 76-98). Chicago: Open Court.

Scharff, R., & Dusek, V. (2002). *Philosophy of Technology: The Technological Condition - An Anthology.* Blackwell Philosophy Anthologies.

Schneider, A., Wilhelm, D., Bohn, U., Wichert, A., & Feussner, H. (2005). An evaluation of a surgical telepresence system for an intrahospital local area. *J Telemed Telecare, 11*(8), 408-413.

Scholes, M., & Barber, B. (1980). *Towards nursing informatics.* In Lindberg, D.A.D., & Kaihara, S. (Eds.) *MEDINFO: 1980.* Amsterdam, Netherlands: North-Holland, 7-73.

Schwirian, P., Malone, J., Stone, V., Nunley, B., & Francisco, T. (1989). Computers in nursing practice. A comparison of the attitudes of nurses and nursing students. *Computer Informatics Nursing, 7*(4), 168-177.

Scollin. P., Healey-Walsh. J., Kafel. K., Mehta. A., & Callahan. J. (2007). Evaluating students' attitudes to using PDAs in nursing clinicals at two schools, *Computers, Informatics, Nursing, 25*(4), 228-35.

Scuffham, P. (2006). Economic evaluation. In: Wootton R, Dimmick S, Kvedar J, editors. *Home telehealth: connecting care within the community.* London: Royal Society of Medicine Press Ltd, 21-35.

Seitzinger, J. (2006). *Be Constructive, Blogs, Podcasts, and Wikis as Constructivist Learning Tools.* Retrieved May 2, 2007 from http://www3.griffith.edu.au/03/ltn/docs/Design_Strategies.pdf

Serres, M. (1995). *Conversations on Science, Culture, and Time.* With Latour, B., University of Michigan Press.

Shea, P., Pickett, A., & Pelz, W. (2003). A follow-up investigation of "teaching presence" in the SUNY learning network. *Journal of Asynchronous Learning Networks*, 7(2), 61-80. Retrieved November 7, 2007 from http://www.aln.org/publications/jaln/v7n2/pdf/v7n2_shea.pdf

Shirey, M. (2006). Evidence-based practice: how nurse leaders can facilitate innovation. *Nurs Adm Q, 30*(3), 252-265.

Shortell, S. M., & Kaluzny, A. D. (2006). *Health care management: Organizational design and behaviour* (5th ed.). New York: Thompson.

Shortis, M., McGovern, J., Berry, M., & Farrell, M. J. (2006). Two case studies on the influence of mobile computing on student learning behaviour. *Proceedings of the 17th Annual Conference of the Australasian Association for Engineering Education: Creativity, Challenge, and Change- Partnerships in Engineering Education*, Auckland, New Zealand.

Shortliffe, E. H., & Cimino, J. J. (2006). *Biomedical informatics: Computer applications in health care and biomedicine*. New York: Springer Verlag.

Shulman, J., Lotan, J., & Whitcomb, J. (1998). *Groupwork in diverse classrooms: A casebook for educators*. New York: Teachers College.

Sibbald, B., Laurant, M. G., & Reeves, D. (2006). Advanced nurse roles in UK primary care. *The Medical Journal of Australia, 185*(1), 10-12.

Silberglitt, R., Anton, P.S., Howell, D.R., & Wong, A. (2006). *The Global Technology Revolution 2020*. Santa Monica, CA: RAND Corporation, National Security Research Division.

Simpson, G., & Kenrick, M. (1997). Nurses' Attitudes Toward Computerization in Clinical Practice in a British General Hospital. *Computers in Nursing, 15*(1), 37-42.

Simpson, R. L. (1959). Vertical and Horizontal Communication in Formal Organizations. *Administrative Science Quarterly*, *4*(2), 188 – 196.

Sit, J. Chung, J., Chow, C., & Wong, T. (2005). Experiences of online learning: Students' perspective. *Nurse Education Today, 25*, 140-147.

Skiba, D. (2006). The 2005 Word of the Year: Podcast. *Nursing Education Perspectives, 27* (1).

Skiba, D. (2007, November). Engaging students through on-line learning. Paper presented at the meeting of the American Association of Colleges of Nursing, Leadership Networks, New Orleans, LA.

Skiba, D. J. (2006). Web 2.0: Next Great Thing or Just Marketing Hype. *Nursing Education Perspectives, 27*(4), 212-214.

Slagter van Tryon, P.J. & Bishop, M.J. (2006). Identifying "E-mmediacy" strategies for web-based instruction: A Delphi study. *The Quarterly Review of Distance Education, 7*(1), 49-62.

Smedley, A. (2005). The importance of informatics competencies in nursing: an Australian perspective. *Computer Informatics Nursing, 23*(2), 106-110.

Smith K, Smith V, Krugman M, & K, O. (2005). Evaluating the impact of computerized clinical documentation. *Computer Information Nursing, 23*(3), 132-138.

Smith, A. C., Scuffham ,P. & Wootton, R. The costs and potential savings of a novel telepaediatric service in Queensland. *BMC Health Services Research* 2007, 7:35, available online at http://www.biomedcentral.com/1472-6963/7/35

Smith, E. L., Cronenwett, L., & Sherwood, G. (2007). Current assessments of quality and safety education in nursing. *Nursing Outlook, 55*(3), 132-7.

Smith-Stoner, M., & Willer, M. (2003). Video streaming in nursing education: Bringing life to online education. *Nurse Educator, 28*(2), 66-70.

Snow, C. P. (1959). *The Two Cultures*. Cambridge University Press. Reissued 1993.

Sovie, M. D. (1988). Variable costs of nursing care in hospitals. *Annual Review of Nursing Research, 6*, 131-150.

Speziale, H. J., & Jacobson, L. (2005). Trends in registered nurse education programs 1998-2008. *Nursing Education Perspectives*, *26*(4) 230-235.

Spouse, J. (1998a). Learning to nurse through legitimate peripheral participation. *Nurse Education Today, 18*, 35 - 39.

Spouse, J. (1998b). Scaffolding student learning in clinical practice. In Entwistle, N. J. (1995). Frameworks for understanding as experienced in essay writing and in preparing for examinations. *Educational Psychologist, 30*, 47 - 54.

Spradley, J. P. (1979). *The Ethnographic Interview*. New York: Holt, Rinehart, Winston.

St. George, I., Cullen, M., Gardiner, L., & Karabatsos, G. (2008). Universal telenursing triage in Australia and New Zealand - A new primary health service. *Aust Fam Physician., 37*(6), 476-9.

Staggers, N., Bagley Thompson, C., & Snyder-Halpern, R. (2001). History and trends in clinical information systems in the United States. *Journal of Nursing Scholarship, 33*(1), 75-81.

Stamper, R. K. (1985). Towards a Theory of Information: Information: Mystical Fluid or a Subject for Scientific Enquiry. *The Computer Journal,* 28, 195-199. BCS, Oxford Journals.

Stead, W. W., Kelly, B. J., & Kolodner, R. M. (2005). Achievable Steps Toward Building a National Health Information Infrastructure in the United States *Journal of the American Medical Informatics Association, 12*(2), 113-120.

Stengel, D., Bauwens, K., Walter, M., Kopfer, T, & Ekkernkamp, A. (2004). Comparison of handheld computer-assisted and conventional paper chart documentation a randomized controlled trial. *Journal Bone and Joint Surgery of America, 86-A(3),* 553-560.

Stohl, C. & Redding W. C. (1987). Messages and Message Exchange Processes. In Jablin, F., Putnam, L., Roberts, K. & Porter, L. (Eds.) *Handbook of Organizational Communication: An Interdisciplinary Perspective*. Newbury Park, CA: Sage, 451 – 502.

Stolworthy, Y.(2003). *RNs are mobilizing*. Retrieved, June 17, 2004 from www.pdacortex.com/RNs_are_Mobilizing.htm.

Stone, W. F., & Schaffner, P. E. (1997). The Tomkins Polarity Scale: Recent Developments. *Bulletin of the Tomkins Institute, 4*, 17-22.

Straus, S.E., Takeshita, H., Davis, D., & Rodrigues-Gianolli P. (2001). *Bringing evidence to the point of care*. Retrieved June 27, 2002 from http://www.cs.toronto.edu/~prg/

Stuart, G. W. (2001). Evidence-Based Psychiatric Nursing Practice: Rhetoric or Reality. *Journal of the American Psychiatric Nurses Association, 7*(4), 103-114.

Sullivan, M. (2003). The New Subjective Medicine: taking the patient's point of view on health care and health, *Social Science & Medicine, 56*(7), 1595-604.

Sutton, J., Stockton, L., McCord, G., Gilchrist, V. J., & Fedyna, D. (2004). Hanheld computer use in a family medicine clerkship. *Academic Medicine,* 79, 1114-19.

Swenson, S., Zettler, P., & Lo, B. (2006). She gave it her best shot right away. Patient experiences of biomedical and patient-centred communication. *Patient Educ Couns. 61*(2), 200–211.

Tanis, M. (2008). Organizational Identification and the Communication of Identity: Effects of Message Characteristics. Paper presented at the annual meeting of the *International Communication Association,* New York City, NY Retrieved 2008-04-22 from http://www.allacademic.com/meta/p14490_index.html.

Tanner, J., & Hale, C. (2002). Developing research capacity: Identifying and quantifying nursing research activity in the NHS. *Journal of Research in Nursing, 7*(3), 212-221.

Tassani, S., Baruffaldi, F., Testi, D., Cacciari, C., Accarisi, S., & Viceconti, M. (2007). Personal digital assistant in an orthopaedic wireless ward: The HandHealth project. *Computer Methods & Programs in Biomedicine, 86*(1), 21-29.

Taylor, S. J., & Bogdan, R. (1998). *Introduction to Qualitative Research Methods*. New York: John Wiley & Sons.

The Biggest –Invasion –Since 1066 (2007).Retrieved on May 22, 2008, from http://bookwormroom.wordpress.com/2007/11/15/biggest-invasion-since-1066/.

The International Council of Nurses (2004). Scope of Nursing Practice.Retrieved June 16, 2008, from http://www.icn.ch/psscope.htm

Thiele, J. (2003). Learning patterns of online students. *Journal of Nursing Education, 42*, 364-366.

Thomas, D., Heinemeier, D., & Breedt, L. (2007). *Agile Web Development with Rails*, Pragmatic Bookshelf; 2nd Revised edition.

Thompson B.W. (2005). The Transforming Effect of Handheld Computers on Nursing Practice. *Nurse Admin Q., 29*(40), 308-314.

Thompson J. D. (1967). *Organizations in Action.* New York: Mac Graw Hill.

Thomson, P. (2000). Implementing evidence-based healthcare: the nurse teachers' role in supporting the dissemination and implementation of SIGN clinical guidelines. *Nurse Education Today, 20*, 39 - 40.

Thurmond, V.A. (2003). Defining interaction and strategies to enhance interactions in web-based courses. *Nurse Educator, 28*, 237-241.

Tilson, H., & Berkowitz, B. (2006, July/August). The public health enterprise: Examining our twenty-first century policy challenges. *Health Affairs, 25*(4), 900-910. Retrieved August 10, 2007, from http://content.healthaffairs.org/cgi/content.full/25/4/900

Tinetti, M. E. (1986). Performance-oriented assessment of mobility problems in elderly patients. *J Am Geriatr. Soc, 34*, 119-126.

Tips to increase success for teaching online: Communication! (2002). *CIN Plus,5*(1), 1, 3-4, 6.

TrendCare (2008). www.trendcare.com.au/trendcare/documents/TrendCare_2008.pdf

TrendCare Systems Pty Ltd (2007). *Training Manual Queensland.*

Trist, E. L., & Bamforth, K. W. (1951). Some social and psychological consequences of the longwall method of coal getting. *Human Relations, 4*, 3-38.

Tumulty, G. (1980). The relationship of heal nurse role characteristics, job satisfaction and unit outcomes, Unpublished doctoral dissertation, University of Texas, Austin.

Turpin, C. (2007). Feminist praxis online teaching and the urban campus. *Feminist Teacher: A Journal of the Practices, Theories, and Scholarship of Feminist Teaching, 18*(1), 9-27.

Tynjala, P. (1997) Developing education students' conceptions of the learning process in different learning environments, *Learning and Instruction, 7*, 277-292.

Underhill, A. (2006). Theories of learning and their implications for on-line assessment. *Turkish Online Journal of Distance Education, 7*(1), 165-174.

United States Department of Health and Human Services (USDHHS). (2007, June 20). *Medicare preventative services: A healthier US starts here.* Retrieved May 25, 2008, from http://www.medicare.gov/Health/Overview.asp

Ure, J., Procter, R., Lin, Y., Hartswood, M., & Ho, K. (2007). *Aligning Technical and Human Infrastructures in the Semantic Web: A socio-technical perspective,* e-Social Science 2007 Conference, Ann Arbor, Michigan. Retrieved June 8, 2008 from http://ess.si.umich.edu/papers/paper188.pdf

Van de Castle, B., Kim, J., Pedreira, M. L. G., Paiva, A., Goossen, W., & Bates, D. W. (2004). Information technology and patient safety in nursing practice: an international perspective. *International Journal of Medical Informatics, 73*, 607-614.

Vangen, S., & Huxham, C. (2003). Nurturing Collaborative Relations: Building Trust in Inter-organizational Collaboration. *Journal of Applied Behavioral Science, 39*(1), 5-31.

Varcoe, C. (1996). Disparagement of the nursing process: the new dogma? *J Adv Nurs, 23*(1), 120-125.

Veterans Evidence-Based Research Dissemination Implementation Center (VERDICT). (2007). Retrieved

August 19, 2007, from http://verdict.uthscsa.edu/verdict/default.htm

Vicente, K. J. (2003). Less is (sometimes) more in cognitive engineering: the role of automation technology in improving patient safety. *Quality & safety in health care, 12*(4), 291-294.

Victorian Centre for Nursing Practice Research. (2001). *National Review of Nursing Education: Aspects of Nursing Education: The Types Of Skills And Knowledge Required To Meet The Changing Needs Of The Labour Force Involved In Nursing - Literature Review* The University of Melbourne

Villa, V. (1984). *Teorie della scienza giuridica e teorie delle scienze naturali: modelli ed analogie.* Milano: Giuffrè.

Villa, V. (1999). *Costruttivismo e teorie del diritto.* Torino: Giappichelli.

von Glasersfeld, E. (1987). *The construction of knowledge: Contributions to conceptual semantics.* Seaside, CA: Intersystems Publications.

von Glasersfeld, E. (1999). How do we mean? A constructivist sketch of semantics. *Cybernetics and Human Knowing, 6* (1), 9 – 16.

Vygotsky, L. S. (1978). *Mind and society: The development of higher mental processes.* Cambridge, MA: Harvard University Press.

Wahlberg, A., Cedersund, E., & Wredling, R. (2005). Bases for assessments made by telephone advice nurses. *J Telemed Telecare., 11*(8), 403–407.

Walcott, J. (2005). Opening Address to Commonwealth Secretariat Seminar on managed migration of nurses. 30-31 March 2005. Sherbourne Conference Centre, Barbados.

Wallace, P., & Clariana, R. B. (2005). Perception versus Reality—Determining Business Students' Computer Literacy Skills and Need for Instruction in Information Concepts and Technology. *Journal of Information Technology Education, 4.*

Walsh SH. (2004). The clinician's perspective on electronic health records and how they can affect patient care. *BMJ, 328,* 1184-1187.

Wang, C., & Burris, M. (1997). Photovoice: Concept, methodology, and use for participatory needs assessment. *Health Education Behavior, 24,* 369-387.

Wang, C., Burris, M., & Xiang, Y. (1996). Chinese village women as visual anthropologists: A participatory approach to reaching policymakers. *Sac Sci Med, 42,* 1391-1400.

Waton, K. (2007, June 11). Corporate Wellness. *Advance for nurses, 5*(13), 31-32. King of Prussia, PA: Merion Publications, Inc.

Watson, J. (2000*). Australian Industrial Relations Commission – Record of Proceedings*, Melbourne AG2001/771423

Watzlawick, P. (1984). *Invented Reality: How Do We Know What We Believe We Know? (Contributions to constructivism).* New York: W.W. Norton & Co Inc.

Watzlawick, P., Beavin, J. H., & Jackson, D. D. (1967). *Pragmatics of Human Communication.* New York: W.W. Norton & Co Inc.

Weber, S. (2007). Clinical decision support systems and how critical care clinicians use them. *Journal of Healthcare Information Management, 21*(2), 41-52.

Weick, K. E. (1996). *Sensemaking in organizations.* Newbury Park, CA: Sage.

Weick, K. E. (1979). *The social psychology of organizing* (2nd ed.). NY: McGraw-Hill, Inc.

Weick, K. E., & Roberts K. H. (1993). Collective mind in Organizations: Heedful interrelating on Flight Decks. *Administrative Science Quarterly, 38,* 357 – 381.

Weir, C. R., Nebeker, J. J. R., Hicken, B. L., Campo, R., Drews, F., & Lebar, B. (2007). A Cognitive Task Analysis of Information Management Strategies in a Computerized Provider Order Entry Environment. *Journal of the American Medical Informatics Association: JAMIA., 14*(1), 65.

Welch, R. L. (1980). Vertical and Horizontal Communication in Economic Processes. *The Review of Economic Studies*, *47*(4), 733 – 746.

Weller, D. P. (2006). Workforce substitution and primary care. *Medical Journal of Australia, 185*(1), 8-9.

Werley, H. H., Devine, E. C., Zorn, C. R., Ryan, P., & Westra, B. (1991). The nursing minimum data set: abstraction tool for standardized, comparable, essential data. *American Journal of Public Health, 81*, 421-426.

Westberg, S., Bumgardner, M., & Lind, P. (2005) Enhancing Cultural Competency in a College of Pharmacy Curriculum. *American Journal of Pharmaceutical Education* 2005 (6) 211-222.

Westbrook, J. I., Braithwaite, J., Georgiou, A., et al. (2007). Multimethod Evaluation of Information and Communication Technologies in Health in the Context of Wicked Problems and Sociotechnical Theory. *Journal of the American Medical Informatics Association, 14*, 6, 746-755.

Westbrook, J. I., Gosling, A. S., & Coiera, E. (2004). Do Clinicians Use Online Evidence to Support Patient Care? A Study of 55,000 Clinicians. *J Am Med Inform Assoc, 11*(2), 113-120.

White, A., Allen, P., Goodwin, L., Breckinridge, D., Dowell, J., & Garvy, R. (2005). Infusing PDA technology into nursing education. *Nurse Educator, 30*(4), 150-154.

White, A., Roberts, V., & Brannan, J. (2003). Returning nurses to the workforce: Developing an online refresher course. *The Journal of Continuing Education in Nursing, 34*, 59-64.

Wilber, K. (2000). *Integral Psychology: Consciousness, Spirit, Psychology, Therapy*. Shambhala Publications.

Wilkinson, J.M. (2006). *Nursing Process and Critical Thinking*, 4th Edition, Prentice Hall.

Williams, A. F. (1999). An antipodean evaluation of problem-based learning by clinical educators. *Nurse Education Today, 19*, 659 - 667.

Williams, A., & Cutchin, M. (2002). The rural context of health care provision. *Journal of Interprofessional Care, 16(2)*, 107-115.

Wilson, B. (1984). *Systems: Concepts, methodologies and applications*. Chinchester: Wiley.

Wilson, E.O. (1998). *Consilience: The Unity of Knowledge*. Abacus.

Wilson, R. M., Harrison, B. T., Gibberd, R. W., & Hamilton, J. D. (1999). An analysis of the causes of adverse events from the Quality in Australian Health Care Study. *Med J Aust, 170*(9), 411-415.

Wilson, S., Dignam, D., & Hay, E. (2002). *Addressing the digital divide between nursing practice and education using a personal digital assistant (PDA)*. Winds of Changing in the Sea of Learning, Proceedings of the 19th Annual Conference of the Australian Society for Computers in Tertiary Education (ASCILITE), Auckland, New Zealand.

Winkelman, W. J. (2003). Evaluating computerised health information systems: Opportunities were missed. *BMJ: British medical journal*(327), 162-163.

Winn, W. (1993). Instructional design and situated learning: paradox or partnership. *Educational Technology*, March, 16 - 21.

Wolf, E. J. (2001). Healthcare's New Tools of the Trade: How to Gain Physician Buy-in. *Healtcare Executive*(Sep/Oct), 14-16.

Wood, S. (2001). *National nursing workload measurement*. Wellington, Ministry of Health, New Zealand.

Woods, R. & Baker, J. (2004). Interaction and immediacy in online learning. *International Review of Research in Open and Distance Learning*. Retrieved November 2, 2007 from http://www.irrodl.org/content/v5.2/woods-baker.html.

Woodward, J. (1965). *Industrial Organization: Theory And Practice*. London: Oxford University Press.

Woolrych, R. (2004). Empowering images: Using Photovoice with tenants with special needs. *Housing, Care and Support, 7*(1), 31-36.

Wootton, R. (2008). Telemedicine support for the developing world. *J Telemed Telecare., 14*(3), 109-14.

Wootton, R., & Craig, J. (eds.). (1999). *Introduction to telemedicine.* London, UK: Royal Society of Medicine Press Ltd.

Wootton, R. & Patterson, V. (Eds.). (2006). *Introduction to Telemedicine* (2 ed.). London: Royal Society of Medicine Press.

Wootton, R., Kvedar, J., & Dimmick. S. L. (2006). *Home Telehealth: Connecting care within community.* RSM, London.

Work, Stress and Health: Findings from the Whitehall 11 study. (2004). Retrieved September 1, 2007, from http://www.workstress.net/downloads/whitehall_11_study.pdf

World Bank. (2001). *World Development Indicators.* Washington, DC: Office of the Publisher, World Bank.

World Bank. (2008). *Global Economic Perspectives: Technology Diffusion in Developing World.* Washington, DC: Office of the Publisher, World Bank.

World Health Organization (2003). World Health Report. Geneva: WHO.

World Health Organization. (2006). The World Health Report 2006 - working together for health. Retrieved May 20, 2007 from http://www.who.int/whr/2006/annex/06_annex4_en.pdf

Wrenn, C. B. (2001). *Truth and the normativity of naturalistic epistemology.* PhD Thesis, from http://bama.ua.edu/~cwrenn/work/DissBody.pdf

Wynne, M. K. (2000). Going mobile: An introduction to hand-held PCs. *Hearing Journal, 53(2),* 10; 12; 14.

Xiao, Y., Schenkel, S., Faraj, S., Mackenzie, C. F., & Moss, J. (2007). What whiteboards in a trauma center operating suite can teach us about emergency department communication. *Ann Emerg Med, 50*(4), 387-395.

Yacci, M. (2000). Interactivity demystified: A structural definition. *Educational Technology, 40*(4), 5-16.

Yerrell, P. (2000). The practitioner-researcher in nursing: there won't be too many. Kilgore Trouts. *Nurse Education Today, 20*, 36 - 38.

Zhang, D. (2005). Interactive multimedia-based E-learning: A study of effectiveness. *The American Journal of Distance Education, 19*(3), 149-162.

Zubin, J., & Spring, B. (1977). Vulnerability - a new view of schizophrenia. *Journal of Abnormal Psychology, 86*, 2, 103-124.

Zuboff, S. (1988). *In the age of the smart machine: The future of work and power.* BasicBooks: United State of America.

About the Contributors

Bettina Staudinger is associate professor at the Institute of Applied Systems Research and Development, University for Health Sciences, Medical Informatics and Technology, Hall in Tyrol, Austria. She took her master's degree (Mag.) in medical informatics (information management) as well as a master's and PhD in health sciences at the University for Health Sciences, Medical Informatics and Technology, Tyrol, Austria. Her field of research interest encompasses data organization and data management especially in the field of nursing.

Victoria Höß, PhD, has been a senior research assistant at the Institute for Human and Economic Sciences, University for Health Sciences, Medical Informatics and Technology since 2007. She obtained a master's degree (Mag. rer. soc. oec.) in studies of international business and economics and a master's degree (Mag. rer. soc. oec.) in studies of economics both from the University of Innsbruck, Austria. She took her PhD in health sciences at the University for Health Sciences, Medical Informatics and Technology. Her research encompasses financing and cost structures in the health care sector.

Herwig Ostermann, PhD, is associate professor at the Institute for Human and Economic Sciences at the University for Health Sciences, Medical Informatics and Technology, Hall/Tyrol, Austria. His research interests encompass the field of public administration and management especially focusing on health care delivery and long-term care structures. He received a master's degree in International Business Administration from Innsbruck University, Austria, a master's degree in Health Sciences and a PhD in health sciences from UMIT, Hall/Tyrol, Austria.

* * *

June Anonson has an extensive background in nursing practice, administration and education. She is currently the assistant dean of nursing at the University of Saskatchewan (Prince Albert Campus). Previously she was the dean of health sciences and social services at the College of New Caledonia (Prince George, BC). Her focus has been in leadership and excellence in nursing. Since 2002, she has been involved in South Korea and China helping to educate nurses about the Canadian health care system.

Nigel Armfield PhD (candidate), MSc, senior research assistant (telepaediatrics), The University of Queensland Centre for Online Health, is involved in developing, managing and evaluating the use of mobile telemedicine within the telepaediatric service. His research interests include neonatal and paediatric intensive care telemedicine, mobile telemedicine and developing scalable approaches to telemedicine service management. As a PhD candidate, he is researching a novel real-time telemedicine application to support consultation between a tertiary neonatal intensive care unit and distant referring hospitals within Queensland. Nigel's previous roles have included communications engineering, management and research. He is also a former president and committee member of SANDS (Stillbirth and Neonatal Death Support) Queensland.

Sandra Bassendowski is an associate professor in the College of Nursing, University of Saskatchewan. She holds a Diploma in Nursing, Bachelor of Education (Regina), Master of Education (Regina) and EdD (Nova Southeastern). Her focus is on adult teaching and learning, technologies in education, and faculty development. She is an innovator in the uptake and development of unique learning strategies in the classroom such as Wikis, blogs, podcasting, and Second Life. She carries research grants in the areas of inter-professional education and educational innovations (i.e., NurseONE).

Mark Bensink PhD (candidate), MEd(leadership), BNurs, RN, senior research assistant (telepaediatrics), The University of Queensland Centre for Online Health is a registered nurse who has worked clinically in a number of different areas including general medical, paediatric intensive care and outpatients. He has also had experience as a nurse educator. Mark's general area of interest revolves around home telehealth. He has been working with the Royal Children's Hospital Paediatric Oncology, Haematology and Stem Cell Transplant Unit since 2003 investigating the use of Internet technologies in the home. The main focus of this work has been to improve the support provided to children and their families from regional and remote areas dealing with childhood cancer. He is currently coordinating a number of trials investigating the cost effectiveness of home telehealth in different areas of paediatric oncology including support for families returning home after diagnosis, families involved in bone marrow transplantation and palliative care.

Elizabeth M. Borycki is an assistant professor in the School of Health Information Science and an adjunct assistant professor in the School of Nursing at the University of Victoria, Canada. Elizabeth has a unique blend of nursing, industry, consulting and academic experience. She has been involved in the implementation and redesign of electronic health record systems in several hospital settings, and has worked in the fields of nursing, health and nursing/health informatics for over 15 years. Elizabeth holds master's of nursing, and a PhD in management and organization from the Department of Health Policy, Management and Evaluation from the University of Toronto. Elizabeth is currently involved in several national and international research projects in health informatics, with a focus on understanding the impact of information technology and devices used in clinical settings upon healthcare work and information processing in nurses and other health professionals.

Daniel Carbone is a lecture/research coordinator for the Rural Health Academic Network (RHAN), University of Melbourne; where he facilitates research capacity in health care settings across north-western state of Victoria, Australia. He is also a health information systems consultant at Central Highlands General Practice Network where he facilitates general practices to adopt relevant information system to improve patient care outcomes. Daniel is also completing a PhD in information systems at Victoria University which focuses on systematic approaches to chronic conditions care models and has been training nurses and doctors in computer and information literacy for over ten years.

Roberta Cuel graduated in 1999 in economics at the University of Trento, received a PhD in Organization and Management from the University of Udine and a Post Doc position at the Computer Science Dept. of the University of Verona. She is currently Assistant professor at the Computer and Management Science Dept. at the University of Trento. Her research interests are aimed at discovering the interdependencies between technology and organizations, such as the impact of innovative technologies on teams, communities, and organizational models, the study of distributed tools and processes that allow organizational learning and knowledge management, and knowledge representation systems (such as ontologies, classifications, taxonomies) as mechanisms for knowledge reification processes. She has written a number of chapters in books, articles in international journals, and has served as the PC member for various interdisciplinary conferences. For further information, please see http://www.disa.unitn.it/net-economy/cuel/.

Daniela Deufert has been a research and teaching assistant at the Institute of Nursing Science, University for Health Sciences, Medical Informatics and Technology, Hall in Tyrol, Austria since 2006. She is also a doctoral candidate. She obtained the master`s degree (MScNH) in studies of nursing and health sciences at the Martin-Luther-University Halle-Wittenberg, Halle/Saale, Germany.

Dawn Dowding is a senior lecturer at the Hull York Medical School and Department of Health Sciences, University of York. She has a background in nursing and psychology, has carried out a number of research studies examining how nurses use information to inform their judgement and decision making, and the development and evaluation of decision support systems in nursing practice. She has co-edited/authored two books in clinical decision making and judgement in nursing and is a member of the MRC College of Experts and the Nursing Times Editorial Board.

Sisira Edirippulige's PhD (Moscow), PhD (Auckland), MSc (Moscow), lecturer/coordinator - graduate programmes in e-health care, The University of Queensland Centre for Online Health main responsibilities involve teaching and include the coordination of all undergraduate and graduate courses in e-health care and continuing professional development courses in telehealth. His research interests include the development, promotion and integration of telehealth education and telemedicine applications into the health care sector. Before joining the University of Queensland, Sisira taught at Kobe Gakuin University in Japan and at the University of Auckland in New Zealand. He has extensive experience in development studies working in number of countries including Russia, Sri Lanka, South Africa, Japan and New Zealand.

Margaret Edwards is a professor and coordinator of graduate programs in the Centre for Nursing and Health Studies at Athabasca University (CNHS), which offers the interdisciplinary master's of health studies (MHS) and the master's of nursing (MN), generalist and advanced nursing practice. Her research interests are in the areas of healthcare informatics, online education, and exemplary care of the elderly.

Efthimis Efthimiadis, PhD is associate professor at the University of Washington Information School. His research interests include information retrieval and user-centered design.

Maureen Farrell, PhD, has a distinguished record in health care education and practice and her innovation are numerous. In education she piloted the use of hand held computers in the education of undergraduate nursing students and is the editor/contributing author of the Australian and New Zealand adaptation of the Smeltzer and Bare textbook of medical surgical nursing, 2nd edition due in 2009. A clinical preceptorship course designed for industry partners and a health care leadership course for Open Universities Australia are also major innovations that Dr. Farrell led. Research publications focus on nursing informatics, education and leadership.

Roberta Ferrario graduated in 1998 in philosophy of science at the University of Milan, then she moved to Trento in order to work with the research group led by Fausto Giunchiglia. In 2003, she received a PhD in Philosophy both at the University of Milan and at the University Marc Bloch of Strasbourg (Italy-France co-tutorship program), with a dissertation on counterfactual reasoning. In 2003-2004 she was visiting scholar at the EPGY centre in Stanford, invited by Patrick Suppes. Currently, she cooperates with the Laboratory for Applied Ontology of the Institute of Cognitive Sciences and Technologies of the Italian National Council in Trento and she's mainly working on e-Government, social ontology, ontology of mental attitudes and intentional agents in general. For further information, http://www.loa-cnr.it/ferrario/.

Elfriede Fritz is associate professor at the Institute of Nursing Science, University for Health Sciences, Medical Informatics and Technology, Hall in Tyrol, Austria. She obtained the master`s degree (Mag. phil.) and the doctorate degree (Dr. phil.) in education from the University of Innsbruck, Tyrol, Austria.

Rebecca Foster is a research assistant in the School of Health Sciences at the University of Southampton. She began her research career with a study of computer use amongst community pharmacists. She has also worked on an investigation of patterns of cocaine and crack use in the UK. She is currently involved in projects to evaluate interprofessional learning among health and social care students and to track the career pathways of health and social care graduates.

Kenric W. Hammond, MD is a staff psychiatrist at VA Puget Sound Health Care System, Seattle Washington. He has worked with the VA CPRS since 1979. He is a clinical associate professor of psychiatry and behavioral sciences and medical education and biomedical informatics at the University of Washington.

Johannes Hilbe is research assistant and doctoral candidate at the Institute of Nursing Science. He obtained the baccalaureate degree in nursing science at the University College of Dublin (UCD) and the master's degree of medical informatics at the University for Health Sciences, Medical Informatics and Technology, Tyrol.

Victoria Hoess, PhD, has been a senior research assistant at the Institute for Human and Economic Sciences, University for Health Sciences, Medical Informatics and Technology since 2007. She obtained a master's degree (Mag. rer. soc. oec.) in studies of international business and economics and a master's degree (Mag. rer. soc. oec.) in studies of economics both from the University of Innsbruck, Austria. She took her PhD in health sciences at the University for Health Sciences, Medical Informatics and Technology. Her research encompasses financing and cost structures in the health care sector.

Thomas James is technical advisor in the area of information and communications technologies for development (ICT4D). He is the principal of Apogia Networks, Ltd. And has overseen the development, coordination, and evaluation of health and education related innovations. His background as a transportation economist has provided him with research and project management skills necessary to strengthen and lead a variety of ICT4D initiatives. His specific interest is in the role of the diaspora in furthering and sustaining the ICT4D agenda.

Peter Jones, RMN, RGN, CPN(Cert.), BA(Hons), PGCE, PG(Dip.) COPE began his nursing career in the UK in 1977 and continues to work in the NHS. Professional qualifications include community mental health and general nursing plus informatics. In the 1990s Peter was awarded BA(Hons.) in computing and philosophy. Independent studies during the past decade have publicised Hodges' model, a conceptual framework to communities beyond health and social care. This effort is ongoing through a website, blog and the chapter to be found in this volume. Peter is married to Christine; they have three children Daniel, Matthew and Bethany.

Professor **Boris Arkadievich Kobrinskiy**, MD, PhD, DSC (b. 1944), graduated from II Moscow Medical Institute in 1970 (MD), PhD in paediatrics, DSC in medical informatics. Author of more than 400 works (including 7 monographs), devoted to the problems of environmental medicine, medical informatics, telemedicine, artificial intelligence in healthcare. During last decades Prof. Kobrinskiy was responsible for a number of federal level and international projects in the mentioned areas. Since 1983 Prof. Kobrinskiy is the head of Medical Centre for New Information Technologies at Moscow Research Institute for Paediatrics and Children's Surgery.

Andre W. Kushniruk is an associate professor and the director of the School of Health Information Science at the University of Victoria, Canada. Andre conducts research in a number of areas including: evaluation of the effects of technology, human-computer interaction in health care, and other domains as well as cognitive science. His work is known internationally and he has published widely in the area of health informatics. He holds undergraduate degrees in psychology and biology, as well as an MSc in computer science and a PhD in cognitive psychology. He focuses on developing new methods for the evaluation of information technology and studying human-computer interaction in health care and he has been a key researcher on a number of national and international collaborative projects.

Shigeki Kuwata has a PhD from Osaka University in Japan, where he had conducted research on healthcare databases, inter-hospital networking and their related security issues as staff of a Department of Medical Information Science at Osaka University Hospital. Since 2003, he has been an assistant professor in Tottori University as well as a deputy director of the Division of Medical Informatics at Tottori University Hospital. His major research interests include development of hospital information systems, implementation of electronic patient records and risk/quality management in the hospital.

Val Lattimer is professor of Health Services Research in the School of Health Sciences at the University of Southampton. Her research interests are in applications of technology designed to improve access to health care, particularly in urgent care and in the management of long term conditions. Previous work has examined the safety, effectiveness and costs of CDSS used by nurses. Current research is addressing how new decision technologies are shaped as they become adopted in practice and the impact of workforce and skill mix change, in systems using new technologies, on patient experience, staff practice and health system performance.

Linda Martindale leads on e-learning in the Distance Learning Centre (nursing and palliative care), University of Dundee. She has worked in research in medical education and has a strong interest in research teaching and in carrying out educational research, particularly in the area of e-learning in health care education. In recent years Linda has been involved in a number of e-learning developments, including development of an international digital repository in nursing education and designing e-study guides for use in continuing education. She has worked in national and international collaborations developing and researching e-learning.

Nikolay Valentinovich Matveev, MD, MPH, PhD, DSC (b. 1962) – graduated from Gorky Medical Institute in 1988 (now Nizhny Novgorod State Medical Academy). Since 1988 until 2004 he worked in Nizhny Novgorod Research Institute for Hygiene and Occupational Diseases (in 1998-2004 –as a Research Director). Dr. Matveev actively worked in sphere of medical informatics and telemedicine and their use in occupational medicine. Since 2004 until 2008 Dr. Matveev was a head of Telemedical Centre at Moscow Research Institute for Paediatrics and Children's Surgery, actively working in sphere of medical image processing for telemedicine. Dr. Matveev obtained his PhD degree in hygiene/dermatology in 1995 at F.F. Erisman Federal Scientific Centre for Hygiene (Moscow, Russia). MPH degree was earned in 2006 at Harvard School of Public Health (Boston, MA, USA). In 2007 Dr. Matveev earned his DSC degree in medical informatics in Tula Research Institute for New Medical Technologies (Tula, Russia). In 2008 Dr. Matveev became professor of The Chair of Medical Cybernetics and Informatics at Russian State Medical University (Moscow, Russia).

Natasha Mitchell is a researcher and trial coordinator at the York Trials Unit at the University of York. Natasha has a background in health psychology and has worked on various projects, covering a number of areas in healthcare including myocardial infarction and the self-regulation model and nurses use of new technology. At present, she is working on a trial assessing the effectiveness of screening older women for osteoporosis.

Mary Oriol, PhD, is an associate professor of nursing in the Health Care Systems Management (HCSM) Master of Science in Nursing Program at Loyola University New Orleans. She was a charter faculty member in the transition of the HCSM on-campus curriculum to that of online delivery. She holds a master's of science degree with a major in mental health nursing from University of Southern Mississippi and a doctor of public health degree in health care systems from Tulane University School of Public Health. She has extensive experience in leadership positions in health care organizations and in nursing education. Her research interests and publications include quality management, patient safety, and health systems.

Beth Perry Mahler is an associate professor in the Center for Nursing and Health at Athabasca University. Beth is a registered nurse and has her PhD in Educational Administration and Policy Studies from the University of Alberta. Beth's research interests in exemplary online teaching and career satisfaction in nursing. Beth teaches in the undergraduate and graduate nursing and health studies programs focusing on leadership courses.

Pammla Petrucka is an Associate Professor in the College of Nursing, University of Saskatchewan. Dr. Petrucka holds a BScN and MN (Saskatchewan), PhD (Alberta) and a Post-Doctoral Fellow (Indigenous People's Health Research Centre). She leads/co-leads various community based research projects with three Aboriginal groups in Saskatchewan. Her work in the Caribbean supported by IDRC focuses on PDAs and nursing in development. Her work in Africa involves pregnant and post-partum women in Kibera, Kenya and Arusha, Tanzania and is funded by a fellowship (Association of Commonwealth Universities) and granting from Social Sciences and Humanities Research Council. further work in Africa. She is supported by the Saskatchewan Health Research Foundation in work considering the needs of Aboriginal and rural people with kidney diseases.

Virginia Plummer has 30 years experience in health services and is an early career researcher. In 2005, she was awarded a PhD entitled 'An analysis of patient acuity data, utilizing the TrendCare system'. The research was supported by a scholarship from the Centre for Health Services Operations Management within the Faculty of Medicine, Nursing and Health Sciences and the Faculty of Information Technology at Monash University. The Department of Human Services Victoria also provided some funds. Dr Plummer was supervised by Dr. Liza Heslop and Dr. Lee Seldon of Monash University and Emeritus Professor Donna Diers of Yale University. Dr Plummer is a registered nurse who has additional qualifications in midwifery, critical care, health service administration and a Master's Degree in Health Policy. In 1998, she was admitted as fellow to the Australian College of Health Services Executives. Her hospital management experience is in both public and private sectors, including board membership for several health care organizations. Experience in casemix funding in the compensation arena was gained in her role as Senior Policy Advisor, Acute Care, Transport Accident Commission, Victoria. Dr Plummer's clinical experience and interests are in acute care, critical care, accident and emergency, midwifery and aged care, and her research interests for the past ten years have been in the areas of nursing costs and nursing resource allocation. She is deputy director of the Mobile Health Research Group of Monash University.

Rebecca Randell is a researcher in the Centre for HCI Design at City University. Although she has a background in software engineering, her research is very much focused on the social, concerned with the design and evaluation of technology within healthcare through the use of qualitative research methods. In 2004, she was awarded the Diana Forsythe Prize by the American Medical Informatics Association. She is on the Executive Committee of the British Computer Society Health Informatics (Nursing) Specialist Group. At present, she is working on a project which aims to design innovative technologies to support the handovers of a range of healthcare professionals.

Hazel Williams-Roberts graduated from the University of the West Indies with an MBBS in 1997. She also holds a master's of science degree in health services and public health research. She currently manages the division of Community Based Health Services in the Ministry of Health in St Kitts. Her responsibilities include oversight of three departments (Family Health, Environmental health and Health Promotion) that execute the public health function for the island.

Elizabeth Rogerson is head of the Distance Learning Centre (Nursing and Palliative Care), University of Dundee. She has practised in the UK and USA in different clinical settings, and since 1982 has been a nurse educator in the UK, gaining her PhD in distance education in nursing. Dr. Rogerson led the Distance Learning Centre to become the first institution outside North America whose programmes are accredited by the National League for Nursing Accrediting Commission. Recently Dr. Rogerson has been involved in e-learning developments and has worked in international collaborations to promote excellence in e-learning.

Jerono P. Rotich is an assistant professor and has been teaching in the Human Performance and Leisure Studies Department at North Carolina A & T State University. Her research interests include: Cross-cultural and multicultural issues; service learning; cultural competency in Health care, wellness and education; and obesity and behavior modification among underserved communities. She is originally from Kenya.

Anthony C. Smith PhD, MEd. (Adult & Workplace Training), BNurs., RN, Senior Research Fellow – Telepaediatrics, The University of Queensland Centre for Online Health is the Senior Research Fellow at the Centre for Online Health at the University of Queensland. He completed a doctorate degree in the field of medicine in 2004 examining the feasibility and cost-effectiveness of a novel telepaediatric service in Queensland. His principal role in the Centre for Online Health includes the management, coordination and evaluation of telepaediatric services. Dr Smith has made a substantial contribution to the literature on telepaediatrics publishing articles in peer-reviewed journals and five book chapters on the subject. Dr Smith assists with the supervision of a broad range of telemedicine projects and teaching programmes in the Centre for Online Health and also provides consultancy services to other university departments and external organisations.

Wanda Sneed is an Assistant Professor at Tarleton State University, Department of Nursing, USA. She has a PhD. in Information Science from the University of North Texas, Denton, Texas and a Master's in Nursing from Emory State University, Atlanta, Georgia. Dr. Sneed has held positions in administration, education and clinical practice since 1964. The Tarleton State University nursing program focuses on rurality and rural health nursing practice. Dr. Sneed has expertise in nursing informatics and rural public health nursing.

Christa Them is the head of the Institute of Nursing Sciences at UMIT. In addition to having built up and chairing the Nursing Institute, in existence now since the past two years, she is a member of several national and international working groups that are responsible for further developing the field of nursing sciences.

Carl Thompson is a nurse, researcher and educator interested in healthcare decision making and judgment. He has co-edited/authored three books on evaluation and clinical decision making in nursing and more than 100 book chapters, refereed research and conference papers, and journal articles. He is editor of Evidence Based Nursing (BMJ publications) and on the Editorial Advisory Board of the British Medical Journal. He is a member of the MRC's College of Experts and adjunct professor at the University of Alberta, Canada. Dr Thompson currently leads a 5 year NIHR research programme evaluating knowledge translation strategies in the North of England.

Gail Tumulty RN, PhD is a professor and interim director of the School of Nursing as well as coordinator of the Health Care Systems Management Program (HCSM) at Loyola University New Orleans. Dr. Tumulty spearheaded the design and development of the HCSM program on-campus and online. She teaches human resources, health policy, and research. She received her master's and bachelor's degrees from Saint Louis University and her PhD in nursing from the University of Texas at Austin. She is certified in nursing administration, advanced, and is noted for her international work to improve the profession of nursing, particularly with developing countries in the Middle East. Her research interest is health care system and work redesign and she has numerous publications on this topic, presenting both nationally and internationally.

Carolyn F. Waltz, PhD, RN, FAAN is professor and director of international activities at the University of Maryland School of Nursing. Dr. Waltz is an internationally recognized expert in the development of outcomes evaluation in clinical and educational settings. She has published extensively including award winning books and articles on research, measurement, nursing outcomes, program development and evaluation. She has provided numerous outcomes evaluations, consultations, presentations, and workshops to varied health care audiences nationally and internationally and is widely acknowledged as a pioneer in outcomes evaluation and research.

Hiromi Watanabe is a registered head nurse at Tottori University Hospital and has been in charge of its nursing information systems for 6 years. She also teaches nursing informatics at the School of Health Science at the Tottori University, Faculty of Medicine. She has conducted research on intensive care, nursing process support systems and nursing management systems. She received the Encouraging Paper Award from the Japanese Society of Intensive Care Medicine in 1999, regarding a risk scoring system for ICU patients.

Charlene R. Weir, PhD, RN is associate director of the Geriatrics Research Education and Clinical Center at the Salt Lake City VA Medical Center. She is associate professor of Medical Informatics at the University of Utah. She has pioneered ethnographic study of implementation of computerized information systems in health care.

Richard Wootton DSc, PhD, MSc, BSc, director of research, The University of Queensland Centre for Online Health, is a recognised leader in the field of telemedicine and telehealth. He has over 200 articles in peer-reviewed journals and a series of textbooks on telemedicine, published by Royal Society of Medicine Press. The eighth in this series, *Home Telehealth* (eds. Wootton, Dimmick, Kvedar), was published in 2006. He is a regular invited speaker at telemedicine conferences around the world. He was a visiting scholar at the Health Telematics Unit at the University of Calgary in 2002. Professor Wootton is the editor of the *Journal of Telemedicine and Telecare*, an international peer-reviewed journal. He was the founder chairman of the UK's academic Telemedicine and e-Health Section of the Royal Society of Medicine and was the government's representative to the G8 telemedicine project.

Index

V

W